TREATMENT OF COMPLEX TRAUMA

ALSO FROM CHRISTINE A. COURTOIS AND JULIAN D. FORD

For more information, visit the authors' websites:
www.drchriscourtois.com and *www.advancedtrauma.com*

Treating Complex Stress Disorders:
An Evidence-Based Guide
Edited by Christine A. Courtois and Julian D. Ford

Treating Complex Traumatic Stress Disorders
in Children and Adolescents:
Scientific Foundations and Therapeutic Models
Edited by Julian D. Ford and Christine A. Courtois

TREATMENT *of* COMPLEX TRAUMA

A Sequenced, Relationship-Based Approach

Christine A. Courtois
Julian D. Ford

Foreword by John Briere

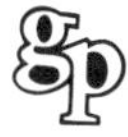

THE GUILFORD PRESS
New York London

A Division of Guilford Publications, Inc.
72 Spring Street, New York, NY 10012
www.guilford.com

Printed in the United States of America

This book is printed on acid-free paper.

Last digit is print number: 9 8 7 6 5 4 3 2 1

Library of Congress Cataloging-in-Publication Data

Courtois, Christine A.
Treatment of complex trauma : a sequenced, relationship-based approach / Christine A. Courtois, Julian D. Ford ; foreword by John Briere.
p. cm.
Includes bibliographical references and index.
ISBN 978-1-4625-0658-3 (hardcover : alk. paper)
1. Post-traumatic stress disorder—Treatment. 2. Psychic trauma—Treatment. I. Ford, Julian D. II. Title.
RC552.P67C69 2013
616.85′2106—dc23

2012036473

To Mom and to Tom,
my most stalwart supporters
—CAC

For Judy, my cotherapist,
coparent, and life partner
—JDF

About the Authors

Christine A. Courtois, PhD, ABPP, is a counseling psychologist in private practice in Washington, DC. She is immediate past president of Division 56 (Psychological Trauma) of the American Psychological Association (APA) and past Clinical and Training Director and cofounder of The CENTER: Posttraumatic Disorders Program, also in Washington. Dr. Courtois is a recipient of the Outstanding Contributions to Professional Practice Award from APA Division 56, the Lifetime Achievement Award from the International Society for the Study of Trauma and Dissociation (ISSTD), and the Sarah Haley Award for Clinical Excellence from the International Society for Traumatic Stress Studies (ISTSS), among other honors. She has published numerous books, book chapters, and articles on trauma-related topics.

Julian D. Ford, PhD, a clinical psychologist, is Professor of Psychiatry at the University of Connecticut School of Medicine, where he is also Director of the Child Trauma Clinic and of the Center for Trauma Response, Recovery, and Preparedness. He is Associate Editor of the *Journal of Trauma and Dissociation* and serves on the board of directors of the ISTSS. With Dr. Courtois, Dr. Ford is a recipient of the Print Media Award from the ISSTD for their coedited volume *Treating Complex Traumatic Stress Disorders*; he has also published several other books on trauma-related topics. Dr. Ford developed and conducts research on the Trauma Affect Regulation: Guide for Education and Therapy (TARGET®) psychosocial intervention for adolescents, adults, and families.

Foreword

Over the last several decades we have witnessed a huge amount of progress in our understanding of psychological trauma, its many forms, its immediate and lasting effects, and how it can be treated. This book is an excellent representation of this progress and, I will suggest, a further step forward.

It wasn't that long ago that those alleging interpersonal trauma were likely to be disbelieved, or at least viewed with suspicion. Similarly, expressions of posttraumatic distress were frequently seen as fabrications, or the effects of other, far more ominous things that were the "real" source of the victim's complaints, including pre-Oedipal psychopathology, hysteria, personality disorder, psychosis, or an easily overwhelmed psychology or neurobiology (Briere & Scott, 2006; Herman, 1992). As a result, therapies were offered that attempted to (1) uncover and resolve unconscious conflicts and hysterical symptoms that were believed to masquerade as posttraumatic distress; (2) strengthen the psychological mettle of individuals whose assumed inherent weakness caused them to overreact to events; or (3) teach the client how to suppress, deny, or otherwise avoid symptoms in order to adjust to life's challenges.

Slowly, however, historical events changed these societal and professional perspectives. One of the most significant of these was the Vietnam War, which confronted the world with the horror of combat and its obvious effects on survivors. These impacts were manifestly real, as repeatedly seen on television sets worldwide, and as witnessed personally in the return of affected relatives, spouses, and friends. Importantly for the time, those impacted could not be dismissed as "merely" women complaining of questionable sexual events, or a small number of individuals inventing psychological symptoms for secondary gain. They were red-blooded soldiers and sailors, and there were a lot of them: Almost 20% of American Vietnam veterans returned home with posttraumatic stress disorder (PTSD; American

Psychiatric Association, 1980; Dohrenwend et al., 2006)—a diagnosis newly coined to categorize veterans suffering from combat trauma.

With the coining of PTSD, a new paradigm was introduced, suggesting that one could have significant psychological problems and symptoms for reasons other than the previously assumed etiologies, such as aberrant neurobiology or having been raised by a psychologically disturbed mother. Apparently, encountering bad things in one's life could produce lasting psychological outcomes, in and of themselves.

The years following the Vietnam War became a time of both professional foment and growth. Although the shift was not instantaneous, the psychological world was changing: graduate students were generating a flood of thesis and dissertation research on trauma, brain researchers were finding neurobiological substrates for a variety of different trauma conditions and symptoms, and clinicians were developing interventions to treat posttraumatic stress. Probably not inconsequentially, new forms of trauma were being uncovered; clergy sex abuse cases began to appear regularly in the newspapers, and wars in Iraq and Afghanistan produced a whole new generation of psychologically injured men and women. Trauma was no longer avoidable as a concept, and the impacts of posttraumatic stress on society became much clearer.

What also became clear, over the years, was that PTSD-based models could not explain the full range of psychological outcomes found in many individuals presenting for treatment. Because many of these people had been exposed to early and severe child abuse and neglect, as well as, in many cases, later adult traumas, their difficulties were quite complex, often involving not only the symptoms of PTSD, anxiety, and depression, but also problems with identity, affect regulation, and relationships, as well as substance abuse, dissociation, somatization, and self-injurious behaviors (Briere, 2004; van der Kolk, 2005). These "complex trauma" effects, in turn, had significant implications for treatment, since a single intervention strategy and short treatment interval were rarely sufficient to address the panoply of trauma symptoms and problems experienced by many clients (Courtois & Ford, 2009).

So, here we are. Currently, there are a number of empirically validated treatments for those who have been traumatized, many trauma-specific professional organizations, conferences presenting cutting-edge trauma research, and large government entities funding trauma research. Trauma and its effects are now increasingly (although far from universally; Courtois & Gold, 2009; DePrince & Newman, 2011) taught in professional curricula, and a subset of clinicians formally specialize in treating traumatized children and adults.

This book exemplifies this new cutting edge in trauma awareness and intervention. Yet, and quite excitingly, Courtois and Ford lead us to a new point as well. As the technology of trauma treatment has burgeoned, and as empirical, laboratory-based interventions have been developed and tested, there has been an understandable assumption that such methodologies represent the general answer to trauma-related pain and disability. To some extent, this is true. The scientist-practitioner approach and its exemplars, such as cognitive-behavioral therapy (CBT), treatment outcome research, and fidelity to manualized treatment procedures, have led to many positive advances in the field. They have given us, among others, therapy models such as prolonged exposure (Foa, 2011), cognitive processing therapy (Resick & Schnicke, 1993), dialectical behavior therapy (Linehan, 1993), eye movement desensitization and reprocessing (Shapiro, 1995), and, for children, trauma-focused cognitive-behavioral therapy (Cohen, Mannarino, & Deblinger, 2006). These treatment packages have helped untold thousands of people who otherwise would have suffered more and longer.

Yet, as noted in this book, there is clearly a need for more. As our profession advances, we are, ironically, rediscovering treatment components that were first developed in nonscience contexts, and that are sometimes rejected by empirically focused clinicians and researchers. Often considered *psychodynamic, client-centered,* or, more recently, *relational*, these components stress the importance of a positive therapeutic relationship, a caring, empathic psychotherapist, and attention to the ebb and flow of the therapy session, including client–therapist attunement and connection, transference and countertransference, boundary negotiations, and attachment-level response. Despite their "softer" foci, these interpersonal elements represent some of the most consistently supported findings of the therapy outcome literature. Research indicates, for example, that therapy in the context of a caring and supportive relationship is considerably more likely to be successful, especially when the clinician exhibits qualities of empathy, self-awareness, compassion, and positive regard (Gilbert, 2009; Lambert & Barley, 2001; Martin, Garske, & Davis, 2000; Norcross, 2011). Furthermore, therapy that activates beliefs, expectations, and perceptions formed early in life appears to support cognitive and emotional processing of important clinical phenomena (Rholes & Simpson, 2004). Whether called *transference* or *activated relational schema*, this process can be as easily viewed as a cognitive-behavioral phenomenon as a psychodynamic one (Briere & Scott, 2006).

Unfortunately, the use of relational principles and techniques is not yet common in cognitive-behavioral trauma therapy, nor are therapist attunement and empathy always highly valued. Similarly, although psychodynamic therapists often titrate or time ("stage") exposure to historical material during treatment as a function of the client's distress level and affect-regulation capacities, many modern evidence-based approaches to trauma do not consider titration or staging important. This is unfortunate, since recent attempts to integrate these approaches and techniques into empirical trauma therapy appear to be quite successful in well-controlled treatment outcome research—see, for example, Cloitre and colleagues'

(2010) skills training for affect and interpersonal regulation (STAIR), and the other interventions outlined in this book.

What we need at this point, and what is demonstrated by Courtois and Ford, is a way to bridge the gap between classic CBT and relational psychotherapy, because neither side of this equation, alone, is likely to be optimally helpful. The classic, empirically focused approach, although useful in many ways, runs the risk of being less responsive to the specific difficulties, capacities, and interpersonal/attachment needs of the client with complex posttraumatic outcomes. Thus, it may help in some ways (e.g., processing explicit trauma memories, intervening in cognitive distortions), but not others (e.g., processing attachment schemas, developing affect- and self-regulation skills). So, too, may the relational psychotherapy approach fall short, especially by not integrating current knowledge on the importance of therapeutic exposure and cognitive interventions in trauma treatment.

Because this book does these things, balancing relational interventions with classic evidence-based principles, it serves as an excellent example of what is likely to be the next stage in the evolution of trauma therapy. We have validated the reality—in fact, the ubiquity—of psychological trauma in our society; we are becoming much better at devising diagnostic and theoretical models of trauma impact; and we have invented a number of therapies that are seemingly quantum leaps from what was available just 20 or 30 years ago. Now, as evidenced by this volume, we are doing the hard work of synthesis and refining the fruits of synthesis; we are creating remedies for survivors that relate both to posttraumatic stress and altered interpersonal functioning, to capacities as well as injuries. In this process, and with this book, trauma treatment moves yet another step forward.

JOHN BRIERE, PHD
Department of Psychiatry and the Behavioral Sciences
Keck School of Medicine
University of Southern California

REFERENCES

American Psychiatric Association. (1980). *Diagnostic and statistical manual of mental disorders*. Washington, DC: Author.

Briere, J. (2004). *Psychological assessment of adult posttraumatic states: Phenomenology, diagnosis, and measurement* (2nd ed.). Washington, DC: American Psychological Association.

Briere, J., & Scott, C. (2006). *Principles of trauma therapy: A guide to symptoms, evaluation, and treatment*. Thousand Oaks, CA: Sage.

Cloitre, M., Stovall-McClough, K. C., Nooner, K., Zorbas, P., Cherry, S., Jackson, C. L., et al. (2010). Treatment for PTSD related to childhood abuse: A randomized controlled trial. *American Journal of Psychiatry, 167*, 915–924.

Cohen, J. A., Mannarino, A. P., & Deblinger, E. (2006). *Treating trauma and traumatic grief in children and adolescents.* New York: Guilford Press.

Courtois, C. A., & Ford, J. D. (Eds.). (2009). *Treating complex traumatic stress disorders: An evidence-based guide.* New York: Guilford Press.

Courtois, C. A., & Gold, S. N. (2009). The need for inclusion of psychological trauma in the professional curriculum: A call to action. *Psychological Trauma: Theory, Research, Practice, and Policy, 1*(1), 3–23.

DePrince, A. P., & Newman, E. (2011). The art and science of trauma-focused training and education. *Psychological Trauma: Theory, Research, Practice, and Policy, 3*(3), 213–214.

Dohrenwend, B. P., Turner, J. B., Turse, N. A., Adams, B. G., Koenen, K. C., & Marshall, R. (2006). The psychological risks of Vietnam for U.S. veterans: A revisit with new data and methods. *Science, 313*, 979–982.

Foa, E. B. (2011). Prolonged exposure therapy: Past, present, and future. *Depression and Anxiety, 28*, 1043–1047.

Gilbert, P. (2009). Introducing compassion-focused therapy. *Advances in Psychiatric Treatment, 15*, 199–208.

Herman, J. L. (1992). Complex PTSD: A syndrome in survivors of prolonged and repeated trauma. *Journal of Traumatic Stress, 3*, 377–391.

Lambert, M. J., & Barley, D. E. (2001). Research summary on the therapeutic relationship and psychotherapy outcome. *Psychotherapy, 38*, 357–361.

Linehan, M. M. (1993). *Cognitive-behavioral treatment of borderline personality disorder.* New York: Guilford Press.

Martin, D. J., Garske, J. P., & Davis, M. K. (2000). Relation of the therapeutic alliance with outcome and other variables: A meta-analytic review. *Journal of Consulting and Clinical Psychology, 68*, 438–450.

Masson, J. M. (1984). *The assault on truth: Freud's suppression of the seduction theory.* New York: Farrar, Straus & Giroux.

Norcross, J. C. (Ed.). (2011). *Psychotherapy relationships that work* (2nd ed.). New York: Oxford University Press.

Resick, P. A., & Schnicke, M. K. (1993). *Cognitive processing therapy for rape victims: A treatment manual.* Newbury Park, CA: Sage.

Rholes, W. S., & Simpson, J. A. (Eds.). (2004). *Adult attachment: Theory, research, and clinical implications.* New York: Guilford Press.

Shapiro, F. (1995). *Eye movement desensitization and reprocessing: Basic principles, protocols, and procedures.* New York: Guilford Press.

van der Kolk, B. A. (2005). Developmental trauma disorder: Toward a rational diagnosis for children with complex trauma histories. *Psychiatric Annals, 35*(5), 401–408.

Preface

More than two decades ago, van der Hart, Brown, and van der Kolk (1989), followed by Herman (1992b), described a three-stage psychotherapy for clients suffering from complex traumatic stress disorders that elaborated a model formulated a century earlier by the French psychiatrist Pierre Janet (1889/1973). Since its reintroduction, Janet's sequenced treatment model, designed to stabilize the client before reworking and resolving the trauma and its effects, has been applied fairly extensively to the treatment of complex developmental trauma and related dissociative disorders. A clinical consensus and evidence base for this approach and associated techniques are currently under development (Cloitre et al., 2011; Courtois & Ford, 2009). In this book, we build on the foundation of this earlier work and incorporate newly available scientific data and technical innovations in clinical practice to further advance a phase-based treatment model. In addition, we address challenges and nuances in the treatment of complex trauma that require creative and sensitive application of clinical concepts and techniques that must be tailored to the needs of the individual client.

Although the sequenced (or phased) model described here is linear on paper, it is dynamic in practice and not applied in a lockstep fashion; rather, tasks and techniques of each phase are organized on the basis of a number of factors, primarily the client's clinical status, emotion-regulation capacity, motivation, and response to treatment. Client resilience and strengths are assessed and built upon right from the start; however, many clients can be expected to have difficulties learning and applying new skills. Accordingly, relapse planning is built into the model, and setbacks are not considered failures but rather indications of the need to revisit therapeutic tasks and to relearn or burnish recently attained skills. From this perspective, the sequenced model can be conceptualized as an upward spiral of therapeutic tasks that are completed progressively. It is simultaneously a recursive model in which clients routinely return to earlier learning tasks and in which various skills are learned and challenged and then revisited, reworked, and solidified in an ever-progressive way through all three treatment phases. The upward spiral is hierarchical, built on a foundation of improved and newly attained skills in emotion regulation and on greater life stability, and the secure base of the therapy relationship. These, in turn, can lead to enhanced self-esteem, better relationships, and overall life improvement. Initially, progress often is of the "two steps forward, one step back" variety; subsequently, it becomes more steps forward and fewer steps back as the client gains mastery and achieves therapeutic goals.

The book begins with two chapters that describe complex forms of psychological trauma and associated complex traumatic stress symptoms and disorders. We highlight the importance of utilizing a comprehensive diagnosis such as complex posttraumatic stress disorder/disorders of extreme stress not otherwise specified (DESNOS; Herman, 1992a) or developmental trauma disorder (DTD; van der Kolk, 2005) in order to fully address the range of "complex traumatic stress disorders" (Courtois & Ford, 2009). We next devote two chapters to the practical preparations necessary to work with complex posttraumatic conditions, including practice tools and policies to reasonably manage risk, the establishment of a strong therapeutic alliance, crisis prevention and management, and initial assessment. In Chapter 5 we introduce the three phase model of treatment, and discuss Phase 1 emphases—safety, client engagement and education, and skill building. Chapter 6 continues with an in-depth discussion of the nuances of Phase 2—trauma processing with clients who have complex traumatic stress disorder—and concludes with a description of Phase 3 interventions that assist the client in applying therapy gains to daily life. Chapter 7 introduces the use of three systemic treatment modalities: group, couple, and family therapy. Chapter 8 addresses advanced issues related to treating severe affect dysregulation and dissociation and their many associated identity, somatic, behavioral, and relational manifestations. Chapter 9 challenges therapists to attend scrupulously to their own emotion regulation and to the management of professional boundaries and limitations, in order to be therapeutically available but "not too close and not too distant." The book concludes by addressing some of the complex transference and countertransference dilemmas encountered by therapists treating clients with complex trauma histories.

For readers interested in deepening their exploration of complex PTSD and its treatment, we have created self-reflection questions to accompany each chapter, as well as lists of additional resources for professionals, clients, and students. These are available in downloadable form from Guilford's website at *www.guilford.com/p/courtois*.

SIX TAKE-HOME POINTS

We emphasize the following half-dozen key points for the therapist to keep in mind in treating complex trauma.

First, even today, the professional training of most therapists unfortunately does not include attention to trauma and posttraumatic responses, despite the fact that traumatized individuals make up high percentages of clinical caseloads. Not infrequently, this circumstance has led to a mismatch in terms of the needs of these clients and the availability of trauma-informed therapy and trauma resolution, resulting at best in modest and short-lived progress and at worst in tragic consequences, including ongoing posttraumatic stagnation, decline, and death. Specialized information, training, and skills are needed to work with clients who have been traumatized, whether the trauma was short term and circumscribed or was more extensive and complex, as described in this volume. Special issues may arise for both the client and the therapist during this treatment; we point these out and discuss them for the reader to anticipate. Even highly experienced therapists can fall into the various "treatment traps," impasses, and traumatic reenactments that occur routinely in the treatment of this population (Chu, 1988, 2011). Despite their experience, these therapists may feel as though they have few therapeutic skills and nothing helpful to offer. For this and other reasons, trauma-informed consultation and supervision and other forms of professional and personal support are well warranted. This is especially the case for novice therapists or those new to working with this population, but it applies to more experienced therapists as well.

Second, we have articulated a relationship-based treatment of the most interpersonally distressed clients, those with multiple and often entrenched posttraumatic adaptations and self-concepts, whose relationships with caregivers (or responsible others) have been compromised by abuse, neglect, and other forms of insecure attachment. Successful treatment is predicated on a trustworthy and secure relationship between therapist and client that simultaneously serves as a catalyst for unresolved relational issues to emerge. The treatment that is proposed is eclectic, multitheoretical, integrative, and evidence and consensus based. It integrates a variety of techniques and tasks that are approached in hierarchical fashion within an established sequence of treatment. It focuses initially on safety and personal and life stabilization and later on processing and resolution of the trauma. The overall aim is the alleviation of posttraumatic and other onerous symptoms that, once achieved, leads to a healthier and more satisfying future.

Third, the three-phase sequenced model is elegant and parsimonious in theory but much less so in practice. The phases are eminently logical, moving in a rational sequence from laying a foundation (pretreatment and Phase 1) to clearing away the rubble of past traumas (Phase 2) to building a new life or doing an extensive remodeling that makes a formerly compromised and dysfunctional life worth living (Phase 3). And indeed, in some cases, psychotherapy for complex PTSD does progress in precisely this sequence, usually when the client has limited traumatic exposure and has a secure or "earned secure" attachment style and a number of personal resources to draw on. Unfortunately, this does not describe the average client with complex trauma. Although the three phases look simple, as treatment progresses there can be countless variations and complications as a result of severe crises, apparent dead ends, relapses, relationship issues, and missed, misunderstood, or mistaken directions. Even when therapy is progressing smoothly, the three phases are not neatly subdivided but tend to overlap, and treatment tasks may need to be repeated numerous times before emotions, beliefs, and cognitions are sufficiently reprocessed and integrated. As often noted, the map is not the territory: The actual trajectory of treatment rarely mimics the ideal sequence. Thus the map—the assumptions and tactics the therapist relies on for guidance—often must be modified in order to accurately reflect the intricacies of the client's psyche and life and of the treatment process itself.

Fourth, assessment and treatment planning occur before treatment and form its groundwork. Starting from the potential client's initial contact and through the intake process, the therapist seeks to broadly inquire about and assess the individual. Questions about past and present-day trauma are routinely included in the intake, and the therapist understands that disclosure might not readily occur, even when the client has a trauma history. At whatever point disclosure takes place, the therapist must learn about the trauma in some detail and may need to proceed to more in-depth assessment with trauma-specialized instruments. Assessment might be repeated over the course of treatment to check for progress and outcome and to customize and redirect the therapy as needed. It is not unusual in this treatment for the resolution of one problem to lead to the emergence of others.

Fifth, Phase 1 is generally the longest of the treatment phases, "measured in mastery of skills, not time" (Turkus, personal communication, 2002). It involves helping the client to acquire (or strengthen) personal safety and psychological and life skills and to make shifts in attitude, affect, and behavior that undergird subsequent therapeutic activities and gains. Proceeding gradually and systematically in laying this foundation (and specifically encouraging the client who understandably wants it "all to go away" or who wants it "done yesterday") to pace and dose the work in ways that make it tolerable ultimately saves later time and effort. These clients often are trapped in alternating states of posttraumatic hyperarousal (e.g., panic or rage) and hypoarousal (e.g., dissociation, avoidance, or paralyzing shame) at the start of treatment. They need a solid foundation of personal safety and emotion-regulation skills and resources to engage in therapy without avoidable crises or regressions.

Sixth, and finally, although Phase 1 does not specifically focus on trauma processing and resolution, much of the work in this phase relates, either directly or indirectly, to traumatic antecedents and posttraumatic reactions and to secondary elaborations (described further in Chapter 1). In Phase 1, the traumatic material is addressed predominantly from an educational/cognitive perspective. The client is educated about trauma and its short- and long-term posttraumatic consequences and developmental adaptations. The client's ongoing safety, symptom severity and duration, functional stability and skills, and engagement in self-reflective processing of relevant current experiences become the basis for determining whether more directed work with the trauma (Phase 2) is required. For some clients, direct trauma processing is contraindicated for a variety of reasons, discussed in Chapters 5 and 6. For others, however, trauma processing sometimes has to occur in Phase 1 and "out of order." Indicators for earlier processing include a client's not being able to stabilize and achieve a modicum of safety because he or she is reexperiencing or reenacting trauma memories to such an extent that it results in ongoing risk. If, after Phase 1 work, the client's overall life has improved but symptoms continue to be troubling, treatment proceeds to Phase 2 and the reworking and emotional processing of the trauma.

Trauma memory processing often is misunderstood as either a revivification or a cathartic release of the recollections and feelings from past traumatic events. This viewpoint omits the crucial ingredient of "processing." Phase 2 involves more than the recollection or simple retelling of the trauma or a cathartic "venting" of the pain those experiences and memories have caused. Therapeutic processing intentionally focuses on many formerly unacknowledged, unconscious, and unintegrated feelings, thoughts, and beliefs so that the client can gain (or regain) the ability to regulate emotions and to think more clearly. It is focused on building increased emotional tolerance that, in turn, promotes emotional processing to the point of resolving onerous symptoms. Clients may need to move back and forth between Phases 1 and 2, especially in times of crisis and/or when they need to refresh skills or apply or reformulate elements of their safety plan. In Phase 3 the gains of Phase 2 processing are applied to current and future life issues and decisions.

In summary, the goal of this book is to provide practicing therapists with information and pragmatic guidance in the treatment of complex traumatic stress disorders. Treatment rests on the foundation of viewing past and current trauma as a primary source of distress and of educating clients about how posttraumatic reactions develop into symptoms and other adaptations that extend into many life domains, causing major developmental and life interruptions and impediments (as well as challenges and specialized skills and resources). Because the lives of survivors extend beyond trauma and encompass many other personal and interpersonal domains, treatment is configured to attend to other life issues and "not trauma alone" (Gold, 2000). Victims and survivors are viewed as resilient, capable, and resourceful, although injured by what has befallen them; their strength is tapped and built on over the treatment's entire course. The treatment is likely to be complicated and is at times discouraging for client and therapist alike, yet change is possible and even probable when a road map and specific directions are available. The task is great, but so are the rewards, as many therapists and clients can attest.

Acknowledgments

Books are written as a result of the authors' interest in the subject matter and in the context of support from those around them. This book is no exception. We are fortunate that both of us have been immersed in learning about the issues raised by complex trauma and its consequences for many years; moreover, we have found ourselves to be highly compatible as coauthors (and, in our past and upcoming edited books on the topic, as coeditors as well). Our interests lie in understanding complex traumatic stress disorders and the criteria by which they are defined, and in discovering how they can best be treated from the perspective of both the therapist and the client. We each have seen clients whose symptoms match those associated with histories of complex trauma and who were misunderstood, misdiagnosed, and mistreated (in all senses of the word). These problems can arise despite genuine positive intent on the part of therapists as a result of gaps in the professional knowledge base and the training available with regard to complex trauma and its sequelae. On the other hand, we have seen in our own practices and those of colleagues many examples in which knowledge of complex trauma has provided a foundation for attention to clients' correspondingly complex issues and to the sequential treatment for these clients that can result in healing—hence, the focus in the title and subtitle of this book on the crucial importance of a sequential approach to treating clients who have complex trauma based on an understanding of treatment's effects on relationships (and relatedness).

Our intent in writing this book is to inform and guide therapists and clients alike about what is involved in the successful treatment of complex traumatic stress disorders. In the approach we describe, the client is provided with a foundation of education, self-management, and life skills that serves as the base for therapeutically addressing the troubling memories and problems with self-regulation that arise in the wake of complex trauma. We consider the relationship (or alliance) developed between the therapist and the client as the essential bedrock of the healing process, and we therefore discuss relational issues and their management in considerable detail. We also view successful engagement in relationships and self-regulation as universal challenges from which therapists are not exempt. We therefore explicitly suggest that therapists "practice what they preach" by applying the same principles to themselves in their professional and personal lives that they teach to their clients, regardless of whether they have a trauma history.

In this, we have sought to do the same. We consider ourselves very fortunate to have the supportive connections and role models for self-regulation that we do. We wish to acknowledge those in our primary professional and personal support systems who provide us sustenance as well as diversion from the "daily grind" required in writing a book. They have allowed us the time away from them (even when we are physically in the same room but our minds are elsewhere, focused on the next phrase or sentence or the appropriate citation) and have done so with great forbearance, grace, and understanding. Before we identify our personal lists, we want to particularly acknowledge the ongoing support of the members of the Complex Trauma Task Force of the International Society for Traumatic Stress Studies, which we co-chair: Drs. Pamela Carlson Alexander, John Briere, Marylene Cloitre, Bonnie Green, Judith Lewis Herman, Laurie Anne Pearlman, Joseph Spinazzola, Bradley Stolbach, Onno van der Hart, and Bessel van der Kolk. In addition to these colleagues, we have been fortunate to learn from the wisdom and inspiration of other professionals from around the globe, including Ellert Nijenhuis, Kathy Steele, Annemiek van Dijke, Nexh Morina, Danny Brom, Ruth Pat-Horenczyk, Jon Elhai, Gil Reyes, Chris Frueh, Frank Putnam, Ruth Lanius, Diana Fosha, Keri Gleiser, Julia Seng, Scott Henggeler, Judy Cohen, Tony Mannarino, Steven Marans, Steve Berkowitz, Bob Pynoos, John Fairbank, Harold Kudler, Nancy Kassam-Adams, Jeff Sugar, David Pelcovitz, Nnamdi Pole, Kathy Kendall-Tackett, Terry Keane, Catherine Classen, Clare Pain, Laura Brown, Judie Alpert, Sandy Bloom, Sandra Paivio, Steve Gold, Constance Dalenberg, Mark Schwartz, Lori Galperin, Pat Ogden, Francine Shapiro, Jim Chu, Jennifer Freyd, Daniel Siegel, Alan Schore, and Colin Ross, among the many professional friends and colleagues who form a list too long to fit in these pages but for each of whom we have the greatest admiration and appreciation. We also acknowledge the collegial support we have received from many members of our primary professional organizations, the International Society for Traumatic Stress Studies, the International Society for the Study of Trauma and Dissociation, the Division of Psychological Trauma (Division 56) of the American Psychological Association, and the National Child Traumatic Stress Network.

Chris acknowledges the following additional professional and personal supports: the therapists affiliated with her private practice, Courtois & Associates, PC: Drs. Lisa Ades, Emily Bauman, Nancy Hensler, Nicole Kaib, Sylvia Marotta, and Kelli Sanness, along with extern Alisa Breetz,

MA, and group co-leader Joanne Zucchetto, LICSW, offered substantial clinical and emotional support over the last year of writing. Additionally, Drs. Leslie Jadin, Jeffrey Jay, Philip Kinsler, Cathi Sitzman, Laurie Pearlman, Deborah Stokes, and Joan Turkus, along with Ruth Anne Koenick, MA, were especially important professional colleagues in terms of ongoing emotional support. Members of her ongoing and years-long professional consultation groups also deserve thanks. Special appreciation goes to Drs. Pat Ogden and Kikuni Minton for getting her started on somatosensory psychotherapy and to Dr. Sue Johnson for teaching her about emotionally focused couple therapy. Chris also salutes family members and close friends who, although they routinely worry about the extent of her workload and greeted the writing of this book with a collective "Not again!!," nevertheless are always there, led by her mother, Irene Courtois, and her husband, Tom.

Julian gratefully acknowledges the mentoring, role modeling, and professional and personal support he has received from colleagues in the Department of Veterans Affairs and its National Center for PTSD (including Matt Friedman, Paula Schnurr, Terry Keane, Jozef Ruzek, Bruce Hiley-Young, Patricia Watson, Annmarie McDonagh-Coyle, Kim Mueser, Elana Newman, Bob Rosenheck, Steve Southwick, and many wonderful colleagues at the Portland, White River Junction, Boston, and New Haven VA Medical Centers) and subsequently at the University of Connecticut (including Leighton Huey, Margaret Briggs-Gowan, John Chapman, Dan Connor, Keith Cruise, Bob Franks, Linda Frisman, Victor Hesselbrock, Ron Kadden, Hank Kranzler, Jason Lang, Judith Meyers, Geri Pearson, Nancy Petry, Karen Steinberg, Howard Tennen, Bob Trestman, and other valued faculty and research team colleagues and trainees). Closer to home are the family and friends who tolerate his workaholism and have made increasingly great strides in teaching him how to focus on the main goals in life, including Jim and Phyllis Ford, Julie and Todd, Lindy, Jessa, and Zack, six beautiful grandchildren (and counting), Allison, David, Elizabeth, Leighton, and most especially Judy.

Senior Editor Jim Nageotte at The Guilford Press suggested this book, and we are grateful to him for his insight and view of the publishing world. Senior Assistant Editor Jane Keislar has again kept us organized and on track. Alisa Breetz, MA, and Lenka Glassman, MA, worked diligently on researching related articles and books and organized the references, the bibliography, and the resources in the online supplement. Thank you all!

Contents

I. OVERVIEW OF COMPLEX TRAUMATIC STRESSORS AND SEQUELAE

1. Complex Trauma and Traumatic Stress Reactions 3

2. Complex Traumatic Stress Reactions and Disorders 28

II. TREATMENT OF COMPLEX TRAUMATIC STRESS REACTIONS AND DISORDERS

3. Preparing for Treatment of Complex Trauma 53

4. Treatment Goals and Assessment 88

5. Phase 1: Safety, Stabilization, and Engagement—Measured in Skills, Not Time 120

6. Phases 2 and 3: Trauma Memory, Emotion Processing, and Application to the Present and Future 144

7. Systemic Therapy across Phases: Group, Couple, and Family Modalities 190

III. ADVANCED TREATMENT CONSIDERATIONS AND RELATIONAL ISSUES

8. Into the Breach: Voids, Absences, and the Posttraumatic/Dissociative Relational Field 235

9. Walking the Walk: The Therapeutic Relationship 269

10. Transference and Countertransference in Complex Trauma Treatment 298

Postscript 329

References 333

Index 366

Self-reflection questions to accompany each chapter, as well as lists of self-help resources and workbooks, resources on the treatment of dissociation and complex trauma, and resources for therapist self-care, are available in downloadable form at *www.guilford.com/p/courtois*.

PART I

OVERVIEW OF COMPLEX TRAUMATIC STRESSORS AND SEQUELAE

CHAPTER 1

Complex Trauma and Traumatic Stress Reactions

Individuals with complex trauma histories pose some of the most difficult challenges and dilemmas faced by therapists and other helping professionals. The traumas they first experienced often date back to the earliest days of childhood, and the problems they experience in their current lives may have been relatively continuous from that time, may have emerged periodically and then remitted, or were mostly absent and emerged in delayed fashion in response to triggering events, experiences, or feelings. These clients typically have coped with several forms of interpersonal trauma—including abuse, neglect, exploitation, betrayal, rejection, antipathy, and abandonment—committed by other human beings. When their primary caregivers (such as parents, other relatives, health care providers, child care workers, or others in positions of authority) were the ones who engaged in these behaviors and mistreated them, the traumatic experiences were a violation of the universal expectation that children should be able to count on their caregivers to be trustworthy, nurturing, and protective. Such betrayals (Freyd, 1994) undermine the child's healthy development by leading to starkly negative beliefs about self and others and to corresponding behavior patterns based on facing a life in which the main priority is to survive overwhelming threats without help or protection. When life is a test of survival from the earliest days of infancy or childhood, the child adapts by anticipating and being prepared for the worst. Thus survival-based beliefs and behavior patterns become symptoms when they persist, even when circumstances no longer warrant them.

Individuals with complex trauma histories often remain in a biological and psychological survival mode (Osterman & Chemtob, 1999), even when they are no longer subject to the same risk of danger. Quite routinely, what were initially "normal reactions and adaptations to abnormal and recurring traumatic circumstances and experiences" (American Psychiatric

Association, 1980, p. 238) become problems over the long term because survival defenses are incompatible with a less dangerous or stressed life. Yet research has demonstrated that adults with complex trauma histories are at considerable risk for retraumatization across the entire lifespan (Duckworth & Follette, 2011; Widom, Czaja, & Dutton, 2008). When victimization continues unabated or recurs, survival reactions become ingrained, leaving their imprint on the individual's physiological and personality development. Survival can come to define a person's entire sense of self and his or her ability to self-regulate and to relate well and intimately with others. These reactions then tend to spawn defenses and coping mechanisms—or what have been identified as *secondary elaborations* of the untreated original effects (Gelinas, 1983)—including such problems as addictions, self-injury, and suicidality, which, paradoxically, may have been first used in the interest of self-soothing.

Many survivors of relational and other forms of early life trauma are deeply troubled and often struggle with feelings of anger, grief, alienation, distrust, confusion, low self-esteem, loneliness, shame, and self-loathing. They seem to be prisoners of their emotions, alternating between being flooded by intense emotional and physiological distress related to the trauma or its consequences and being detached and unable to express or feel any emotion at all—alternations that are the signature posttraumatic pattern. These occur alongside or in conjunction with other common reactions and symptoms (e.g., depression, anxiety, and low self-esteem) and their secondary manifestations. Those with complex trauma histories often have diffuse identity issues and feel like outsiders, different from other people, whom they somehow can't seem to get along with, fit in with, or get close to, even when they try. Moreover, they often feel a sense of personal contamination and that no one understands or can help them. Quite frequently and unfortunately, both they and other people (including the professionals they turn to for help) do misunderstand them, devalue their strengths, or view their survival adaptations through a lens of pathology (e.g., seeing them as "demanding," "overdependent and needy," "aggressive," or as having borderline personality).

Yet, despite all, many individuals with these histories display a remarkable capacity for resilience, a sense of morality and empathy for others, spirituality, and perseverance that are highly admirable under the circumstances and that create a strong capacity for survival. Three broad categories of survivorship, with much overlap between them, can be discerned:

1. Those who have successfully overcome their past and whose lives are healthy and satisfying. Often, individuals in this group have had reparative experiences within relationships that helped them to cope successfully.
2. Those whose lives are interrupted by recurring posttraumatic reactions (often in response to life events and experiences) that

periodically hijack them and their functioning for various periods of time.

3. Those whose lives are impaired on an ongoing basis and who live in a condition of posttraumatic decline, even to the point of death, due to compromised medical and mental health status (Felitti, Anda, Nordenberg, Williamson, Spitz, et al., 1998) or as victims of suicide of community violence, including homicide.

At the present time, no percentages are available for these three categories, but it is clear that for many (if not the majority of complex trauma survivors), their lives are interrupted and encumbered on a periodic or ongoing basis, and many of them seek relief from their symptoms from medical and mental health professionals.

What can helping professionals do to assist these individuals (hereafter identified as "complex trauma survivors" or "survivor clients") to overcome the correspondingly complex traumatic stress symptoms that once helped them to survive and to capitalize on their strengths and add to their resources? This is the question we address in this book, fully acknowledging that any answer is at best partial given the complexity of the challenge and the limitations of the evidence base of practice for this population. We believe that despite the complexities and challenges involved in their treatment, with appropriate and knowledgeable assistance many of these wounded yet spirited individuals can move beyond the point of survival to develop a greater capacity for a satisfactory life.

We begin with two composite case descriptions (both of fictional individuals) that capture many of the challenges and dilemmas that face complex trauma survivors and the helping professionals who seek to support them. The starting point for recovery from complex trauma is an understanding of how crucial experiences (including but not limited to trauma) have uniquely shaped the life and self of each individual.

Doris Hurley

Doris Hurley, a Caucasian woman in her 40s, sought psychotherapy because her husband gave her an ultimatum: "If you don't find a therapist who can make you stop hounding me and driving me crazy, I'm going to leave." Doris has long been unable to trust anyone close to her, yet she also is terrified of being abandoned. She vacillates between being highly dependent on her husband, pursuing him for emotional and physical closeness, and distancing and pushing him away. His resulting confusion and frustration led him to withdraw, confirming her belief that she will never find anyone trustworthy—and her unspoken fear that she is unlovable. This pattern was not limited to her marriage. Doris has a history of first charismatically ingratiating herself with family members and acquaintances and then rejecting or alienating them. Anyone who tried to get to know her usually drifted (or ran) away after they tired of her (largely unspoken) demands and "tests" and her anger. Over time, Doris became increasingly despondent, enraged, and desperate.

Doris's early experiences included numerous abandonments by her parents. From a young age, her mother was repeatedly in and out of state psychiatric hospitals, suffering from schizophrenia. During these periods, she and her siblings, individually or in pairs, were sent to stay with different relatives who were welcoming and emotionally available only to varying degrees. When her mother was at home, she was quite unstable and highly medicated and, as a result, was inconsistent in both her emotional states and parenting behaviors. Her father was sometimes attentive, but he used his wife's illness and protracted absences as an opportunity to rationalize his sexual abuse of the girls and physical abuse of the boys. Doris often witnessed her father's abusive episodes when he was drinking and tried to protect her siblings by "allowing" her father to abuse her rather than them. At times, her father treated Doris with loving care and attention and as his special confidante. Yet he also berated Doris for causing all of her mother's problems and told her she could never do enough to make up for her "sins." By age 11, Doris felt a deep sense of self-loathing and a guilty obligation to take care of her mother and siblings. She had no one (other than her sometimes responsive but abusive father) available to nurture, encourage, or protect her. Doris came to believe that she ruined every relationship and harmed every person she cared about and that she had to make up for this by denying her own needs and doing everything for other people because they could not be trusted to take care of themselves. She continues to feel unloved and unlovable, a source of anguish and mounting frustration, feelings that she sometimes manages with alcohol.

Hector Alvarez

Hector Alvarez is a 21-year-old Latino male, the oldest of three children. When he was 4 years old, his parents sought asylum in the United States from their home country in Central America, where his father had been tortured for his political beliefs. As his next of kin, the family fled the country fearing for their lives. Once in the United States, Hector's parents took low-income jobs that required both to work full time and long hours. He began kindergarten the year they immigrated and learned to speak English reasonably quickly. As a result and as often happens in immigrant families, his parents came to rely on him to serve as their interpreter. They also relied on him to care for his two siblings when they were working—he was essentially a full-time after-school babysitter for both siblings by the time he was 7 or 8 years old.

Hector's father suffered from terrible nightmares of his torture experience that would routinely awaken family members. He was often irritable due to lack of sleep and would take his anger and irritability out on Hector and his mother, both of whom he regularly physically assaulted, especially after he had been drinking (he drank more and more heavily over the years, in a futile effort to make the nightmares go away). Hector tried to protect his mother but to no avail, and both often had cuts and bruises that they hid from outsiders.

Hector's mother was very passive and deferential in response to her husband, suffered from major depression, and coped by turning to her Catholic faith or by sleeping, while Hector took care of his siblings.

Hector was a shy child who was quiet and reserved at school—he never "made waves" and was not rambunctious like the other boys in his class. Over time, other boys made fun of him, taunting him for being a "teacher's pet" and a "sissy" (and worse) and for always having to go home right after school instead of being able to play. They also teased him about being Latino and for his shabby clothing. Over time, he became more and more isolated and seemed to his teachers to be "in his own world." Some teachers tried to connect with him but found him frustrating because he was so hard to reach. His school performance was subpar, and some of his teachers wrote him off as being slow.

Hector was dutiful in his religious studies, mostly in an effort to spend time with his mother and to get her approval. In seventh grade, his attentiveness and piety were noticed by the parish priest, who began to think Hector might have a religious calling. The priest befriended him and gave him extra attention, something that made him feel better about himself even as it brought more derision from his peers. The priest began to visit his home and became friends with both of his parents, who were thrilled to have the attention of "God's representative on earth." They often invited him to share a meal with them and to spend his free time at their home. Over time, this priest became someone Hector could share his problems with and someone who intervened with his parents on his behalf. In efforts to foster Hector's vocation, the priest offered to take him on trips to visit various seminaries. Some of these trips required overnight stays. During these trips, the priest encouraged Hector to sleep in his bed and over time began to sexually molest him. Hector liked the attention but was confused about the sexual contact; he didn't know what it was, though he knew it was wrong when the priest told him not to disclose "their little secret," but he also knew it felt good. Over time, he came to dislike it, especially when it involved anal intercourse and not just mutual fondling and fellatio. The relationship and the abuse continued until Hector graduated from high school. He never told anyone what was happening with the priest, but the amount of time they spent together was noticed and whispered about. The priest had warned him that no one would understand their "special relationship from God" and that he would be punished by God if he ever disclosed it to anyone.

When Hector turned 18, instead of going to the seminary, as had been the plan, he joined the military to get away from his family and from the priest. Both his parents and the priest were furious with him, feeling let down and betrayed by what they described as "his selfishness." His mother grieved that he had given up his faith and his true vocation. His father railed that he had joined an arm of the government that would engage him in killing and torturing others, as he had been tortured. Hector went to boot camp, where he did well. He was deployed to Iraq, where he killed civilian combatants (including women and children) and witnessed the deaths and dismemberments of several other soldiers. While deployed, he was sexually gang-raped by a group of soldiers who had noted that he did not have a girlfriend and therefore assumed him to be gay. Again, Hector told no one. Afterward, he became verbally abusive and started getting into physical brawls, as well as using drugs when he could get them. Hector returned home from his first tour of duty a changed man. At first, he was depressed and withdrawn, not wanting to tell anyone about his military duties. He was ashamed at the homecoming reception, believing himself to be "a monster" and "disgusting." He started drinking heavily. He became disruptive in his unit and was ordered to get a mental health evaluation. When he was diagnosed with depression and posttraumatic stress disorder (PTSD), as well as alcoholism, he was separated from his unit and the military, leaving him even more bereft and betrayed. He was also isolated from his family, who felt they no longer knew him and kept their distance. Over time, he became homeless and relied on military buddies for a place to stay and for support. They would routinely dry him out and keep an eye on him when he became suicidal. One day, they dropped him off at the Community Mental Health Crisis Center, where he was evaluated and admitted to an inpatient unit, where he reluctantly began treatment.

These two very different cases illustrate what is often the case for complex trauma survivors: the shock of multiple, repeated, and overlapping victimizations and traumatic exposures beginning in childhood in insecure and/or abusive attachment relationships; the child or adolescent's initial reactions that were either unrecognized or given no explanation, support, or intervention; longer term reactions in late adolescence or adulthood that occurred in conjunction with the age and life stage issues of the individual; and the development of coping mechanisms and defenses (including cognitions and beliefs rooted in the trauma) that then created additional problems for the individual. What was often life-sustaining or life-saving at the time of the repeated trauma (e.g., dissociation, denial, repression, forced silence) paradoxically interfered with the later ability to function in life and to relate to others in ways that are healthy and satisfactory.

This book is designed to provide practicing psychotherapists and clinical researchers with detailed information about complex traumatic stress disorders, along with state-of-the-art best practices and protocols for conceptualization, assessment, treatment, policy, and research. In the remainder of this chapter, we provide additional description of what has come to be known as *complex trauma* or *complex traumatic stressors*, including those that begin early in life, those that occur in adulthood, and those that overlap and are cumulative over the lifespan. Adult-onset complex trauma can occur in an individual without a previous history yet nevertheless cause complex reactions. More commonly, adult traumatic stressors consist of additional exposures and victimizations that build on, add to, or exacerbate the effects of earlier traumas. In Chapter 2, we describe how, over time, these adaptations to exposure to complex trauma can become persistent *complex posttraumatic reactions, adaptations, and disorders*. Many of these problems have long gone unrecognized or untreated in mental health (and medical) practice, usually because the most apparent symptoms were treated without regard to the posttraumatic origin and adaptations that contributed to or perhaps even caused them (Gelinas, 1983).

Available clinical consensus (supported by emerging empirical data) endorses the use and sequencing of treatment strategies that go beyond those that have proven effective in treating the symptoms of "classic" PTSD as currently defined in the *Diagnostic and Statistical Manual of Mental Disorders* (DSM-IV-TR; American Psychiatric Association, 2000; Adults Surviving Child Abuse, 2012; Arnold & Fisch, 2011; Chu, 2011; Cloitre et al., 2011; Courtois, 1999, 2010; Courtois & Ford, 2009; Courtois, Ford, & Cloitre, 2009; Ford, Courtois, Van der Hart, Steele, & Nijenhuis, 2005; Herman, 1992a, 1992b; Ogden, Minton, & Pain, 2006; Paivio & Pascual-Leone, 2010; Van der Hart, Nijenhuis, & Steele, 2006). As discussed in the Preface, these additional strategies include a preliminary focus on safety, increased life stabilization, and the development of emotional regulation and life skills (among others) offered in a progressive and hierarchical sequence and applied according to the client's emotional capacity and resources.

DEFINING COMPLEX TRAUMA

Traumatic events as defined in DSM-IV-TR involve death and threat of death, exposure to the grotesque, or violation of bodily integrity. In the proposed forthcoming new version of the DSM—DSM-5—the definition of traumatic stressors has been streamlined by dropping the requirement that the individual must experience intense subjective distress (i.e., fear, helplessness, or horror) during or soon after the event (*www.dsm5.org/ProposedRevision/Pages/proposedrevision.aspx?rid=165*). This change is consistent with research indicating that those subjective reactions exclude some peritraumatic responses that are associated with PTSD (e.g., amnesia and dissociation; O'Donnell, Creamer, McFarlane, Silove, & Bryant, 2010) and are better understood as "risk factors rather than diagnostic requirements for PTSD" (Karam, Andrews, Bromet, Petukhova, Ruscio, et al., 2010, p. 465). Two other proposed changes in the DSM-5 definition of traumatic events are that they may include (1) learning of a violent or accidental death or threat of death that happened to a close relative or close friend or (2) "repeated or extreme exposure to aversive details of the event(s) (e.g., first responders collecting body parts; police officers repeatedly exposed to details of child abuse)." These two additions are consistent with a more complex view of traumatic stressors that includes a relational component—the traumatic impact of an actual or potential loss of a primary attachment relationship or the vicarious impact of learning of something terrible happening to key people or to other vulnerable persons, such as children.

In addition to those classic criteria, complex traumatic stressors involve relational/familial and interpersonal forms of traumatization and exposure that are often chronic and include threats to the integrity of the self, to personal development, and to the ability to relate to others in healthy ways. They include abandonment, neglect, lack of protection, and emotional, verbal (including bullying), sexual, and physical abuse by primary caregivers or others of significance or loss of these primary attachment figures through illness, death, deployment, or displacement of some sort. Although these stressors more commonly occur during childhood and adolescence, some occur in adulthood in such forms as domestic violence, kidnapping, war, torture, genocide, human trafficking, and sexual or other forms of captivity or slavery.

Additionally, complex trauma may be based on and associated with the victim's very identity, including such immutable characteristics as race, ethnicity, skin color, gender, genetic and medical conditions and physical limitations, family/tribal/clan background and history, and other factors, such as religious and political orientation, class, economic status, and resultant power or lack thereof (Kira et al., 2011). Traumatic victimizations based on these characteristics can literally begin pre-birth and be life-long or can occur primarily in adulthood. They may result in both individual victimization and in the persecution of entire communities or populations who share characteristics that lead their members to be deemed suspect, inferior, or of sufficient threat to warrant their eradication. Kira and colleagues (2011) have described the violence perpetrated in the name of these types of prejudices or political and economic motives as "identity trauma" because they are based on the intent to discredit and destroy the personal and cultural identity of victims.

Complex trauma, whatever its type or whenever it begins, is usually not a one-time occurrence. Instead, it is most often recurring, escalating in severity over its duration. One type of trauma may "layer" on top of another, a pattern found in family abuse victims who are multiply victimized in the family by more than one member (poly- or multiple victimization) and who are more vulnerable to abuse outside of the family (revictimization) in many life domains such as school, work, the military, religious congregations and groups, and so forth. The result is what has been identified by Ford and Courtois (2009), Duckworth and Follette (2011), Follette, Polusny, Bechtle, and Naugle (1996), and Kira and colleagues (2010) as cumulative forms of trauma and retraumatization that deprive victims of their sense of safety and hope, their connection to primary support systems and community, and their very identity and sense of self. Such compounded stressors are the norm rather than the exception for any number of complex trauma survivors. Treatment must therefore be correspondingly complex, multifaceted, and yet individualized in order to fully address the scope of the traumatic experiences and their multiple life impacts (Briere & Lanktree, 2011; Courtois, 2004; McMacklin, Newman, Fogler, & Keane, 2012).

COMPLEX TRAUMA IN CHILDHOOD

Child psychiatrist Lenore Terr distinguished two main types of children's exposure to psychological trauma that also apply to adults (Terr, 1991). "*Type I*" *single-incident trauma* refers to a one-time or short-term event that occurs suddenly and "out of the blue" and is thus unexpected and profoundly shocking: a traumatic motor vehicle accident; a natural disaster; a terrorist bombing, an episode of abuse, assault, or rape; a sudden death or displacement; or the witnessing of violence or something overwhelming that is highly out of the ordinary. In terms of causation, this type of trauma may be *impersonal* (i.e., not caused by another person but rather a true random event or accident, often labeled an "act of God") or it may be *interpersonal* (i.e., caused or carried out by another person or persons, sometimes with intention, other times not). In contrast, "*Type II*" *repetitive or complex trauma* refers to ongoing physical, sexual, and emotional abuse and neglect and other forms of maltreatment in the nuclear or extended family (or quasi-family); domestic violence; community danger and violence; cultural, gender, political, ethnic, illness and religion-based oppression, violence, and physical and geographic displacement; refugee status; terrorism; torture; war; and genocide. These are all interpersonal, involving intentional acts by, or the failure to act by, other human beings.

Although Type I traumatic stressors are typically one time or very time limited, they can range from relatively mild to those of high-magnitude intensity that cause enough distress in the short-term aftermath to meet criteria for what is listed in DSM-IV-TR as acute stress disorder (ASD) and PTSD, acute type (American Psychiatric Association, 1994, 2000). On average, children are more easily stressed or traumatized than adults due to their immaturity and dependence on adults for response and protection. Children place their own age-related interpretations on events especially when they receive no explanation or soothing. Yet, both children and adults have an easier time recovering from Type I traumas (even of high intensity) than from those of the Type II variety. This is especially true when Type I traumas (such as a weather event or other natural disaster or an industrial, ecological, or transportation accident) occur within and affect an entire community or country. They constitute public events that require public emergency response and that are openly discussed in the broader community. Type I traumas typically do not recur, at least not with the same unexpectedness or strength as the original event, or they do so after a period of relative calm, as in the case of recurrent natural or weather-related disasters. However, their influence may be felt for years and beyond. In consequence, Type I trauma victims may remain vigilant to the possibility of recurrence, a response that tends to (but does not always) diminish over time as life returns to normal or a "new normal" is established for individuals, families, and entire communities (Shapiro, 2012).

Although Type II trauma might be expected to be less common than its Type I counterpart, it unfortunately appears to be much more common and prevalent than previously recognized, especially in children, adolescents, and others in conditions of dependency and disempowerment (such as females in patriarchal cultures; the politically oppressed; refugees and others who are displaced; the unemancipated, or those who lack basic resources; the emotionally, intellectually, or physically ill or disabled; the infirm and the elderly). Kaffman (2009) described childhood victimization as a "silent epidemic," and Finkelhor, Turner, Ormrod, and Hamby (2010) reported that children are the most traumatized class of humans around the globe. The findings of these researchers are at odds with the view that children have protected status in most families, societies, and cultures. Instead, Finkelhor reports that children are prime targets and highly vulnerable, due principally to their small size, their physical and emotional immaturity with its associated lack of control, power, and resources; and their related dependency on caregivers. They are subjected to many forms of exploitation on an ongoing basis, imposed on them by individuals with greater power, strength, knowledge, and resources, many of whom are, paradoxically and tragically, responsible for their care and welfare. These traumas are *interpersonal* in nature and involve personal transgression, violation, and exploitation of the child by those who rely on the child's lesser physical abilities, innocence, and immaturity to intimidate, bully, confuse, blackmail, exploit, or otherwise coerce.

In the worst-case scenario, a parent or other significant caregiver directly and repeatedly abuses a child or does not respond to or protect a child or other vulnerable individual who is being abused and mistreated and isolates the child from others through threats or with direct violence. Consequently, such an abusive, nonprotective, or malevolently exploitive circumstance (Chefetz [personal communication] has coined the term "attack-ment" to describe these dynamics) has a profound impact on the victim's ability to trust others. It also affects the victim's identity and self-concept, usually in negative ways that include self-hatred, low self-worth, and lack of self-confidence. As a result, both relationships and the individual's sense of self and internal states (feelings, thoughts, and perceptions) can become sources of fear, despair, rage, or other extreme dysphoria or numbed and dissociated reactions. This state of alienation from self and others is further exacerbated when the occurrence of abuse or other victimization involves betrayal and is repeated and becomes chronic, in the process leading the victim to remain in a state of either hyperarousal/anticipation/hypervigilance or hypoarousal/numbing (or to alternate between these two states) and to develop strong protective mechanisms, such as dissociation, in order to endure recurrences. When these additional victimizations recur, they unfortunately tend to escalate in severity and intrusiveness over time, causing additional traumatization (Duckworth & Follette, 2011).

In many cases of child maltreatment, emotional or psychological coercion and the use of the adult's authority and dominant power rather than physical force or violence is the fulcrum and weapon used against the child;

however, force and violence are common in some settings and in some forms of abuse (sometimes in conjunction with extreme isolation and drugging of the child), as they are used to further control or terrorize the victim into submission. The use of force and violence is more commonplace and prevalent in some families, communities, religions, cultural/ethnic groups, and societies based on the views and values about adult prerogatives with children that are espoused. They may also be based on the sociopathy of the perpetrators.

Unfortunately, Type II traumas such as childhood sexual or physical abuse, neglect, and family violence frequently occur concurrently or in succession. Such "cumulative trauma" (Cloitre et al., 2010; Kira et al., 2010) or polyvictimization (Finkelhor, 2008; Finkelhor, Ormrod, Turner, & Hamby, 2005) is associated with particularly severe and complex symptomatic problems (Arnold & Fisch, 2011). In such cases, survival adaptations can become habitual and persistent, interwoven in complex ways with the child's developing body, emotions, personality, mental processes, and relationships (Ford, 2005).

Type II trauma also often occurs within a closed context—such as a family, a religious group, a workplace, a chain of command, or a battle group—usually perpetrated by someone related to or known to the victim. As such, it often involves a fundamental betrayal of the relationship between the victim and the perpetrator and within the community (Freyd, 1994). It may also involve the betrayal of a particular role and the responsibility associated with the relationship (i.e., parent–child, family member–child, therapist–client, teacher–student, clergy–child/adult congregant, supervisor–employee, military officer–enlisted man or woman). Relational dynamics of this sort have the effect of further complicating the victim's survival adaptations, especially when a superficially caring, loving, or seductive relationship is cultivated with the victim (e.g., by an adult mentor such as a priest, coach, or teacher; by an adult who offers a child special favors for compliance; by a superior who acts as a protector or who can offer special favors and career advancement). In a process labeled "selection and grooming," potential abusers seek out as potential victims those who appear insecure, are needy and without resources, and are isolated from others or are obviously neglected by caregivers or those who are in crisis or distress for which they are seeking assistance. This status is then used against the victim to seduce, coerce, and exploit. Such a scenario can lead to *trauma bonding* between victim and perpetrator (i.e., the development of an attachment bond based on the traumatic relationship *and* the physical and sexual contact), creating additional distress and confusion for the victim who takes on responsibility and guilt for what transpired, often with the encouragement or insinuation of the perpetrator(s) to do so.

It is for all of these reasons that Type II or complex forms of trauma that involve interpersonal violation and disregard have been found to be associated with a much higher risk for the development of PTSD (acute, chronic, and delayed variants) than Type I trauma (e.g., 33–75+% risk vs.

10–20% risk, respectively; Copeland, Keeler, Angold, & Costello, 2010; Kessler, Sonnega, Bromer, Hughes, & Nelson, 1995) and to result in additional effects beyond the standard criteria for PTSD (Cloitre et al., 2009; Finkelhor, 2007). Thus polyvictimization or complex trauma are "developmentally adverse interpersonal traumas" (Ford, 2005) because they place the victim at risk not only for recurrent stress and psychophysiological arousal (e.g., PTSD, other anxiety disorders, depression) but also for interruptions and breakdowns in healthy psychobiological, psychological, and social development. Complex trauma not only involves shock, fear, terror, or powerlessness (either short or long term) but also, more fundamentally, constitutes a violation of the immature self and a challenge to the development of a positive and secure self, as major psychic energy is directed toward survival and defense rather than toward learning and personal development (Ford, 2009b, 2009c). Moreover, it may influence the brain's very development, structure, and functioning in both the short and long term (Lanius et al., 2010; Schore, 2009).

Complex trauma often forces the child victim to substitute automatic survival tactics for adaptive self-regulation, starting at the most basic level of physical reactions (e.g., intense states of hyperarousal/agitation or hypoarousal/immobility) and behavioral (e.g., aggressive or passive/avoidant responses) that can become so automatic and habitual that the child's emotional and cognitive development are derailed or distorted. What is more, self-integrity is profoundly shaken, as the child victim incorporates the "lessons of abuse" into a view of him- or herself as bad, inadequate, disgusting, contaminated, and deserving of mistreatment and neglect. Such misattributions and related schema about self and others are some of the most common and robust cognitive and assumptive consequences of chronic childhood abuse (as well as other forms of interpersonal trauma) and are especially debilitating to healthy development and relationships (Cole & Putnam, 1992; McCann & Pearlman, 1992). Because the violation occurs in an interpersonal context that carries profound significance for personal development, relationships become suspect and a source of threat and fear rather than of safety and nurturance.

In vulnerable children, complex trauma causes compromised attachment security, self-integrity, and ultimately self-regulation. Thus it constitutes a threat not only to physical but also to psychological survival—to the development of the self and the capacity to regulate emotions (Arnold & Fisch, 2011). For example, emotional abuse by an adult caregiver that involves systematic disparagement, blame, and shame of a child ("You worthless piece of s—t"; "You shouldn't have been born"; "You're the source of all of my problems"; "I should have aborted you"; "If you don't like what I tell you, you can go hang yourself") but does not involve physical or sexual violation or life threat is nevertheless psychologically damaging. Such bullying and antipathy on the part of the primary caregiver or other family members, in addition to maltreatment and role reversals that are found in many dysfunctional families, lead to severe psychobiological dysregulation and reactivity (Teicher, Samson, Polcari, & McGreenery, 2006).

Complex Trauma in Infancy

When trauma occurs in infancy, the immediate aftereffects are consistent with the developmental conditions of this earliest phase of life, as well as the infant's limited capacities for response (Scheeringa & Zeanah, 2001). The infant's sense of self is somatosensory and preconscious and is based on developing the capacity to organize the flood of sensory inputs and whatever support and security are available. The infant's interactions with caregivers, such as reciprocal gazing, the physical sensations of being held, fed, clothed, toileted, and communicated with through vocalizations and gestures, are critical to the organization and management of this sensory input. Emotion regulation is largely derived from caregiver responses that provide physical contact and soothing with emotional comforting and the identification of emotional states. Competent caregiver behaviors balance the amounts of pleasurable or dangerous multisensory stimulation that the infant is exposed to and function as outside regulators. Over time and with repeated experiences of modulation by and with the caregiver, the infant begins to learn self-regulation of physical and emotional states and develops security with the caregiver.

When traumatic stressors occur during infancy, they are often due to neglect and lack of appropriate and needed care resulting in understimulation on the one hand, to gross exposure and overstimulation with inadequate response or protection on the other, or to physical injury (or all of the above). It takes little to traumatize an infant due to his or her physical and psychic immaturity and extreme state of helplessness and dependence on caregivers for food, shelter, protection, nurturance, response, and stimulation. In consequence, infants are traumatized more readily and by less intense events than are older children or adolescents. The infant's reactions to trauma may emerge as problems in achieving core developmental milestones, such as nursing or bottle feeding (and, later, eating), speech, and a regular sleep cycle. Or they may appear in the form of unpredictable fussiness or insatiability, as well as difficulties in nutrition and digestion. Toileting may be delayed or complicated by excessive or restricted elimination or emotional distress in response to needing or having diaper changes or (later) encouragement to independently "use the potty." The traumatized infant may have emotional outbursts such as rageful protests, a separation cry, inconsolable crying, or withdrawal and despair. If the traumatic circumstances persist and if help or comfort is not forthcoming, the infant may "fail to thrive" and detach from and appear indifferent to the external world, even when caregivers are available. If traumatic injury, emotional intrusion, and neglect/lack of stimulation are of sufficient severity or duration, the infant is at risk of becoming physically ill and even of dying.

Because these self-regulatory, behavioral, social, and emotional problems can occur for many reasons in infancy and early toddlerhood, they should not be assumed to be necessarily or exclusively due to trauma. Yet trauma may be involved—for example, due to direct exposure to physical violence or intrusions (including but not limited to physical and sexual molestation) or to indirect exposure (seeing or hearing family violence, war violence, a natural or human-made accident or disaster) or to profound neglect or sudden catastrophic loss of a primary caregiver (or all three). Under conditions of great danger and insecurity, survival replaces the exploration and growth experiences associated with secure attachment and relational security. Rather than seeking out stimuli, as seems to be the hardwired tendency for most infants, the trauma-exposed infant or young child is likely to experience stimuli as terrifying and overwhelming, anxiety-provoking, painful and frustrating, or confusing and meaningless. This is true of both internal stimuli (such as bodily feelings or newly emerging emotions) and external stimuli (such as new sights, sounds, smells, and touch). What ordinarily would be exciting opportunities to explore, organize, and gain a sense of mastery in relation to one's own body and the external world instead become experienced as threats, as a condition of psychic discomfort and pain, and as confusing and indecipherable "noise." The self-regulatory, relational, and emotional problems that emerge are the direct result of having the developing body and brain's self-protective stress response systems hijacked by the basic imperative—survival—in the absence of adequate nurturing and soothing.

Complex Trauma in Toddlerhood through the Elementary School Years

As the child grows, he or she develops a foundation of basic identity and sense of self, self-regulatory capabilities, and the ability to use language to verbally organize and orchestrate these core capacities. When complex forms of traumatic victimization or loss begin in this stage, the impact can still be severe. This is especially the case if the traumatic shock or the sudden loss of primary attachment figures overwhelms the child's ability to sustain organized self, relational, and emotion regulation, disrupting normal developmental tasks and causing symptoms of distress. As an example: a toddler who has well-developed self-regulatory skills and a consistently responsive and available caregiver may recover from some traumatic experiences without lasting aftereffects or harm. On the other hand, if that same toddler experiences prolonged exposure that extends over many months or years, and if either the toddler's or the caregivers' (or both) ability to self-regulate and maintain relational security are overwhelmed, then the child is likely to develop bodily, behavioral, emotional, or social problems that reflect regression to an earlier level of functioning similar to that of a traumatized infant.

Furthermore, when a toddler or even an older (early elementary school-age) child has not developed a sense of optimism, agency, and security in primary relationships, that child is particularly at risk for experiencing profound "regression" in self-regulatory capacities if subjected to any type of abuse, violence, neglect, or loss. This may not actually be regression as commonly understood, but instead an unfortunate highlighting and exacerbation of the child's poorly developed self-regulatory and relational capacities. Any residual deficits might not become apparent until many years later, especially if caregiver relationships and the environment provide consistency and security and the child does not experience additional traumatic stressors; these children are often identified as asymptomatic. The deficits often become apparent when the normal challenges of adolescence or young adulthood trigger reminders of the trauma or overwhelm self-regulatory or relational capacities. The deficits are akin to a "crack in the foundation" or a "fault line," a vulnerability that can lead to a major loss of personal psychosocial functioning. Thus it is understandable that a child or adolescent who seemed to be well adjusted could develop problems with self-regulation that seem "infantile," such as bedwetting, encopresis, temper tantrums, difficulty delaying gratification, depression, major fears and anxiety, and reactive attachment disturbances involving withdrawal from close relationships after exposure to a reminder of the original trauma(s).

The initial reactions of victimized toddlers and school-age children also involve newly developed or intensified problems with emotion regulation and sense of self. Feelings (such as anxiety, terror, confusion, guilt, rage, shame, despair, or loss and grief reactions) and predominantly negative self-perceptions (such as a sense of being abnormal, bad, stupid, ugly, or deserving of mistreatment and nonresponse) may develop in the aftermath of abuse. Yet, in some cases, feelings such as these may be absent especially when the abuse involves grooming and seduction of the child into a special relationship involving excessive attention that over time, includes sexual activities. In relationships involving *traumatic bonding*, the child's attachment system is invoked, and the resultant feelings of being special are likely to continue and compound over time. This may also occur when the child has been misled or blamed by a perpetrator or a misguided caregiver.

Even when a perpetrator is excessively cruel or uncaring toward the victimized child, the child may still seek contact due to the need for attachment and attention. This paradoxical response is likely when the child needs and depends on the perpetrator even in the face of the abuse or believes that this is a person who, by virtue of his or her authority or status, should be mollified or even loved or respected. Moreover, the child may feel a sense of protectiveness, loyalty, and devotion to the perpetrator that can effectively split the child's awareness into structurally dissociated mental states: simultaneously or alternately feeling loved and special or loyal, responsible, and guilty while also feeling terrified or enraged (Freyd, 1994; Van der

Hart, Nijenhuis, & Steele, 2006). If other children or loved ones (e.g., a battered parent) are victimized, the child may develop a similar dissociation between feeling developmentally appropriate fear and helplessness and feeling an age-inappropriate parentified sense of responsibility (and failure) to protect loved ones, including, in some cases, the perpetrator.

At the opposite end of the spectrum, when victimization is sudden in onset and forcefully committed by a stranger or by someone with no tenderness or desire to cultivate a pseudo-relationship, the child is likely to experience a more immediate sense of shock, disbelief, fear, terror, anxiety, and helplessness (as described earlier as Type I trauma; Terr, 1991). Whatever the case, the child will probably show effects at the time, such as emotional shock and a look of being stunned or distracted and withdrawn. If the traumatic abuse or violence continues or if the child feels too frightened or confused to seek help, the initial shock and fear reactions tend to metastasize psychologically, spreading into many areas of the child's psyche and emotional and interpersonal life. Within a matter of weeks, this can lead to the development of severe symptoms of depression (emotional numbing, dysphoria), anxiety (including behavioral regressions, phobias, panic, obsessive rumination), dissociation, hypervigilance and startle reactions, and related debilitating feelings of shame, guilt, and worthlessness. Family members and others, such as teachers or friends, often notice such changes. However, in the absence of disclosure by the child and without actually witnessing or having other evidence of the victimization (or because of naivete about, minimization of, or unwillingness or inability to believe that a traumatizing event—especially abuse by a family member—could have occurred), they may not understand these reactions or what they represent.

Thus, children's posttraumatic responses may show up in a number of symptoms that frequently are not recognized as being driven by the anxiety, fear, or terror associated with victimization/trauma. These can include:

- Compulsive or ritualized behavior and phobias.
- Sleep disturbances, such as nightmares, night terrors, and fear of sleeping or of sleeping alone, refusing to sleep in a bed, sleeping in a closet or on the floor between the bed and the wall, sleeping with lights on or in layered clothing.
- Excessive worry about family's or loved ones' safety.
- Perceptual distortions, such as hearing sounds and feeling physical sensations.
- Dissociative reactions, such as losing time, personal discontinuity, splitting from or disowning reality, going into a trance, or feeling like several different persons.
- Difficulty recalling events or information, mood swings, sudden episodes of apparent paralysis ("frozen watchfulness").
- Emotional "meltdowns" or "blow-ups"; a tendency to be defiant

and oppositional; or, at the other end of the spectrum, to be excessively detached, passive and compliant with the demands and wishes of others, especially authority figures.

None of these problems is intrinsically associated with trauma, but all of them reflect adaptations that may result from experiencing traumatic threats or harm in the absence of adequate protection or caring. When these patterns begin during complex trauma exposure in childhood and are not recognized or treated, they unfortunately tend to persist into adolescence and adulthood as pervasive difficulty with identity development and self-worth, with the regulation of bodily functions, emotional states, and mental processes, and with maintaining healthy relationships. Thus the common denominator across all developmental epochs is a loss or distortion of normal self-regulatory abilities. Early childhood and preadolescence are crucial developmental periods for the consolidation of these abilities—ideally to provide the child with a solid foundation on which to create a positive and organized sense of self and an integrated personality during the next tumultuous developmental period, adolescence.

COMPLEX TRAUMA IN LATENCY AND ADOLESCENCE

When traumatic victimization or other traumatic exposure begins, continues, or remains unresolved in latency and adolescent years, the youth's immediate reactions tend toward desperate attempts to cope, a despairing sense of shame and self-blame, or angry protest and resistance. Briere and Elliott (2003) helpfully point out that although many activities (e.g., substance use, bingeing and purging, self-mutilation, suicidal attempts, impulsive and high-risk behavior, and indiscriminate sexual behavior) are counterintuitive, as they seem to be self-destructive, they often serve to maintain a sense of self by serving as *tension-reduction behaviors*. These behaviors usually begin in later childhood or adolescence as attempts to distract from, reduce, or manage the emotional pain and confusion elicited by victimization. They offer a short-term solution to overwhelming emotional distress by providing a sense of physical or emotional relief, or escape. Some behaviors may amplify physical arousal, whereas others may numb it, and both may be needed by the adolescent in the throes of polarities of reexperiencing/hyperarousal and numbing/dissociation. These strategies are generally effective in providing some relief or a sense of being in control rather than helpless. Moreover, as adolescents get physically bigger and stronger and have more opportunities for independence, they may engage in behaviors that were not possible previously, such as fighting back, resisting, running away, and so on. Although frequently labeled as "acting-out" or "externalizing" behaviors driven by impulse or addiction, in this population, these tactics are more helpfully seen as attempts at problem-solving and emotional regulation in the face of painful emotions. As effective (but problematic) coping strategies, these also can be defined as secondary elaborations of the original untreated effects that were mentioned earlier, first identified by Gelinas (1983). In other words, these are new development-related problems that have emerged in an attempt to cope with the traumatic aftermath that often require treatment above and beyond the direct posttraumatic aftereffects.

A primary task of the adolescent years is the development of personal identity and a sense of self-worth. Not surprisingly, it is in adolescence that previous feelings and thoughts about what being victimized says about "who I am as a person" may take center stage and result in the development of a negative identity and exceedingly low self-esteem. The seeds for such pervasive and damning self-perceptions may be found in earlier victimization; in adolescence, self-scrutiny and self-awareness become so developmentally urgent that any lasting sense of helplessness, complicity, guilt, shame, or failure can expand into a full-blown view of oneself as dirty, disgusting, worthless, stupid, deformed, or otherwise shameful and permanently damaged. Traumatized adolescents often feel different from their peers and like outsiders who do not fit the norm. Some develop secondary sex characteristics earlier than their peers, also making them look and feel different from others in their peer group (Trickett, Kurtz, & Noll, 2005).

In contrast, some adolescent survivors describe feeling special, powerful, and sometimes entitled. This is especially true of those for whom excessive attention was part of the abuse relationship by virtue any power they held over the abuser or members of the family—especially their mothers in some cases of father–daughter incest—and of any affection or sexual pleasure they experienced. All of these feelings can coexist with self-loathing and shame or might alternate with them. Some victims experience this power as personally affirming, resulting in feelings of grandiosity, whereas others believe themselves to be malignantly powerful and defective. As children, these victims may have developed the belief that they could willfully manipulate others and "make or break" the family or their peer group (or the broader community setting) with their terrible powers or the secrets they hold. In adolescence these largely implicit ideas no longer manifest mainly or only as the egocentrism associated with early childhood. A more pervasive form of narcissistic entitlement and power and an apparently callous indifference to and contempt for others can lead to conduct disturbances and the victimization of others. Many individuals with apparent sociopathic tendencies and conduct disorders were victimized as children. Such individuals at some point had the capacity for respect, empathy, and genuine social responsibility that was lost and corrupted in the struggle to survive, to make sense of, and to remove themselves from the receiving end of victimization. Identification with the perpetrator and the victimization of others is specifically included as a core feature of complex PTSD (see the following sections). Thornberry, Henry, Ireland, and Smith (2010) discussed the causal impact of early maltreatment on early adulthood adjustment. (For a highly descriptive and moving discussion on the impact of complex trauma on development, see Arnold and Fisch [2011]).

COMPLEX TRAUMA IN ADULTHOOD AND ACROSS THE LIFESPAN

Complex trauma that begins in adolescence or adulthood may have a profound impact, but in a different way than does repetitive and untreated trauma over the course of childhood. By later adolescence and adulthood, the individual has matured in body, personality, identity, and ability to relate to others and so has many more resources than the immature, developing child. Nevertheless, experiences of complex trauma during these later years can have great impact and can even break down key developmental achievements at any point in the lifespan. For example, an individual who had a fairly sheltered life and security of attachment growing up may become caught in community or political violence up to and including genocidal conflicts as an adult. Thereafter, he or she may become phobic about being out in public and withdraw from interactions with others. Whatever their origin, the common thread that makes these traumas complex is that they are overwhelming in their threat or harm, not only to the individual's personal safety but also to his or her identity, relationships, and overall security and that they negatively impact or reverse the individual's development.

Kira (2010) discussed how some of the distinguishing and immutable characteristics of an individual's very being and identity can cause him or her to be targeted for ongoing persecution and even attempts at systemic eradication. Other personal characteristics or group affiliations that are not inborn or unchangeable but nevertheless are central to the individual's sense of self and community—such as religious or political affiliations, belief systems, and practices—may be used by adversaries to single them out for imprisonment, forced evacuation and relocation, torture, or other forms of violence and cruelty, including genocide.

Chu, Frey, Ganzel, and Matthews (1999) described the phenomenon of *chronic disempowerment* that so often accompanies ongoing victimization and entrapment. Violence that terrorizes or attempts to destroy a gender, culture, religion, or generation or that violates fundamental human values is disempowering because it destroys victims' core source of personal power: their sustaining beliefs, guiding principles, and essential hopes. Colonialism, torture, captivity, genocide, "gendercide," terrorism, and other atrocities are purposefully disempowering because they shatter victims' sense of personal safety, their identity, and the meaning and value of their lives and their communities. In the face of such terror and the helplessness associated with ongoing entrapment, only survival may seem possible, and that may even seem of questionable desirability (Kira et al., 2010). The result is not just shock and anxiety but also the loss of trust in—or even the ability to recognize—oneself and the hopes that had been one's foundation and compass for years or even decades before the trauma. Thus complex trauma can destroy not only families, communities, and cultures but also the ability of each affected individual to maintain an intact personality, sense of self, and body and to maintain hope and a sense of agency.

Additional forms of complex traumas in adulthood can include:

- War and combat, as either a warrior or a noncombatant.
- Intractable poverty or homelessness.
- Inescapable exposure to community violence or terrorism.
- Political, ethnoracial, religious, gender, and/or sexual identity persecution.
- Incarceration and residential placement involving ongoing threat or actual assault.
- Human trafficking, forced prostitution, and sexual enslavement.
- Involvement in authoritarian groups or cults (some with a religious basis, others based in political or other closed beliefs), some involving mind control perpetrated by a charismatic leader and/or group influence and control mechanisms.
- Political repression involving genocide or "ethnic cleansing," and torture.
- Violence or exploitation due to displacement, refugee status, and relocation.
- Physical enslavement.
- Witnessing gruesome injury or death in the line of police and emergency response work.

Kira and colleagues (2010) suggested that these types of traumas constituted another two categories, in addition to the types identified by Terr (1991) described earlier in this chapter: *Type III*, having to do with one's identity, and *Type IV*, having to do with community membership. They also noted that complex traumas need not be of the catastrophic sort; rather, they may occur in the form of daily microaggressions that gradually break down an individual's (and a community's) spirit and the will to live and resist. Prior to Kira's suggestion, Solomon and Heide (1999) had suggested that *Type III* trauma consisted of multiple, pervasive, and violent events beginning at an early age and continuing over a long period of time. Both of these suggested types (III and IV) refer to the unfortunate fact that some victims routinely or sporadically experience all four types of victimization over their entire life course, making their traumatization that much more complex and compounded.

COMPLEX TRAUMA, COMPLEX TREATMENT

When psychotherapy begins, a therapist has no way of knowing what hidden forces are driving the individual to seek treatment. At first, the difficulties may seem clear-cut, especially when the therapist conducts a detailed psychosocial evaluation, when the individual is articulate in describing his or her past and current needs, or when a referrer or past therapist has not flagged anything out of the ordinary. Yet, as therapy progresses, it is not at all uncommon for therapists to discover that a client suffers from a range of symptoms such as those included in Table 1.1. This partial list is no doubt familiar to many therapists who may have been surprised by the extent of symptomatic distress suffered by some of their clients, even those who "present well" and are apparently well functioning. Whether these impairments emerge sporadically or are chronic, even without a readily discernible triggering event or exposure, it is important for therapists to consider that the client may be suffering from the effects of past or current psychological trauma. This stance is referred to as trauma-reformed orientation on the part of providers (Adults Surviving Child Abuse, 2012; Harris & Follot, 2001; Jennings, 2004; Saakvitne, Gamble, Pearlman, & Tabor, 2000).

Many clients who have had devastating and life-altering traumatic experiences are reluctant to disclose them at the start of therapy. There are a variety of reasons for this reluctance, among them: the painfulness and stigma surrounding them; loyalty to the perpetrator, family, or others; forced silence based on threat or terror; the belief that these experiences are irrelevant to current problems and symptoms; and, in a related vein, the individual's disconnection from the original trauma, lack of trust in the assessor or therapist, or lack of (or incomplete) memory about them. Of particular relevance are traumatic experiences that took place during developmentally formative periods of life (i.e., childhood through adolescence). These include all of the forms of childhood maltreatment and abuse described earlier in this chapter, as well as exposure to and experiencing of ongoing violence or bullying due to group membership (i.e., racial or ethnic group, religion) and exposure to community-based events (i.e., ongoing violence, gangs, war, political conflicts).

Profoundly injurious, terrifying experiences such as these are likely to be psychologically traumatic for any person who experiences them firsthand or who witnesses them. They are particularly likely to be traumatizing if they occur repeatedly and chronically and escalate in severity over time or if they involve multiple occurrences of intentional harm by one or more perpetrators. They can also create conditions of anticipatory anxiety and hypervigilance. As noted previously, the impact of trauma and social maltreatment on children and adolescents can be particularly severe due to their physical and psychological immaturity, and the fact that they are still in the process of personality development.

TABLE 1.1. Potential Sequelae of Exposure to Complex Trauma

- Extreme mood lability (unregulated and dysregulated extremes of emotions and/or cycling between states of manic-like hyper-arousal and severe depression and hypoarousal).
- Social isolation, alienation, and detachment from others.
- Excessive self-sufficiency and fear of intimacy and relationship.
- Excessive dependency, passivity, and superficial compliance with the wishes of others.
- Alcohol or other substance abuse.
- Addictions, including love, relationship and sexual contact.
- Compulsions, including eating disorders (anorexia, bulimia, bulimarexia, binge eating, restricting, and morbid obesity), overwork/workaholism, sexualizing, hoarding, and excessive exercise, gambling, shopping and spending.
- Impulsivity, high-risk behaviors or dangerous thrill-seeking, with disregard for personal welfare and that of others, including children and other dependents.
- Uncontrolled anger or aggression directed toward self or others.
- Episodes of cruelty toward others and toward animals.
- Self-injury ("accidental" or intentional).
- Suicidality (ranging from ideation to parasuicidal or lethal attempts) and parasuicidality.
- Social problems due to persistent suspicion and mistrust of others and lack of social skills.
- Dysfunctional and pathological relationships, including emotionally or physically harmful, exploitive, violent, cruel, and malicious relationships with parents, siblings, partners, peers, employers, mentors, strangers, authorities, or one's own children; sexual, physical, and psychological revictimization or perpetration of victimization.
- Persistent dissociation, including depersonalization, derealization, and loss of personal continuity and awareness, not limited to but potentially including identity alterations.
- Posttraumatic symptoms of intrusive reexperiencing and physiological hyperarousal, alternating with emotional numbing and avoidance of reminders of traumas.
- Medical conditions that cannot be diagnosed or that do not respond to medical treatment.
- Chronic medical conditions, especially autoimmune disorders.
- Chronic low self-esteem, up to and including self-loathing.
- An inability to tolerate or recover from even mild emotional distress.
- Self-blame and self-condemnation, shame, guilt, and unresolved bereavement.
- Primary attachment styles and relationships that are ambivalent, dismissive, dependent, conflicted, anxious, fearful, or disorganized/unresolved.
- Pervasive feelings of helplessness and ineffectiveness.
- Dysfluence and incoherence in discussing personal events and life history.
- Pervasive feelings of hopelessness and despair of ever being understood or of being able to view oneself or be viewed by others as "normal."
- Alienation from or rejection of spirituality and spiritual/religious beliefs.
- Information-processing problems, including attention deficit, failure to complete or perform consistent with one's innate ability key tasks in work or school, or the opposite, the ability to perform very well but with a sense of being an imposter who is actually incompetent.
- Conduct disorders, including oppositional defiant disorder and hyperactivity.
- Psychotic-like experiences of command hallucinations or intrusive negative voices or images that alternately threaten, denigrate, or urge self-harm or the harm of others.
- Psychosis and hallucinations.

We define "complex trauma" as traumatic attachment that is life- or self-threatening, sexually violating, or otherwise emotionally overwhelming, abandoning, or personally castigating or negating, and involves events and experiences that alter the development of the self by requiring survival to take precedence over normal psychobiological development. Note that traumatic events experienced in adulthood may have similarly complex adverse effects by severely damaging or destroying a person's previously formed self, beliefs, and perceptions, for example, when torture, genocide, or extended abusive captivity are inflicted on individuals or entire populations.

Although knowledge of details of the traumatic stressors (the "who, what, when, where," or the objective dimensions) can be very important in treatment, it is sometimes less important than understanding the immediate and longer term reactions, meanings, coping strategies, or survival tactics that currently persist (the subjective and personal dimensions) (Wilson, Drozdek, & Turkovic, 2006). The events may be of subjective importance to the survivor (so as to create a coherent narrative of "what happened to me"), but it is the survivor's biological, emotional, cognitive, behavioral, and relational adaptations that must be understood in order to help with recovery. Many traumatized individuals blame themselves for their survival strategies (often in response to blame or criticism from others) and incorporate beliefs about themselves along the lines of "This is just the way that I am, just the flaws in my personality or nature that I was born with and can never change . . . I'm too damaged, I'll never be any good . . . I'll never be loved . . . I'm not capable of love." They often cannot understand how these apparently troublesome and incapacitating reactions could ever make sense, except as a reflection of something repugnant *about them*. Just as most children egocentrically incorporate *what was done to them* as being *about them* and consequently develop a shamed identity, self-loathing, and illogical responsibility for being victimized, adults who experience trauma (especially involving interpersonal victimization by someone known to or related to them in some way) may similarly adopt a sense of self-blame because there seems to be no other reasonable explanation for its occurrence and for their continued suffering.

For some clients, symptoms such as those listed in Table 1.1 are a constant in their lives. For others, symptoms can emerge suddenly in response to one or more experiences or somatosensory states that serve as reminders of the trauma. These "triggers" can include positive as well as negative life events, such as single or accumulated life stressors, anniversaries, births and deaths, other significant transitions, and physical or emotional reactions that in some way serve as reminders of the original traumatic event or experience. Some individuals are adept at hiding these symptoms from others, functioning fairly well and appearing relatively intact, although a great deal of effort might go into producing this effect. Others are not so adept, or their symptoms are not so easily suppressed or disguised, becoming apparent at home or work in erratic or otherwise problematic behavior and changed or charged emotional responses. In either case, the individual may feel as though he or she is going crazy. Although some seek treatment soon after the emergence of symptoms, others cope on their own by self-medicating or self-soothing in ways that can create additional problems (e.g., secondary elaborations such as addictions, workaholic behaviors, procrastination, sexual dysfunction or promiscuity, social withdrawal and personal detachment, eating disorders, compulsive shopping, financial mismanagement and chaos, ongoing self-injury, suicidal ideation or suicidality) and the relationship and family problems that accompany them.

Many complex trauma survivors describe having made multiple attempts at treatment over the years with only transient or negligible progress. Furthermore, they frequently report having been misunderstood, misdiagnosed, medicated (often to excess), and even institutionalized, then stigmatized when they did not get better. The individuals show remarkable perseverance, courage, and hope in making yet another attempt to get help from professionals, even as they might simultaneously hold a number of understandable biases toward treatment, including mistrust of the process and suspicions regarding the motives of the therapist or allied professional. For example, they may have developed a sense of chronic disempowerment and hopelessness—the feeling that nothing will help them and that they can do nothing to get better as they are beyond help—and a corresponding belief that authority figures, including therapists, family members, and friends, are not trustworthy and do not really care. Reactions such as these must be understood by the therapist as resulting from the additional "insult added to injury" that many survivors experienced repeatedly in their lives, whether in the context of therapy or with significant others. Initially, these biases may interfere with developing a therapeutic alliance or with other dimensions of the treatment, a further complication to the process. On the other hand, survivors who are newer to psychotherapy may not have had the same negative treatment history and may not be as jaded, but they are equally desperate for help in quelling their distressing symptoms.

Not every individual with an intractable psychiatric history or personality disorder suffers from a history of complex trauma. However, both clinical observations and research findings suggest that a substantial percentage of mental health clients (as well as persons seeking medical treatment) with a combination of the symptoms and difficulties listed earlier are likely suffering from the aftereffects of trauma exposure (in childhood or later in life, or both) and subsequent reactions. And unfortunately, in many of those cases, it is rare that the posttraumatic origin and nature of their problems have been recognized or addressed in psychotherapy. A posttraumatic or trauma-informed lens is helpful in conceptualizing the client and these symptoms: It is less pathologizing or stigmatizing but does not reduce the clinical relevance of other potential biological or environmental sources of distress or impairment. Instead, when symptoms are viewed as posttraumatic stress reactions in a context, they can be treated as cumulative adaptations that an individual has made over time, largely or entirely without awareness, in order to survive repeated experiences of overwhelming harm, danger, or loss.

CONCLUSION

Complex trauma prevents, disrupts, or shatters the victim's ability to develop a sense of self and to trust self and others. Knowing when complex trauma occurred in a client's life can provide a basis for understanding—and helping the client to understand—how symptoms were developmentally appropriate and adaptations that were necessary or functional at that age and stage of development. If problematic symptoms can be traced back to how the individual coped with and survived trauma—and how those adaptations altered or disrupted healthy development—then therapy can provide clients with a basis for both empathy for themselves and for hope that it is possible to rework developmental challenges that were derailed or had to be abandoned to survive. This developmental reworking does not involve regressing to childhood; rather, it is designed to help clients draw on their strengths and capacities as adults in the interest of developing skills and diminishing symptoms. The reworking of trauma to the point of resolution is in the interest of healing past injuries and creating healthier present-day coping and relationships that are less imbued by trauma. It is clearly also in the interest of an improved future.

CHAPTER 2

Complex Traumatic Stress Reactions and Disorders

In this chapter, we discuss the nature of and the clinical difficulties posed by three core domains of complex traumatic stress reactions and disorders: (1) emotion dysregulation, (2) the loss of self-integrity, and (3) disturbances in the ability to relate to and be intimate with others. These three form the basis of the array of symptoms experienced by complex trauma clients. Before we discuss these three domains and their associated symptoms, we return to the lives of the two composite clients who are seeking, albeit reluctantly and with great pessimism and skepticism, therapeutic help for symptoms that began as ways of coping with their traumatic experiences that have become sources of day-to-day distress in their lives.

Hector

Hector entered treatment unwillingly and in a highly hypervigilant, untrusting state of mind that was substantially compounded by his chronic use of drugs and alcohol. He initially refused to disclose much about himself, fearing that he would be "turned over to the authorities and tortured." He answered questions monosyllabically and offered few details about himself. The therapist had to resort to interviewing the buddies who had dropped him off and then to reviewing his service records in order to gain more background information. He also requested to speak to Hector's parents and siblings, but Hector would not allow it. In this vacuum of information and verbal interaction, the therapist worried about Hector's degree of suicidality and his ability to stay safe and found himself pulled into Hector's hopelessness and powerlessness. As a means of quelling his own trepidation with this difficult start and to begin to forge a preliminary connection with Hector, the therapist decided to accept him as he was and took to doing most of the talking during their sessions. He learned that, even as he continued to be noncommunicative, Hector paid careful attention to everything he said. The therapist provided education about trauma and traumatic stress reactions, depression, anxiety, and substance abuse and then introduced concrete treatment tasks. He helped Hector to find safe housing and then to begin the process of detoxification from alcohol and drugs and attendance at Alcoholics Anonymous (AA) and Narcotics Anonymous (NA) meetings. He also suggested that Hector be evaluated for medication to address his depression, anxiety, and sleep disturbance. Although Hector was highly mistrustful, he was also quite used to being deferential to authority figures, and so he usually complied with the various tasks suggested by the therapist. In turn, the therapist reinforced this behavior by stressing Hector's courage in addressing rather than running from his problems and continuously told him that he had the potential to heal, that is, to feel and to function better. It took several months to "break the ice," but Hector became a bit more verbal at each subsequent session (although the therapist continued to do the bulk of the talking but was also careful to ask questions of Hector and to "make space" for the time it took for him to respond).

Doris

Doris's reactions from her childhood replayed throughout her life. She had limited ability to tolerate strong emotions, evident in her tendency to either dissociate or blow up, responses that emerged in any situation in which she felt she might be unable to influence or control others' behaviors or when she became emotionally threatened by their withdrawal from her. Understandably, these reactions had developed from the time she was abused by her father and in response to her mother's vacillating availability. Doris could not express what she needed in words but became verbally abusive or withdrew when threatened. She flew into rages and, on some occasions, hit her husband when she felt frustrated beyond her tolerance. At times, she would go on drinking binges that also served to fuel her anger and to limit her ability to control her outbursts against others. After such episodes, she would feel additionally shamed, desperate, and rejected by others.

Because Doris was so experienced at putting up a false front and masking her real feelings, it was not evident how frightened she was at the start of treatment. In the first session, the therapist conducted herself in her usual way, careful to be inquisitive, responsive, and supportive. Doris returned for the second session and told the therapist that she felt "disgusted" by herself and by the therapist and didn't think she could continue. After much patient questioning on the therapist's part, it became clear that Doris's fears of connection were almost inexplicably transformed into feelings of disgust when people were kind to her. She was disgusted—and even shamed—by the very thing she sought and needed. Doris's therapist was obviously confused at her statement of disgust, as she thought the first session had gone relatively well and had difficulty reconciling the warm client she had met with the contemptuous person who now sat before her. She was to experience this masked presentation of self and relational discontinuity repeatedly in the early years of treatment and learned to "read" Doris's subtle cues to her distress and help her put them into words rather than act them out precipitously or in delayed fashion. Doris experienced enormous relief as she learned to identify and name her mixed relational messages and their precipitants and to ask for clarification when she was confused by a response, rather than going away and making assumptions, usually at her own expense.

Doris's adaptations exquisitely but tragically illustrate another path that those with disorganized (and also fearful/anxious and dismissing) attachment problems can take even decades later. She both yearned for and feared the therapist's caring, and, as she did with her husband and others, she engaged in a confusing relational push–pull. In the early years of treatment, her mood instability was extreme and her ability to manage it limited, especially during episodes of binge drinking. In addition, she engaged in a variety of self-injurious behaviors and began to tell the therapist about them only after 2 years of treatment.

COMPLEX TRAUMATIC STRESS DISORDERS: THREE PRIMARY DOMAINS

As discussed in Chapter 1, children's immediate reactions to traumatic victimization and associated stressors are complicated and can go well beyond the triadic categories of symptoms that make up classic or traditional PTSD. Many events and experiences that potentially traumatize children do not meet the current DSM-IV-TR criteria for a traumatic event, such as graphic/grotesque events involving injury, loss, death, threatened death, and actual or threatened serious injury or sexual violation. Many childhood traumatic events do not meet these specifications because they are more emotionally dysregulating (Ford, 2005) than physically violent or assaultive (Briggs-Gowan, Ford, Fraleigh, McCarthy, & Carter, 2011). Even when prevalent and controversial potentially traumatic events such as emotional abuse or bullying are excluded, children experience many threats to their or their primary caregivers' lives and safety that can result in posttraumatic reactions that persist (in sporadic, chronic, and/or delayed form) and extend into later childhood (Briggs-Gowan et al., 2010), adolescence (Ford & DTD Field Trial Work Group, 2011), and throughout adulthood (Anda, Butchart, Felitti, & Brown, 2010). These reactions and symptoms meet criteria for chronic PTSD; however, they typically exceed them. They tend to be more convoluted and insidious, intertwining with stages of physiological and psychosexual development and interrupting, derailing, and/or accelerating associated developmental tasks. The complex traumatic antecedents and the resultant array of traumatic and developmental symptoms make complex traumatic stress disorders difficult to identify, diagnose, and treat. Bryant (2010) commented on this in his editorial "The Complexity of Complex Trauma."

We now move to a discussion of emotion dysregulation and loss of self-identity and integrity as the core domains of complex trauma. We begin by highlighting some of the most common emotional reactions associated with complex traumatic stress disorders in adults that build on those found in children and adolescents and presented in the previous chapter. Then we incorporate the various adaptations and symptoms into a comprehensive formulation. This formulation makes the symptom more easily understood by mental health practitioners, allied professionals, and clients alike and are further informative in terms of directing the treatment.

Common Emotions and Reactions in Complex Trauma

The following are some of the most common emotions and reactions that are experienced by adult survivors including some of the contradictory or polarized ways in which they can be experienced or expressed.

Anxiety reactions include fear, terror, apprehension, hypervigilance, panic attacks, sleep disturbance, and nightmares, in addition to various phobias (including fear of one's own emotions, of other people, of enclosed places, of leaving home, of the dark, etc.), and span the full range of anxiety disorders. Physiological hyperarousal alternating with hypoarousal are common physical concomitants to feelings of terror, fear, and anxiety.

Depressive reactions show up in a variety of ways: in ongoing diffuse sadness, hopelessness, and despair; in the inability to feel interest in and enjoyment of most life activities; in not feeling close to or safe with other people (social detachment) or not feeling any emotion other than a vague sense of flatness, frustration, or irritability (emotional numbing or alexithymia); in feeling an internal void or absence or feeling tainted and dangerous to others; in self-defeating and self-injurious behavior; in believing one has nothing to live for; and in resultant chronic suicidal ideation that sporadically emerges in gestures and attempts. Major affective disorders are commonly severe and recurrent, becoming chronic over time. At times they may include psychotic features.

Survivors further struggle with intense feelings of anger and rage, ranging from an ongoing sense of irritability, annoyance, disappointment, disgust, contempt, and frustration with themselves and others to episodes of uncontrollable rage that can precipitate impulsive acts of protest and aggression. These can be self-directed in the form of self-defeating behaviors, self-harm through self-mutilation, substance abuse, or the elicitation of reprisals from others or by directing it at others through passive-aggressive, aggressive, and violent behaviors.

A common denominator linking these emotions is a sense of self-estrangement and emotional deadness. Anxiety, depression, and anger tend to be reactions not only to external problems and threats, the basis for all anxiety, affective, and anger-based (e.g., oppositional defiant and conduct) disorders, but also, more fundamentally, to a sense of being threatened, harmed, or held prisoner and tortured by one's own emotions. Anxiety is also based on a fear that, if feelings (especially anger/rage, but also fear/terror, sadness/despair, guilt/responsibility, and shame) were allowed to emerge, they would be so intense that they would result in victimizing others, going crazy, causing others to reject or abandon them, or committing suicide or homicide. Depressive feelings tend to be based on not just feeling down, discouraged, helpless, hopeless, or even worthless but on the experience of a "black hole" or a "yearning void," a sense of being unlovable and of utter emptiness, badness, and resultant despair. It is as if nothing is inside but anguish, pain, and isolation and loneliness; therefore, there is no basis for ever feeling hope, happiness, or positive self-esteem.

In consequence, the survivor is at risk for experiencing not just severe emotional distress but an underlying inability to recognize (or having a phobia about) personal emotions as appropriate, useful, and reliable and as a means of self-understanding and a healthy sense of self. Where the child's attachment figure dismissed or punished emotional displays and the needs they conveyed, emotions were shut down in the interest of self-protection from further rejection and nonresponse. This provides a rationale for being avoidant and emotionally vacant, because no emotion at all is far preferable to the sense of dread, disgust, and shame that can develop when any (even positive) emotion is felt.

The primary challenge of emotion regulation for many survivors is therefore not just to recognize, understand, modulate, and communicate feelings, nor even to recover from intensely distressing emotions. Even before these can be attempted, the survivor must find a way to overcome the phobia of emotions and to begin to recognize, identify, and label visceral sensations that accompany and signal them. Over time and after identification and acceptance (by self and others, including the therapist), he or she can learn to use emotions as a primary means of discerning identity and as a means of self-expression and communication with others. Developing this capacity based on personal self-exploration is an essential task of psychotherapy.

When displays of emotion have been internalized as personally intolerable and even dangerous, it is not surprising that these reactions generalize to a parallel aversion to physical sensations and reactions, cutting off somatosensory information, the physiological basis of emotions. Just as the victimized infant may react not only with inconsolable emotional distress but also with bodily distress, so too the adult may develop a plethora of physical reactions. The extreme demands that persistent stress reactivity place on the body have been implicated theoretically (Friedman & McEwen, 2004) and empirically (Felitti et al., 1998) in adult survivors' somatoform manifestations of distress and their greatly increased risk of medical illness (including cardiovascular, pulmonary, immune, autoimmune, gastrointestinal, genitourinary and endocrinological illnesses, chronic pain and fatigue, diabetes, and cancer; Schnurr & Green, 2004). Somatoform manifestions include conditions that often defy or muddle medical diagnosis but that nevertheless are debilitating and often refractory to treatment. Due to both somatization and actual health impairment and illness, health care utilization tends to be very high in this population.

Adult survivors often feel betrayed and disgusted by their bodies, at times expressing these feelings by mercilessly ignoring, depriving, or injuring their bodies or by putting themselves in harm's way. Some survivors develop phobias not only about their bodies but also about being touched. They may continue the strategies they employed (such as dissociation or learning not to feel physical sensations through depersonalization, self-anesthesia, and analgesia) or the injunctions they learned during episodes of physical and sexual abuse, namely, to disregard their bodies and their associated physical reactions and needs. At the most extreme, some survivors are so body alienated that they do not experience a need to eat, rest, or sleep and do not feel pain or register temperature changes. Adverse physical reactions include discomfort, chronic pain and spasms, wounds, infection, unpredictable and unexplained feelings of stimulation, fears and phobias about body areas, or even organ failure (tending to occur in body areas that were violated or exploited). Long-term physical reactions include dissociative (conversion) reactions that occur spontaneously when specific stimuli or anxiety are experienced.

More generalized physical effects are varied, including gastrointestinal disturbance, respiratory distress, muscular tension, and stress problems such as migraine headaches, temporomandibular joint (TMJ) pain, high blood pressure, frozen joints (e.g., frozen pelvis or clenched fists), ringing in the ears (tinnitus), inability to physically relax due to hyperalertness and hypervigilance, obesity, binge eating, anorexia or restriction, bulimia, and diabetes. Some survivors compulsively seek large amounts and many types of health care—essentially becoming "professional patients," eager and desperate for the attention of authority figures and those charged with caregiving (sometimes leading to a diagnosis of Munchausen Syndrome). Some may have an alternative motivation, of having painful medical procedures as a form of unconscious trauma reenactment. At the other end of the spectrum, those who were humiliated and terrified, shamed, disfigured, or injured during the abuse may routinely avoid preventive or needed medical care due to shame and fear of exposure. This can lead to tragic consequences, as occurs when a sexually transmitted disease (STD) is not diagnosed in a timely way and leads to damage of reproductive or other organs or when physical injury goes untreated and persists and worsens over time. Repercussions of this sort are additionally traumatic for the survivor and for significant others, including therapists in some cases.

Somatic problems are the same or very similar to the symptoms of somatoform disorders. Studies have accumulated suggesting that a large proportion of patients with somatoform disorders have histories of childhood victimization, typically undocumented and unaccounted for in health care records. Although they may be genetic or epigenetic (i.e., changes in the person's core genetic makeup that result from injury or environmental exposures), risk factors for persistent extreme somatic dysregulation represent a potentially treatable contributor to these profound physical health problems. Bodily sensations and feelings are the most common elicitors of emotions; hence the trauma survivor who experiences emotion as harmful and intolerable is likely to experience physical sensations as correspondingly dangerous and toxic. What might otherwise be healthy signs of a well-functioning body or of manageable and treatable physical problems may be interpreted instead as signs of painful, frightening, confusing, or disgusting breakdowns, deformities, medical concerns, or illness. Traumatic victimization in infancy or early childhood that resulted in chronic physical distress can lead to a phobia or intolerance of physical sensations that may have developed simultaneously with emotion dysregulation. In any event, somatic dysregulation in complex traumatic stress disorders involves not only persistent physical and health problems and distress—up to and including a range of medical illnesses—but also an aversion to all kinds of physical sensations.

Emotion Dysregulation

Survivors often have difficulty coping with or recovering from emotional distress that occurs in reaction to daily life events, including seemingly minor stressors or difficulties but also, in apparent contradiction, to positive and celebratory events. It is when these events and their associated reactions and emotions serve as reminders of the trauma (whether they get registered in conscious awareness or at a somatosensory/implicit and unconscious level), they can elicit powerful emotional reactions. These emotions typically exceed the ability to regulate them, because the skills for such modulation were not learned. As a result, emotional reactions tend to manifest in "all or nothing" ways, either full-on or shut-down with little in between, causing self and interpersonal difficulties (Cloitre, Miranda, Stovall-McClough, & Han, 2005). The in-between state has been called the "therapeutic window" (Briere, 1996; Briere & Scott, 2006), the "window of tolerance" (Fisher & Ogden, 2009; Ogden & Fisher, 2013), or the "affective edge" (Olio & Connell, 1993), referring to the capacity for tolerating and modulating various emotional states. In the absence of such capacity, individuals in the throes of strong emotional responses typically avoid them or find other ways to shut them down (e.g., through repression, dissociation, compulsions, addictions). Thus, in the traumatized, this window is typically quite narrow and it takes little to set off major response. This all-or-nothing polarity of emotions (as commonly associated with personality disorder [Linehan, 1993], and similar to the alternating reexperiencing and numbing found in posttraumatic reactions) makes it even more difficult for survivors to discern and regulate them. This, in turn, elicits and reinforces feelings of powerlessness and lack of self-control. The ability to identify and modulate emotional states is an important milestone in human development that undergirds identity development, positive self-control, and relations with others.

If this emotion regulation deficit were not enough, many survivors have little or no conceptualization of physical and emotional boundaries in terms of themselves or in interactions with others. In consequence, they often function in ways that are confusing and seemingly contradictory, either by not having adequate boundaries between self and others (developing intense dependence, getting enmeshed with or preoccupied with others who they expect will define them or explain them to themselves) or by having too-rigid boundaries (developing extreme self-sufficiency and having little or no need of others and dismissing and detaching from others who seek to get close).

The treatment of complex trauma must therefore address these skill deficits in order to help clients understand and manage their various emotional states, as a means for them to learn about themselves and others. The development of these skills assists clients in expanding their emotional repertoire and their capacity. It also attends to the differentiation of self from others and builds skills of assertiveness, collaboration, and interdependence. Techniques for skill building in emotional regulation and boundary development are detailed in Chapter 5.

Loss of Self-Integrity and Self-Integration (Dissociation)

Persistent emotional and somatic dysregulation tend to elicit and intensify dissociative reactions. When there is no practical way to escape from or avoid uncomfortable or painful emotion, knowledge, and physical sensation, the dissociation-prone (and especially the chronically traumatized and terrorized child) separates from them in the interest of suppressing or avoiding the distress they cause; however, emotions and physical sensations do not necessarily diminish when dissociation is used. Increased and repeated use may be needed to manage the split and to keep them from emerging. Over time and with recurrent use, the dissociative process can become automatic and involuntary.

Posttraumatic dissociation is understood as the psychophysiologically based segregation or fragmentation of consciousness or awareness of different emotions, physical sensations, memories, behaviors, and knowledge that occurs in response to psychodynamic triggers (Putnam, 1989). This process leads to an atypical compartmentalization of personal awareness involving either a sharp reduction or a drastic amplification of emotions, physical sensations, knowledge/memory, and associated behavioral impulses. The common denominator is the self-protective fragmentation and compartmentalization of awareness or memory of distressing trauma-related feelings and thoughts.

Van der Hart, Nijenhuis, and Steele (2006) developed the structural theory of dissociation based on French psychiatrist Pierre Janet's original theoretical formulations developed at the end of the 20th century. They posited that dissociation is more than a simply psychological defense. Instead, it involves the splitting of personal experience into divisions in the individual's personality and functioning. What they term the "apparently normal personality" (ANP) develops in the interest of having little or no knowledge of the trauma and its associated reactions, allowing the individual to function well and in an apparently normal way in the absence of this knowledge. The "emotional personality" (EP; otherwise known as the "traumatic personality") holds the split-off knowledge and emotion, keeping it segregated from the ANP. This segregation (that might involve a loss of all or part of the memory of the trauma) literally keeps the trauma out of mind, to function at work, home, and in relationships in ways that appear normal.

In the majority of cases, these structurally dissociated parts of the self are different states of mind rather than the dissociated "identities" or self-states as seen in dissociative identity disorder (DID), in which the person has the experience of having executive control overtaken by separate and distinctly different "selves" for periods of time for which they are later amnestic. Those with DID also experience major time loss, discontinuities in their consciousness, and changes in their sense of self. Most complex trauma survivors do not experience themselves as so distinctly differentiated, but instead as simply (1) unaware for the most part of distressing emotions and sensations related to past traumatic experiences and (2) feeling as if they can be quite different at times (e.g., outgoing and assertive, when usually they are withdrawn and shy although they always have the same core self). The different states of mind are not separate autonomous "selves" with minds of their own, so to speak. Instead, they are expressions of the individual's different feelings that, in a nontraumatized healthy individual, ordinarily are well integrated in the person's overall sense of self (i.e., a fairly constant set of memories, feelings, and thoughts that simply fluctuate in response to changes in mood and circumstances). Dissociation hijacks that normal ebb and flow by splitting off and creating barriers between the person's different "states of mind" so that feelings, thoughts, and memories are distinct rather than shared. Putnam (1997) discussed how the course of a child's normal development, such states become integrated, rather than segregated.

Given the extreme dysregulation of emotion, physical functions, (including sexual functioning) and their relationships and personal awareness and memory can become dominated by dissociated core beliefs about themselves and the world. Most basically, survivors' self-perceptions tend to become, and remain, not only profoundly negative but also extremely fragmented in a manner consistent with structural dissociation. Although many survivors blame themselves and their very existence for having somehow provoked maltreatment, they also have existential questions, such as "Why did it happen to me?"; "How could someone who is supposed to love me do this?"; "Why did God allow this and abandon me?" In the absence of information to the contrary, they often answer this question in their own disfavor: assuming that they were "born bad" or "marked for abuse," that something *about them that they can never change* either causes harm or signals others that they are an easy target for mistreatment. Survivors are often not consciously aware of the extent to which their lives are dominated by such beliefs—and in some cases not even aware of the beliefs at all—or are only aware of them when experiencing certain emotions (i.e., when depressed or enraged). Thus it is not the negative beliefs per se but their compartmentalization in dissociated parts of the self that pose a great challenge in treatment. In Chapter 8, we discuss the structural theory of dissociation in more detail, along with ways therapists can work with dissociative symptoms and parts of self.

Toxic and fragmented beliefs about being damaged or culpable may also be echoes or repetitions of personally disparaging messages communicated by perpetrators or, even more tragically, by other important adults who did not understand the child's distressed or difficult behavior and reacted with criticism, frustration, or disappointment. A perpetrator's insinuations that the child liked, wanted, or caused abuse or an unintentionally insensitive adult's condemnation of the child as irresponsible, stupid, lazy, or unacceptably emotional or oppositional increase the confusion and substantiate the child's negative self-perception. Even in the absence of outright emotional abuse or critical/judgmental adult reactions, the lack of effective assistance and intervention unfortunately provides a great deal of substantiation for this almost inevitable conclusion: "Someone would have helped me if I had not been so reprehensible; therefore, I am at fault and I am deserving of the blame and criticism."

When victimization goes on for prolonged periods within significant relationships without notice or intervention, it negatively affects core schema and attachment "working models," (Bowlby, 1969) that is, beliefs about the self, including spirituality or purpose in life, the safety and trustworthiness of relationships, and the world. These negative cognitions can become not just deeply held beliefs but can actually become the main fabric of the survivor's inner life. Thus, consistent with cognitive models of PTSD (Dalgleish, 2004), increasingly large portions of the survivor's network of mental and emotional associations can become dominated by organizing beliefs ("schemas") that are very difficult to alter or disconfirm because they are based on "data" (i.e., repeated emotionally definitive experiences) that come from the child's adaptations to repeated trauma without recourse, rather than from more benign hopeful and life-affirming experiences.

Although negative schemata may predominate, other, more hopeful responses have been identified. Some individuals who experience extreme traumatization somehow do not show the same pattern of existential anguish and self-condemnation and retain or develop spiritual beliefs to counter their despair. Some have temperaments and physiologies that are resilient even in the face of great adversity. Some are able to get into relationships with emotionally healthy partners through whom they attain "earned security" of attachment, including the ability to trust others and to develop positive self-esteem. As well, some survivors who are able to acknowledge how co-opted their development was by the traumatization are able to cultivate self-compassion and self-forgiveness.

In recent years, researchers have identified patterns of posttraumatic growth (Joseph, 2008, 2011; Linley & Joseph, 2008; Tedeschi & Calhoun, 2004; Werdel & Wicks, 2012) in some trauma survivors who report that, although the experiences were negative, they were nevertheless able to gain strength and wisdom from them. There are also individuals who come to view and take pride in their posttraumatic reactions and adaptations as creative survival strategies. These serve them well in their lives and provide foundations on which they build additional skills and capacities (e.g., hypervigilance that develops into skills of anticipation and planning; sensitivity to the needs of others and a related ability to empathize, both skills that are useful in many occupations). In a similar way, "survivor missions" (Blank, 1994), that is, actions or activities that counteract elements of abuse and trauma that some survivors pursue may be their way to make sense of what happened and to have some influence and control. None of these make up for the losses associated with traumatization, but they form a basis for restoring hope and trust in others, providing other resources on which to build a less trauma-compromised future.

Compromised Relationships with Others

Complex trauma survivors have ample reason to mistrust other people. They are frequently suspicious (sometimes coming across as paranoid, though it is best considered as "realistic paranoia". They expect mistreatment and exploitation and so may be surprised and apprehensive when treated with respect and kindness. In terms of attachment style, many survivors show simultaneous signs of relational withdrawal and excessive self-sufficiency (a "dismissive" or detached style), neediness and dependency (a "preoccupied" attachment style), or both, in unpredictable and inconsistent vacillations (a "disorganized" style). Rather than seeming simply insecure in an obvious sense, they often appear to be conflicted and "disorganized" in their feelings about relationships—torn between avoiding the dangers of being close to others and their desire and underlying need and longing for connection.

Most unfortunately, insecure and disorganized attachment may make victimized children and later adults a target of additional victimization, as their very isolation and neediness, their compromised emotions and ability to protect themselves and their ongoing availability to or repetitive contact with victimizers, make them very vulnerable. This "disorganized" approach may be further complicated by behavior that involves compulsively "seeking out" (in terms of learned behavior, traumatic reenactments, or repeated but futile attempts at mastery) victimizing or risky relationships or using once adaptive defense mechanisms such as dissociation that increase vulnerability. For example, the habitual use of dissociation may interfere with the ability to register threat or may cause the individual to freeze and collapse, rather than fight back or flee, when in situations of danger. As a result of learned patterns of interaction (such as passivity, compliance, helplessness, and surrender) and expectations regarding the motives of others and the inevitability of being treated badly, revictimization can be understood as a means of confirming those expectations, making it useless to fight back and best to surrender to the inevitable. Paradoxically, such behavior may provide a means of achieving a modicum of control and power over the situation ("I will make it happen on my timetable, when I'm ready"), to manage its inevitability ("Hurry up and get it over with"), or to confirm feelings of shame and guilt ("I'm bad and this is what I deserve").

The apparent neediness of many complex trauma survivors may appear abundantly obvious or, in an opposite pattern may be camouflaged by their self-sufficiency or their detached/dismissive, parentified/caretaking, or superficially compliant behaviors and styles. On the surface, detached or caretaking individuals appear to be self-sufficient and highly functional. Many children and adolescents that are in ongoing traumatic family circumstances (usually those that are highly disorganized) learned to cope in two main ways: by caretaking or controlling others. As caretakers, they keep the peace, and the needs of everyone else in the family take precedence over their own, even as these are simultaneously neglected, negated, and dismissed. As controllers, they establish order by being dominant and taking charge, sometimes through outright aggression and coercion. These quite opposite coping styles provides these children with some sense of agency and self-worth. Unfortunately, it further reinforces the belief that their value comes from *what they do* rather than *who they are*.

In the caretaking-based style, compulsive doing for others often began as a means of self-protection in the dysfunctional/abusive family, a way of organizing and managing the chaos of the surroundings while gaining affirmation and acceptance from others. This caretaking and response pattern is also compensatory: "doing" equates with "being," and the intent is to do as much as possible for others in order to gain needed approval and appreciation to offset further hurt, rejection, or abandonment. This pattern of enabling and rescuing usually continues in adult relationships (in families of origin and in intimate and work relationships). Although this pattern would seem to be more common in females than in males, it is common in both genders.

In a variant of this pattern, "doing the impossible" on an ongoing basis becomes the norm, with little or no regard for the personal toll involved. Many survivors strive to be completely self-sufficient and flawless as the "perfect man/woman," "model student, athlete, or leader," or informal "counselor" to whom their peers turn for guidance or a shoulder to cry on. As adults, they perpetuate and receive reinforcement for this persona as self-described fixers, rescuers, codependents, caretakers for the entire world, avengers and "white knights" who are responsible for everyone else's issues and problems. They often believe that it is their responsibility to protect the underdog or the disenfranchised, with whom they identify. Such extensive focus on the needs of others at the expense and exclusion of personal needs is itself a form of dissociation. Beneath the surface, these children (and later adults) tend to feel desperately alone, like frauds or imposters, and may be quite frustrated at not having their own needs met. Their exterior control and perfection are used to paper over these feelings, keeping them secret from others but, more important, keeping them from themselves.

Regrettably, this approach tends to be self-perpetuating, leading to excessive and unrealistic expectations on the part of family members, friends, and coworkers, even as they might be frustrated or annoyed by the survivor's excessive self-sufficiency and need to control. This pattern usually comes under scrutiny and changes when the survivor has a breakdown of some sort due to stress or exhaustion or develops other compulsions or addictions (e.g., infidelity and sex addiction, overspending, hoarding, substance use and abuse) as a means of relief and self-soothing. It may take breakdown or otherwise "hitting bottom" before these behaviors and their underlying dynamics come to light.

The other main pattern of response related to an insecure or disorganized upbringing is at the opposite end of the spectrum, involving hostility and defiance, unmanageability, aggression, coercion, and violence. Feelings and behaviors such as these may be directed primarily toward the perpetrator or displaced onto others (especially authority figures) inside or outside the family, expressed directly or in passive–aggressive ways. They may also be directed toward the self in the form of self-injury, suicidality, risk taking, self-disregard, and self-defeating behaviors. Although responses such as these tend to be more common in males than in females, they are not exclusively so and are best understood as another way for victimized persons to cope, to have a modicum of control, and to express their often otherwise unacknowledged and unspoken rage.

In yet another relational variant, some survivors act out their mistrust by withdrawing from interpersonal and social contact, becoming isolates and loners. This social withdrawal may be a lifelong pattern; it can involve active dissociation; and it is to be expected in those who have suffered the most serious and prolonged forms of victimization with little or no protection, support, or soothing. It may be the only way for children in such circumstances to protect themselves and to self-soothe or the best way to stop being a target of mistreatment by making themselves "invisible." Psychological withdrawal by some traumatized children and adults can be extreme, for example, taking the form of conversion symptoms such as blindness, deafness, muteness, paralysis, and catatonia, and psychotic-like states that are expressed in rocking and self-holding behaviors. At the most extreme, they might result in psychogenic death. As responses of this type can be erroneously diagnosed as psychotic or autism spectrum disorders, they should be reconsidered as posttraumatic or dissociative if a significant trauma history is uncovered.

Another set of relational problems may be manifested in sexual functioning and in behaviors that range from sexual compulsivity to sexual aversion. At one end of the spectrum, children who become eroticized and sexually reactive in response to sexual abuse may relate to others in primarily sexual ways. Long-term sexual problems may begin with compulsive masturbation up to and including physical injury or precocious and promiscuous engagement with others starting at a young age (sexually reactive children) and continuing through adolescence (often involving unprotected sex with older partners). In consequence, their interpersonal relationships may be marked by others' keeping them at a distance due to discomfort or, alternatively, becoming sexually involved with them, resulting in another experience of victimization. As adults, some sexual abuse survivors on this end of the spectrum become trapped in patterns of compulsive exposure or exploitation (i.e., exhibitionism, pornography, prostitution) and other problematic and dangerous sexual behaviors (i.e., sadomasochism and bondage and discipline, serial relationships with victimizers, dangerous and unsafe sex due to intoxication, sex with multiple or anonymous partners, sexual addictions, and so on).

At the other end of the spectrum, childhood sexual abuse survivors report many sexual aversions and phobias. Sex organs and secondary sex characteristics are frequently viewed as ugly, dirty, terrifying, or out of control. Sexual feelings, behaviors, and physical sensations (whether they are self-initiated or in interaction with others) may elicit extreme emotional distress (including anger, as well as fear, guilt, shame, or despair) or avoidance, emotional numbing, and dissociation (see description of criteria for complex PTSD in a later section).

Exposure to complex trauma early in life can cause survivors to be vulnerable to a full range of sexual dysfunctions and disturbances. Therapists should therefore take a trauma history into consideration when any client seeks help for a sexual or intimacy problem. Although focus here is on problematic sexual responses and symptoms, it should be noted that many survivors of childhood victimization (sexual or otherwise) do not exhibit disturbed sexual behaviors or attitudes. Whether this is the result of compensatory defenses or of protective factors such as innate resilience, reparative relationships, or corrective emotional experiences, these individuals function relatively well and seemingly without major impact on their ability to be sexual or to be intimate. However, this sexual adaptation might change in seemingly inexplicable ways at times when life circumstances trigger reminders of victimization.

Survivors of childhood trauma other than sexual abuse also may develop phobic–disgust–avoidance or counterphobic–compulsive–risky patterns of sexualized behavior. Exposure to physical abuse or witnessing domestic or community violence in childhood may lead to chronic fear of others or an avoidance of connection. Dysregulation of anger secondary to physical abuse or witnessing interpersonal violence may lead to extreme difficulty tolerating being emotionally or physically vulnerable or to the development of behaviors that are controlling or aggressive. In reaction, survivors may either avoid or behave in a conflicted or aggressive manner in their interactions with others, sexual or otherwise.

CONCEPTUALIZING AND DIAGNOSING COMPLEX TRAUMATIC STRESS DISORDERS

The issue of diagnosis of complex traumatic stress disorders has been contentious going back to the end of the 20th century when (mostly, if not exclusively) female clients who reported trauma histories and who exhibited symptoms similar to those discussed in this chapter were labeled as hysterics and later as borderline personalities. Although detailed discussion of the politics surrounding diagnosis is beyond the scope of this book, we wish to acknowledge how diagnoses have been used and misused in ways that were perjorative and demoralizing. As mental health practitioners, we utilize diagnoses to identify and organize symptoms and to set the course of treatment. What is offered below is not an attempt to label or pigeonhole the client but rather to follow the lead provided by Herman in her groundbreaking work *Trauma and Recovery* (Herman, 1992b), to offer diagnostic conceptualizations that take into account what happened to the individual that led to the symptoms and secondary elaborations that require treatment. The contemporary discussion of the validity of a complex PTSD diagnosis can be found in a recent issue of the *Journal of Traumatic Stress*, in response to the publication of a clinician survey and preliminary treatment best practices for complex trauma (Cloitre et al., 2011). In the special section on complex trauma, a review article by Resick et al. (2012a) and commentaries by Bryant (2012), Goodman (2012), Herman (2012) and Lindauer (2012) along with a rejoinder by Resick et al. (2012b) give a flavor of the discourse.

Before we move on to discussing the practical aspects of establishing the clinical frame and approaches to assessment and treatment (covered in Chapters 3–7), we consider how clinicians can comprehend complex traumatic stress disorders in light of this varied array of symptoms that span all five axes of the DSM model (symptoms, personality, medical/somatic, degree of functioning past and currently). Recent advances in conceptualization and diagnosis of traumatic stress disorders can assist clinicians in this process. First we consider a version of PTSD that has been incorporated into the World Health Organization's (2005) *International Classification of Diseases*, 10th edition (ICD-10), and recently proposed changes to the PTSD diagnosis in the upcoming revision of the DSM, DSM-5. Then we present current criteria for two diagnostic conceptualizations, proposed to the DSM revision committee: (1) complex PTSD or disorders of extreme stress not otherwise specified (DESNOS) in adults, and (2) developmental trauma disorder in children and adolescents.

PTSD in ICD-10

The best-known system of medical diagnoses is the ICD-10, for which an 11th revision is under development (World Health Organization, 2005). In addition to acute stress disorder and PTSD, the ICD includes an additional diagnosis of "enduring personality change after catastrophic experience" (F62.0), which does not have a counterpart in the current DSM, nor is one expected in the revised DSM-5. The "catastrophic experiences" identified by experts on traumatic stress as most likely to lead to enduring personality changes include torture, being held hostage or held in a concentration camp, war, sexual assault, and domestic violence (Beltran, Silove, & Llewellyn, 2009). The key features of these experiences that experts consider most traumatizing are sustained and repetitive exposure (rather than a single or isolated set of events) to events or experiences that are intentional, malicious, violating, unjust, life threatening, undermining of the individual's personal integrity, and shame and guilt inducing (Beltran et al., 2009, p. 398). Childhood abuse and victimization are not explicitly identified as precursors to enduring posttraumatic personality change, a significant omission since physical, sexual, and emotional abuse and neglect, in addition to other types of traumatic exposure during childhood, reflect these key features.

Per the ICD-10 definition, the specific personality changes following catastrophic experiences include the following:

1. A hostile or distrustful attitude toward the world.
2. Social withdrawal.
3. A constant feeling of emptiness or hopelessness.
4. An enduring feeling of "being on edge" or being threatened without

any external cause, as evidenced by an increased vigilance and irritability.

5. A permanent feeling of being changed or being different from others (estrangement).

Traumatic stress experts surveyed by Beltran and Silove (1999) ranked the first criterion item, a hostile or distrustful attitude toward the world, as the most clinically important feature, although all five criteria were judged to be clinically relevant. In addition, these experts suggested the following additional features: "problems with impulse control, changed perception of self, somatization, survivor guilt, hostility, depression, disturbed emotional reactions, revictimization and passivity, impairment in intimacy, loss of self-esteem, numbing of conscience, . . . anxiety, learning and concentration problems, coping defenses, existential issues, and estrangement" (Beltran & Silove, 1999, p. 398). Taken together, the official features and those added by this panel of experts closely parallel the description of the adverse changes in emotion and somatic self-regulation, sexual functioning, and core beliefs about self, world, relationships, and ethical/spiritual values that occur as consequences of complex trauma. When the ICD-10 is utilized for clinical or research purposes, complex traumatic stress disorders are fairly well represented by the diagnosis of "enduring personality changes after catastrophic experience"; however, the characteristic problems with integration of cognition and consciousness due to dissociation are thus far not included, creating the need for the clinician to make a separate dissociative diagnosis when using the ICD system.

PTSD in DSM-5

At present, the American Psychiatric Association is considering several changes to the definition of PTSD in its next edition of the DSM (DSM-5; *www.dsm5.org*). This is important because most psychiatric clinical and research work in the United States, and in other countries as well, is conducted using the DSM rather than the ICD for diagnostic purposes. The proposed DSM-5 PTSD diagnosis that is currently under discussion disaggregates active avoidance of reminders associated with traumatic events from several types of emotional dysregulation (including but not limited to the DSM-IV focus on emotional numbing). The active avoidance symptoms are now proposed to be included in a separate criterion, and the emotional numbing symptoms have been expanded as follows as another separate feature: "negative alterations in cognitions and mood that are associated with the traumatic event(s) that began or worsened after the traumatic event(s)" (American Psychiatric Association, 1995, p. 210). Three emotions that are common sequelae of complex trauma, anger, guilt, and shame have been suggested in addition to the three emotions that were previously included (fear, helplessness, and horror). As a result of these changes, the PTSD diagnosis may therefore be more applicable to describing the substantial "persistent" emotion dysregulation that often occurs for years or even decades after exposure to complex trauma. This change to PTSD's definition also reflects scientists' and clinicians' observations that complex trauma victims often are too young, too shocked and horrified or demoralized, or too cognitively and behaviorally focused on simply surviving to know or recall what they were feeling at the time of traumatic exposure. When the trauma was prolonged or recurrent, they may have dissociated their emotional reactions at the time (peri-traumatic dissociation) and afterward. Although emotional distress at the time of traumatic exposure may be a risk factor for subsequent persistent posttraumatic impairment, many individuals of all ages (and particularly children) do not have a coherent emotional reaction when still in the throes of psychological trauma. They can nevertheless develop serious emotional difficulties weeks, months, or years later as a result of persistent trauma-related stress reactions.

The revised criteria for DSM-5 reflects emotional dysregulation and altered fundamental beliefs, in addition to the DSM-IV symptoms of emotional numbing, feelings of detachment or estrangement from others, dysphoria, anhedonia, and psychogenic amnesia. Specifically, emotion dysregulation is represented by including a new symptom of "pervasive negative emotional state—for example, fear, horror, anger, guilt, or shame" (DSM-5; *www.dsm5.org*). Altered fundamental beliefs are addressed by adding two symptoms: "persistent and exaggerated negative expectations about one's self, others, or the world and "persistent distorted blame of self or others about the cause or consequences of the traumatic event(s)" (DSM-5; *www.dsm5.org*). Although these posttraumatic affects and cognitions may be experienced by adults who endure catastrophic violence, disasters, or accidents or by children who survive horrific disasters or accidents, they are particularly likely to occur (as we have been discussing) among children who suffer repeated and chronic traumatic victimization and as long-term problems by adults and adolescents who were victimized earlier as children.

Finally, two important changes have been proposed for the symptom cluster that deals with hyperarousal and hypervigilance. First, the symptom formerly described as "irritability or outbursts of anger" has been expanded to include not only irritable but also "aggressive" behavior. Second, a new symptom has been added, described as "reckless or self-destructive behavior" (DSM-5; *www.dsm5.org*). These changes mirror the forms of angry protest and self-defense, as well as self-harm and self-endangerment that are common immediate and long-term aftereffects for people of all ages who experienced traumatic victimization in childhood.

As a consequence of these proposed changes to the criteria for PTSD, individuals diagnosed with PTSD in the future may include those suffering from persistent emotional dysregulation, traumatically impaired core beliefs, and problems with aggressive impulses toward themselves and others, as well as those trauma survivors who primarily suffer from severe anxiety and dysphoria (the essence of prior definitions of PTSD). However, symptoms of somatic (including sexual) dysregulation are not addressed, nor is emotion dysregulation per se. Persistent emotional distress is added, but this does not differentiate clearly between people who are primarily fearful or dysphoric and those who (like many survivors of childhood victimization) have a primary inability to experience or recover from, or a tendency to pathologically dissociate when confronted with, extreme emotional distress.

A dissociative subtype of PTSD is likely to be included in the DSM-5. See the August 2012 issue of the *Journal of Depression and Anxiety* on the topic of focus on dissociation in PTSD.

Complex PTSD

The diagnosis of PTSD first formally included in DSM-III (American Psychiatric Association, 1980) was derived primarily from the study of war trauma. The criteria were applied to other types of trauma (i.e., rape trauma syndrome; post–child abuse syndrome, battered woman syndrome) because they generally fit what clinicians saw in response to them and because a similar diagnosis had not been available previously. Before long, however, clinicians and researchers noted that the fit between the PTSD criteria and the typical consequences of child abuse trauma was not exact, especially as pertained to the developmental effects of chronic child-onset trauma. In 1992, Herman and colleagues developed a new diagnostic conceptualization, complex PTSD/DESNOS, proposed it for inclusion in DSM-IV (Herman, 1992a, 1992b), and field-tested it to establish the preliminary validity of its seven criteria categories (Van der Kolk, Roth, Pelcovitz, Sunday, & Spinazzola, 2005). Field-test results were positive, yet, after having been favorably voted on by the DSM-IV committee for inclusion as a freestanding diagnosis, it was instead listed as an associated feature of PTSD, where it remains today.

Despite the fact that it was not included as a formal diagnosis, complex PTSD/DESNOS was immediately accepted and used by a wide variety of clinicians treating patients with complex trauma histories because it had face validity. Complex PTSD/DESNOS better matched the varied presentations made by their clients and was a more parsimonious and less stigmatizing way to understand and diagnose the symptom constellation than the alternatives provided by the DSM. One of these alternatives has been to diagnose PTSD and several comorbid Axis I disorders, such as bipolar, eating, dissociative, and substance use disorders. This can be problematic when patients with complex trauma histories do not qualify for the PTSD diagnosis because, for example, they had such severe dissociative symptoms that they were largely unaware of their trauma. It also can lead to situations in which patients have so many "comorbid" diagnoses that a large and unwieldy—and clinically questionable—array of diagnoses, medications, and psychotherapy interventions would be necessary to fully address all of the symptoms.

Another DSM-IV alternative to diagnosing or describing complex trauma survivors has been to diagnose Axis II personality disorders as well as or instead of PTSD. The most relevant Axis II diagnoses are from Cluster B, because it includes personality disorders that are defined by symptoms that tend to involve the kinds of problems with self-integration, interpersonal relatedness, and emotion regulation that are characteristic of many adult survivors of childhood victimization. However, as Herman (1992b) cogently noted two decades ago, these personality disorders can be iatrogenic, causing harm to individuals as an inadvertent result of the social stigma they carry and the widespread (but not entirely accurate) belief among professionals and insurers that those with Cluster B personality disorders (especially borderline personality disorder [BPD]), cannot be treated successfully, cannot recover, and are a headache to practitioners. For example, the BPD diagnosis continues to be applied predominantly to women often, but not always, in a negative way, usually signifying that they are irrational and beyond help. Describing posttraumatic symptoms as a personality disorder not only can be demoralizing for the client due to its connotation that something is defective with his or her core self (i.e., personality) but also may misdirect the therapist by implying that the patient's core personality should be the focus of treatment rather than trauma-related adaptations that affect but are distinct from the core self. In this way, both therapists and their clients may overlook personality strengths and capacities that are healthy and sources of resilience that can be a basis for building on and enhancing (rather than "fixing" or remaking) the patient's core self and personality.

An updated proposal for complex PTSD/DESNOS diagnosis was submitted to the DSM-5 revision committee (Herman, Cloitre, & Ford, 2009) and is under review by the committee that will determine the nature and form that traumatic stress disorder diagnoses take in the revision. The seven categories that were proposed remain the same and include:

1. *Alterations in the regulation of affective impulses*, including difficulty with modulation of anger and tendencies toward self-destructiveness. This category has come to include all methods used for emotional regulation and self-soothing, even those that are paradoxical, such as addictions and self-harming behaviors.

2. *Alterations in attention and consciousness* leading to amnesias, dissociative episodes, and depersonalization. This category includes emphasis

on dissociative responses different from those found in the DSM criteria for PTSD. Its inclusion in the complex PTSD conceptualization incorporates recent findings regarding dissociation: primarily, that it tends to be related to prolonged and severe interpersonal abuse trauma occurring during childhood and, secondarily, that children are more prone to dissociation than are adults.

3. *Alterations in self-perception*, predominantly negative and involving a chronic sense of guilt and responsibility and ongoing feelings of intense shame. Chronically abused individuals (especially children) incorporate abuse messages and posttraumatic responses into their developing sense of self and self-worth.

4. *Alterations in perception of the perpetrator*, including incorporation of his or her belief system. This criterion addresses the complex relational attachment systems that ensue following repetitive and premeditated abuse and lack of appropriate response at the hands of primary caretakers or others in positions of responsibility.

5. *Alterations in relationship to others*, such as not being able to trust the motives of others and not being able to feel intimate with them. Another "lesson of abuse" internalized by victim-survivors is that other people are venal and self-serving, out to get what they can by whatever means, including using and abusing others. Survivors may be unaware that other people can be benign, caring, and not dangerous.

6. *Somatization and/or medical problems*. These somatic reactions and medical conditions can relate directly to the type of abuse suffered and any physical damage that was caused or they may be more diffuse. They ave been found to involve all major body systems. These are not specifically mentioned in the current or proposed PTSD criteria.

7. *Alterations in systems of meaning*. Chronically abused and traumatized individuals often feel hopeless about finding anyone to understand them or their suffering. They despair of being able to recover from their psychic anguish and to lead better and more satisfying lives.

If complex PTSD is not included in the DSM-5, the new Dissociative subtype of PTSD may be the formulation that is most similar.

Developmental Trauma Disorder

The extensive clinical and research evidence that victimization in childhood can have adverse effects on not only the functioning but also the core psychobiological and personality development of children (Ford, 2005) resulted in a proposal spearheaded by Van der Kolk (2005) and several investigators in the National Child Traumatic Stress Network (NCTSN) for a new childhood psychiatric diagnosis labeled developmental trauma disorder (DTD). Its criteria were based, in part, on the results of surveys of more than 14,000 abused children, distributed and collected by the NCTSN and identified as the Comprehensive Data Set (Pynoos, 2011). As originally formulated, DTD involved exposure to traumatic victimization, a "triggered pattern of repeated dysregulation in response to trauma cues" (including dysregulation of emotion, bodily functioning, behavior, cognition, relationships, and self-attributions), and "persistently altered attributions and expectancies" in relation to self, caregivers, social systems, and victimizers (Van der Kolk, 2005, p. 404). DTD subsequently has been refined and the traumatic exposure criterion expanded to include major disruptions or losses in primary caregiver relationships (including neglect) and to separately define symptoms into following criterion sets (Ford & the DTD Field Trial Work Group, 2011):

- Emotion dysregulation: temper dysregulation; impaired recovery from dysphoric states; psychic numbing; impaired expressive emotion functions; avoidance of emotion expression.
- Somatic dysregulation: sleep disturbance; dysregulated eating; dysregulated eliminative functions; somatoform dissociation: (1) pain; (2) negative conversion symptoms; (3) positive conversion symptoms. (Note: Conversion symptoms involve the breakdown or loss of bodily functioning whose etiology or degree of extremity are medically inexplicable.)
- Attentional dysregulation: threat-related preoccupation with or avoidance of cues.
- Behavioral dysregulation: threat-related reactive aggression; threat-related reactive avoidance; extreme risk taking; self-harm; maladaptive self-soothing behavior.
- Relational dysregulation: expectancy of betrayal; expectancy of victimization; physical boundary diffusion; emotional boundary diffusion; expectancy of irresolvable attachment loss.
- Self-dysregulation: self-loathing or perception of self as permanently damaged.

DTD currently addresses the most frequently observed and functionally detrimental initial and long-term posttraumatic aftereffects experienced by traumatized children (as well as adolescents whose victimization occurred in childhood). A field trial study led by Van der Kolk and Ford has surveyed several hundred child- and family-serving professionals (including case managers, counselors, family educators, marriage and family therapists, pediatricians, psychiatrists, psychiatric nurses, psychologists, social service program staff, and social workers) nationally to determine their views on whether DTD symptoms are sufficiently clinically important and distinct from those of other psychiatric disorders to potentially warrant the creation of a new DTD diagnosis. In the second phase of the field trial, several hundred structured interviews for DTD and alternative DSM-5 psychiatric disorders were conducted by clinical interviewers with children and their parents or caregivers at eight sites around the United States to determine whether a DTD diagnosis could add to the understanding and effective treatment of victimized children. Results are under analysis and are forthcoming.

CONCLUSION

Therapists working with patients who have experienced complex psychological trauma—particularly (but not exclusively) those who suffered developmentally adverse interpersonal trauma over the course of childhood—must be cognizant of and able to recognize an array of traumatic stress symptoms that go well beyond even the newly reformulated (proposed) diagnosis of PTSD. Seven main categories of additional symptoms currently make up the conceptualization of complex traumatic stress disorders or complex PTSD/DESNOS, and similar criteria are found in DTD. In particular, these include three primary domains: emotions and reactions, emotion dysregulation, and loss of self-integrity, including psychological and somatic dissociation. These diagnostic conceptualizations are quite broad, but, as noted by Herman (2009): "Sometimes the whole is greater than the sum of its parts" (p xiii). In the case of complex trauma, this integrative and coherent formulation helps to make sense of the often confusing symptoms common in the aftermath of repeated and chronic trauma. Moreover, it gives therapists direction in providing effective assistance that enables them to not just cope with but to recover from their ongoing symptoms. We therefore turn next, in Chapter 3, to the preparations necessary for therapists to successfully meet this often daunting—but nevertheless achievable—challenge.

PART II

TREATMENT OF COMPLEX TRAUMATIC STRESS REACTIONS AND DISORDERS

CHAPTER 3

Preparing for Treatment of Complex Trauma

This chapter presents issues that typically arise in the treatment of adults with histories of complex trauma who have an array of symptoms of the type described in the previous two chapters. The major principles of trauma-focused treatment apply, but additional relational and developmental objectives are relevant. We particularly discuss some of the challenges facing therapists treating this population and highlight the clinical, ethical, economic, and professional foundations that should be in place before and during the treatment. These include but are not limited to: general and specialized training; supervision and consultation; self-awareness and maturity, professional judgment, emotional health, and self-care; the ability to consistently relate to and empathize in what are often daunting relational and posttraumatic contexts; and a defined and communicated treatment frame that covers many aspects of informed consent.

FOUNDATIONS OF TREATMENT

Ochberg, in his seminal book on trauma-focused treatment, had this to say about the distinctive properties of this treatment: "The advantages in . . . post-traumatic therapy (PTT) are its assumption of psychological health, its fundamental assumption that the victim is not to blame [*for the victimization, even when it is repetitive and chronic, nor for revictimization, and*] its ability to facilitate a working relationship between victim and therapist through partnership and parity in respect and power" (Ochberg, 1988, p. 10; italicized phrase in brackets added). The treatment of complex trauma is founded on these and on four additional principles articulated by Courtois (2010). The first two are foundational assumptions that must be understood and communicated by therapists: (1) that exposure to and the experiencing of traumatic stressors (especially chronic and complex interpersonal forms) can leave long-lasting and even lifelong negative imprints on the survivor client; (2) that posttraumatic symptoms can be understood as once-adaptive attempts to cope with overwhelming stressors that, when unresolved, later can have the unfortunate effect of undermining the survivor's development and functioning. The third and fourth principles are therapeutic conditions that therapists must provide for all clients but that are particularly salient for complex trauma: (3) personal and interpersonal safety, with special emphasis on (4) safety within the therapeutic relationship with a therapist who is empathic and respectful yet is emotionally regulated with appropriate and defined boundaries and limitations. These foundational principles establish the treatment setting and relationship as a "secure base or safe haven" (Bowlby, 1969) from which clients can explore and come to better understand and regain their emotions, themselves, and their relationships and to resume their interrupted development.

Therapy for the effects of complex trauma has five essential foci: **P**osttraumatic adaptations, **R**elational working models, self-**I**dentity, healthy **D**evelopment, and **E**motion regulation (PRIDE; Ford, 2012). The role of shame in PTSD and dissociation, particularly as a result of emotional abuse, alone or in combination with other forms of chronic victimization recently received increasing attention (e.g., Harman & Lee, 2010; Resick et al., 2008; Teicher et al., 2006). For many survivors, gaining (or regaining) the capacity to feel the opposite of shame (i.e., PRIDE, as described in the preceding acronym defining treatment foci) has been an insurmountable problem most of their lives. Therapy for these survivors therefore provides the interpersonal and educational conditions necessary to understand themselves and their histories in a way that rekindles (or provides for the first time) a sense of pride versus shame.

CHALLENGES OF TREATMENT

Multiple trials await the therapist working with complex traumatic stress reactions. Clients with complex trauma histories often make complex and, at times, seemingly contradictory presentations of themselves and their symptoms. Moreover, symptoms are rarely straightforward in their manifestation and are often compounded, creating an amalgam of posttraumatic, self, and relational issues, usually developed over the course of many years and incorporated into the client's personality and functioning. Awareness of the effects of having experienced chronic interpersonal victimization assists the therapist in understanding the complex interplay of self-impact, ability to self-regulate, relational patterns, and posttraumatic symptoms. Obviously, the therapist who is knowledgeable about and anticipates these varied issues has an easier time contending with them than one who does not. Some of the primary challenges faced by the therapists in this treatment include the following.

Validating the Reality of Complex Trauma

The basic difference between a trauma-informed therapy framework and the traditional perspective taken by professionals and the public is that *the traumatic event or experience is **never** viewed as irrelevant to understanding and treating behavioral or mental health problems.* Reactions are not minimized or discounted as something that will just "go away" with the sufficient passage of time. Nevertheless, it is not assumed that all trauma impact is the same, as victim-survivors have different emotional "thresholds" and constitutions. Similarly, not all trauma—whether it is complex or not—causes the development of PTSD. Yet the research and clinical evidence reviewed in Chapters 1 and 2 strongly suggests that posttraumatic reactions, especially when the traumatic stressors began early in life, were repetitive, escalating and cumulative and occurred within the context of significant relationships and that, without adequate response, they are often persistent, long-lasting, and have a severe impact (usually in detrimental ways but sometimes in ways that are paradoxically beneficial) on the individual's lifelong development and functioning.

The posttraumatic perspective is not an "abuse excuse" and not an attempt to make victims out of everyone or to inflate the severity of all negative or traumatic life experiences by conflating "drama" with trauma. Nor is it an attempt to "infantilize" individuals or make them less responsible for their behavior, nor to homogenize the reactions of survivors by suggesting that all reactions are the same or that reactions are traumatic and devastating for all. Quite the contrary, a complex trauma or traumatic stress perspective provides survivors (and their loved ones and other supporters) with hope and knowledge for understanding what are frequently misunderstood and misattributed traumatic stress reactions and their developmental and secondary elaborations. It is geared to the needs of the individual client, following assessment of salient issues and symptoms. It also provides concrete skills training and tools that enable clients to be active participants in their own psychosocial recovery and growth.

Understanding Symptoms as Coping Skills and Adaptations

The treatment of complex traumatic stress disorders is predicated on understanding traumatic stress symptoms as ***normal** reactions, coping efforts, and adaptations to **abnormal** circumstances and events.* Traumatic stressors occur in the lives of at least half (or more) of the children and adults in relatively privileged nations (and far more often in groups and populations that face severe socioeconomic, cultural, gender, health, and political adversities and prejudices). Of course, most people are *not* routinely exposed to imminent death or other danger or the permanent loss or incapacity of those on whom they depend for security and survival. However, for those who do live in such conditions on an ongoing basis, especially during developmentally formative life periods such as in childhood or transitions from one developmental epoch to another (e.g., adolescence, early adulthood, midlife, old age), getting through these circumstances is likely to require biological shifts that are protection- and survival-based rather than developmental and life enhancing (Ford, 2009b). As a result, although traumatic stress symptoms can express themselves in quite pathological ways, they are not considered to be manifestation of disease or pathology per se. To the contrary, they are viewed as alterations in or derailment of the individual's potential for development (of physical and psychological integrity, sense of identity, core beliefs, ways of being in the world, and relationships with others) that were necessary for psychic if not physical survival. Complex trauma can begin during infancy and impact the earliest developmental phases of childhood, creating major impediments to healthy development. Moreover, as noted earlier, when life-threatening violence, exploitation, subjugation, or betrayal occur and recur across the lifespan, or even when they begin later in life, they can cause significant developmental regression and posttraumatic decline in individuals who had previously been relatively healthy, regardless of whether they had had prior traumatic exposure.

Posttraumatic adaptations also offer explanations for why so many complex trauma survivors are prone to being revictimized. Adaptations present not because victims seek further victimization but rather due to tragic lessons learned—namely, that they expect to be victimized because that is what they experienced repeatedly, usually without adequate protection or response. Their experiences led them to create assumptions about others and related beliefs about themselves such as "this is my lot in life" and "this is what I deserve." Some also learned that personal safety and happiness are of lower priority than survival and that it may be safer to give in than to actively fight off additional abuse or victimization. When abuse is perpetrated by intimates, it is additionally confounding in terms of attachment, betrayal, and trust. Victims may be unable to leave or to fight back due to strong, albeit insecure and disorganized, attachment and misplaced loyalty to abusers. They may have also experienced trauma bonding over the course of their victimization, that is, a bond of specialness with or dependence on the abuser.

Therapy, therefore, must begin with empathy—not a patronizing sympathy, but instead one that is unflinching (Marotta, 2003). Empathy of this sort is highly attuned to the client, no matter the circumstance. The therapist strives to "travel in the client's shoes" or to "view the world from the client's perspective" in order to really understand his or her emotions, cognitions, and beliefs—in short, to understand from the perspective of the other (Wilson & Thomas, 2004). Treatment involves understanding that a client's defeatist and apparently helpless, disempowered, or "masochistic" perspectives can be a logical outgrowth of formative traumatic experiences and, further, may be highly creative means of self-protection. The therapist must not attempt to undo or "make up for" past abandonment or betrayals by their clients' caregivers or in their close relationships, but instead first understand the client's perspective and approach to the world, while working to provide alternative perspectives on both past and present that promote change. We turn again to the case of Hector to make this point.

Hector

Therapy, for Hector, was "something only weak people need—and I don't want anyone to think I'm weak or needy, ever!" He viewed life as a constant struggle to remain "bloodied but undefeated," with such preferred ways of coping as "drinking until I black out," or "picking a fight with someone who'll really put the hurt to me," or "going back to my emotional bunker and building a bigger wall around myself to keep anyone from getting close." Hector viewed dealing with "my demons" as being "the cross that I have to bear." These "demons" were the nightmares that haunted him on the rare nights when he got more than brief snatches of sleep and the daily "torture chamber" he faced due to intense panic attacks, terrifying flashbacks, feelings of rage, self-loathing, hopelessness, and impulses to escape via suicide. Hector understood these symptoms through the lens of his Catholic upbringing. Tragically, the resultant belief that "he was tainted and beyond hope and redemption" was reinforced by the abusive priest who coerced Hector into adopting a position of passive acquiescence to the abuse and who then blamed him. True to his early religious experiences and training, Hector believed that his inner suffering was both a mark of his own "sinful nature" and a kind of purifying vocation to which he had been called by God. However, he took no comfort from this latter belief, as he also believed he was "beyond redemption." His God was one who was unmerciful and unforgiving and who he could never trust. He didn't expect forgiveness or redemption because of all of the "terrible things" that he had done with the priest, but especially what he had done in the course of his wartime service.

Hector's beliefs made it crucial for the therapist to communicate nonjudgmental recognition of his principled rejection of the very idea of therapy and of emotional or spiritual healing or recovery. Although such a stance might seem to reinforce Hector's posttraumatic demoralization and alienation, to the contrary, it was a way for the therapist to join him emotionally. He did this by respectfully acknowledging the importance to Hector of taking a principled stand in the face of his extremely adverse life experiences and his ongoing distress. By agreeing that it would be presumptuous of Hector, and even more so of any therapist, to believe that the emotional burden that he was carrying could ever be put down or released, the therapist paradoxically offered Hector an opportunity to consider whether therapy could be helpful to him *in other ways*.

This stance required the therapist to put aside any preconceptions about how therapy can help, specifically by shifting focus from the conventional "therapy = healing" view to an alternative model more consistent with Hector's outlook. This required careful consideration of what was adaptive in Hector's apparently maladaptive beliefs and coping tactics. Hector had begun treatment very reluctantly, in order to, in his words, "not be put in a straitjacket or loony bin with a bunch of wackos or drunks." The crisis counselor's initial assessment was that, clinically and ethically, Hector could not be considered safe at the time of his unscheduled visit to the mental health center unless he was psychiatrically hospitalized (by involuntary commitment if necessary), placed in an intensive residential treatment for substance abuse, or agreed to and followed through with a plan to attend outpatient psychotherapy regularly (on an at least twice-weekly basis initially) with a therapist experienced in the treatment of severe trauma.

Hector chose psychotherapy "as the lesser of three evils," approaching his sessions as he did other activities in which he felt "exposed and vulnerable." This involved saying as little as possible and not betraying any sign of emotion other than frustration, impatience, contempt, and boredom. To the therapist, he seemed to be assuming the stance of a virtual prisoner under interrogation. The therapist acknowledged this without criticism, stating that it made sense given Hector's past experiences that he might feel that he should share only his "name, rank, and serial number" and not reveal information that he felt might be used against him. The therapist framed this as a validation of Hector's determination to "selflessly protect the people who depend upon you or whom you care about, by making sure that no one feels that they need to worry about you or help you, which might be a burden or upsetting for them."

While fully recognizing that Hector had developed a position of isolated self-reliance as a way of coping with his own internal distress (an insecure-detached attachment style), the therapist chose to focus on the altruism and relational integrity reflected in Hector's willingness to suffer in place of, or at least without indirectly burdening or worrying, others (this is historically what had happened with his parents and siblings, later his mother, and, more recently, with his friends and buddies). This reframing provided a basis for the therapist to suggest that therapy might help Hector to continue to achieve these admirable goals by supporting him in managing his severe symptoms. Consequently, his friends or family would not have to worry so much or work so hard to get him help (as his friends did by bringing him to the mental health center). Thus, by emphasizing the adaptive goals and strengths inherent in Hector's apparently dysfunctional and symptomatic presentation, the therapist was able to establish common ground for collaboration based on recognizing and enhancing his abilities rather than critically highlighting and attempting to "fix" his symptoms or past history.

Creating Safety in the Therapy

Individuals who have been traumatized have been made unsafe, emotionally as well as physically. This fact underscores that treatment must be organized on a philosophical foundation of *safety as essential to the process of healing* (Herman, 1992b). The individual who is still in a hazardous circumstance or condition, because of ongoing danger from others (such as domestic and community violence, emotional abuse, political repression, homelessness, or human trafficking) or from him- or herself (such as danger seeking, risk taking, self-injury, addiction, or suicidality), still needs to retain strong defenses and adaptations to withstand additional traumatic adversity. Therefore, he or she will be hard-pressed to do anything else but survive and will be unable to lower defenses sufficiently to engage in therapy. Therefore, *treatment must have an initial goal of supporting the client in establishing safety in her or his life*, often in direct contradiction to what was previously (or continues to be) experienced or expected. On a short-term basis, this means developing sufficient protection from danger to prevent additional victimization and retraumatization. This may not be a realistic expectation for clients who live in disturbed families or violent communities who have no way to leave or change their circumstances. In such cases, therapy usually is safest and most helpful if it remains focused on education, safety, stabilization, and life skills, all tasks of the first phase of treatment (see Chapter 5) designed to increase the ability to cope with ongoing adversities and possibly to escape them. Therapy can empower clients to make changes that substantially increase their long-term safety, by developing safety and escape plans, reshaping or leaving abusive relationships, becoming clean and sober, finding a safe place to live, and seeking and engaging in relationships and work that do not threaten—but instead support—their security and well-being. Attention to safety by the therapist may itself be a novel experience for the client—someone expresses interest in and caring about her or his welfare. In such a preliminary way, the client begins to discern that something different can happen in his or her life such as being noticed and cared about and receiving support and encouragement in efforts to change.

Co-Creating an Attuned and Secure Therapeutic Relationship

In a parallel manner to the requirement of safety from physical, relational, or other harm, a relationship becomes therapeutic only when the client can count on interactions with the therapist (and the therapeutic setting itself) to be consistent and predictable. The client must be able to feel a degree of sustained empathy from the therapist for trust to grow and a working alliance or partnership to develop. Kinsler, Courtois, and Frankel (2009) commented that the therapeutic relationship is both a *foundation* and a *method* of treatment, a safe "holding environment" (Winnicott, 1963) that functions as a catalyst to the exploration of self and of past and current relationships.

Trust of others is in short supply for many adult survivors, as complex trauma generally involves major relational betrayal. It is, therefore, expectable (although paradoxical) that clients with these histories are predisposed to be mistrustful at the outset of therapy, precisely because of (and in proportion to) the actual trustworthiness of the therapist. When past experiences have taught hard lessons, namely, that one can least afford to trust the people who should be most trustworthy, it stands to reason that confusion about trust results. The therapist must understand and not take offense either personally or professionally and not react judgmentally or defensively. Practically speaking, this involves the therapist being prepared to patiently and empathically respond to active or passive tests or challenges to trustworthiness as legitimate and meaningful communication that deserves a respectful reply in action as well as in words. Doris exemplifies some of these trust issues.

Doris

As the therapist reflected on their first session and Doris's later feedback in their second, she realized that she had registered some subtle cues of distress in Doris despite the fact that Doris had portrayed herself as confident and collaborative. When she closed the session by mentioning that she had enjoyed meeting Doris and looked forward to continuing with her, the therapist had seen a fleeting look on her face that seemed to convey a combination of longing and terror. The therapist realized that she may have ended the session too casually, without communicating her understanding that it had been a highly stressful and personally crucial encounter for Doris due to her deep mistrust of others and her fear of betrayal. Based on this recognition, when in their next session Doris expressed a sense of "feeling sick and tired of relationships that should be trustworthy but can't be trusted," the therapist was able to acknowledge that she may have not have been sensitive enough to Doris's fears and mistrust. Doris was initially taken aback by this response but was later able to say that it was actually a relief that the therapist could understand why she had gone from seeming satisfied with the first session to appalled and disgusted in the second. She added that she had not understood this extreme shift in emotion and attitude previously, but hearing the therapist give a quite reasonable explanation gave her hope that she could understand the "emotional roller coaster" on which she'd felt trapped in every important relationship.

As a client with a disorganized attachment style (who also exhibited fearful/anxious and dismissing characteristics), Doris's shift to disgust and contempt and her resilient ability to take in and utilize the therapist's empathic reframing exquisitely illustrates the "double-edged sword" of complex posttraumatic adaptations. Her survival had depended on shifting rapidly between superficial deference and aggressive fight/flight reactions, and she reenacted that dysfunctional yet highly adaptive scenario at the very outset of therapy.

Although she responded very positively to the therapist's empathic reframing, it is important to note that responses of this sort had to be repeated countless times over the course of a lengthy therapy before Doris was able to access and trust that the empathy was genuine and to self-regulate the intense posttraumatic adaptation of fleeing from and attacking or submissively deferring when someone expressed caring.

As a result of this withholding and detachment associated with mistrust, the therapist frequently felt confused, as if she were missing information or had misunderstood their interactions. However, with regular trauma-responsive consultation regarding these apparent ruptures in the exchanges and the therapist's own feelings in response to Doris, she came to understand the tremendous threat Doris experienced in the process of forming a therapeutic relationship. She also learned to trust her own ability to provide a secure and respectful therapeutic frame for Doris, even when Doris went through periods of emotional intensity and upheaval, then engaged in dissociation, self-medicating, and self-injury used to defend herself, especially in her more desperate times (usually when her husband threatened to leave, when her offers of friendship were rebuffed, or when the therapist was away). The complex trauma perspective enabled the therapist (despite at first feeling off-balance and stunned by the extreme shifts in Doris's presentation) to empathically name and reframe the feelings and explore the behaviors and their self-protective functions. She was also able to initiate "relational repair" by taking responsibility for inadvertently contributing to Doris's distress (i.e., her unintended but very real empathic failure) to prevent it from becoming a lasting "fault line" in Doris's sense of ongoing security and trust.

Doris exhibited a high level of sensitivity to issues of confidentiality and third-party involvement. Practices that the therapist initially took for granted, such as asking Doris to sign a consent form for treatment or a release of information, keeping progress notes, and storing records were matters of great concern. They had to be discussed at length initially and again each time her sense of trust was disrupted. Early on, Doris was verbally accusatory toward her therapist—a resurgence of her sense of posttraumatic threat, which she countered by shifting into a detached aggressive stance of contempt and of being "one up." She softened that stance and did not assume it as regularly or frequently as she learned, through the therapist's willingness to nondefensively discuss issues with her, to rely less on knee-jerk hostility and to trust her own ability to assert herself and negotiate her own needs.

In Doris's case, the greatest progress in healing her attachment wounds was made when the therapist could reopen discussions about whether and how Doris had been offered the opportunity to give informed consent to work on the painful emotions that emerged as she struggled to trust another person—and about Doris's fear that the therapist would not attend to her by focusing on external issues (such as keeping clinical notes) instead of on being focused on Doris. It took many sessions over many months for Doris to have those "looking back" discussions without impatience or foreclosure of options. Eventually Doris was able to say that the most important healing in the relationship came when she could trust that the therapist would respectfully listen to her while recognizing her fears and needs. Doris could recall how that process had started right from the start with her therapist's ability to remain caring the first time she had shown her emotional pain and aloneness in her early outburst of disgust.

As this case illustrates, the assessment and testing of the therapist begins from the earliest contact (including telephone, e-mail, or other interactions before the first in-person meeting) and continues throughout the entire treatment. A crucial first step in developing a working alliance with clients who have complex trauma histories involves making a careful assessment of attachment style and emotion regulation capacities. Although there are universal professional principles regarding the nature of a safe and helpful therapeutic relationship (discussed later in the chapter), each client–therapist relationship can be expected to evolve differently depending on the client's attachment style/security and emotion regulation capabilities and those of the therapist. An intersubjective perspective that stresses the uniqueness of each therapeutic dyad is useful in this regard.

As we discuss in the next chapter, such an assessment enables the therapist to tailor her or his style of interaction to match the client's in two crucial respects: first, not to inadvertently increase the client's sense of attachment insecurity but instead to reinforce secure interactions with the therapist; second, not to inadvertently trigger or exacerbate unregulated emotions. Based on the evidence summarized in Chapters 1 and 2 that complex trauma clients typically suffer from affect dysregulation and disorganized internal working models of attachment (IWM; Bowlby, 1977a, 1977b), their ability to benefit from therapy hinges on the quality of the therapeutic relationship that they and the therapist co-construct. This relational and intersubjective perspective implies that the therapeutic relationship is *both a healing context* ***and*** *a mechanism of therapeutic change*. It is dynamic rather than static and in constant flux, factors that can be disorienting to therapist and client alike, especially initially; yet the quality of the relationship can make this tolerable for both members of the dyad and can encourage and support change (see Gartner, 1999; Kinsler et al., 2009; Pearlman & Courtois, 2005; Perlman, 1999). Per Kinsler et al. (2009):

> *The therapy relationship is itself the vehicle of change*. Optimally, it models secure attachment, provides containment of the patient's anxiety, offers the opportunity for expression of other core emotions, provides a context within which to work out relational issues, and provides a basic *valuing* of *or validation* that the patient may never have had. A healing therapy relationship becomes a model for what can be. . . . As attachment becomes more secure over the course of treatment, emotions become more accessible and less onerous, the client's self-regard increases, and relationship skills develop. As a result, the client has a new template for relationships and new abilities to apply in his or her interpersonal world. (pp. 186–187; italics in original)

The overarching principle of a therapeutic relationship is that therapists should be ever mindful of a variant of the Hippocratic oath and, to the degree possible, strive to "do no *more* harm" (Courtois, 2010). Complex trauma clients have already experienced considerable harm, much of it at the hands of other human beings. As a result of the ubiquitous processes of transference, attachment styles, and IWM, these clients often view the therapist's behavior and their relationship through the lens of their trauma-related negative interpersonal expectancies and unhealed emotional wounds and injuries. Therapists should not be surprised to be "guilty until proven innocent," not because clients with complex trauma histories are "unfair" or "unreasonable" but precisely the opposite—because the most realistic self-protective stance for them (given the fact that betrayal and harm have been more the rule than the exception) is to "distrust first and verify" (or to be hypervigilant) rather than to start with an expectation of safety and trustworthiness.

If the therapist understands and does not take mistrust as a personal affront, the therapeutic relationship can evolve gradually. The client can begin to recognize that the therapist actually "gets" why he or she is initially skeptical, self-protective, or "realistically paranoid" and does not pressure the client to be a "happy camper" but instead works to earn trust by being honorable, reliable, and consistent. This also implies a view of the client's initial mistrust as expectable in light of the client's history—that is, as a strength rather than as a deficiency or pathology.

In an opposite pattern regarding trust, the client might be hypovigilant and quite naive regarding the intentions and trustworthiness of others or might shift between hyper- and hypovigilance. The overtrusting client typically lavishes the therapist with statements of immediate or instant trust that is untested and has been unearned. From this perspective, clients become immediately deferential and superficially compliant in their quest to receive the therapist's approval and unfettered availability. The therapeutic task with those operating from this preoccupied and anxious position is to help them to understand that trust should not be turned over prematurely and certainly without first getting to know the other person and assessing and testing trustworthiness. Although there is no guarantee in terms of the trustworthiness of others, skills development helps clients who are unaware and vulnerable to build their defenses and boundaries and to appropriately test others.

The attunement of the therapist in the form of respectful empathy (described further in Chapter 10) is an essential component in the treatment of trauma, as it is in all psychotherapy. Recent studies in attachment support the necessity of attunement and synchrony on the part of the primary caregiver to healthy physical, psychosexual, and psychosocial development (Ford, 2009b; Fosha, Siegel, & Solomon, 2009; Schore, 2003a). Consistent with this perspective, empathic attunement by the therapist may be the underlying source of a working alliance or bond and the underpinning necessary for the resumption of development interrupted by trauma. In consequence, a basic responsibility of the therapist is to provide enough stability, consistency, and availability to make the psychotherapy a place where clients are increasingly able to experience distressing emotions with response and support, allowing them to build their emotional recognition and tolerance. Therapeutic relational attunement further enables the client to engage in self-reflection that, over time, leads to increased self-esteem and a positive identity. Put another way, the client benefits from the reflection of self-in-relationship, that is, of being attuned to and seen and felt by the therapist, who reflects the client's emotions back to him or her through the processes of attunement, synchrony, and prosody (Chefetz, 1997; Schore, 2003b). The therapy relationship can be analogized to a learning laboratory, a place to experiment with new ways of feeling, being, and relating to others. With heightened access to emotions and improved ability to modulate them, the client can move from an insecure or disorganized attachment style to one of "earned security" that promotes increased personal and interpersonal health and that applies to relationships outside of therapy.

The therapist must create relational conditions in which the client is individually "seen," appreciated, and emotionally validated in ways that counter the invalidiation typically associated with attachment trauma. In short, the therapist functions as an active, empathic, and responsible listener and a guide in working with the emotional material that emerges. The therapist assists the client to examine feelings and thoughts that are spontaneously introduced into the therapy (often nonverbally and without conscious awareness, through somatic reactions and symptoms and through enactments with the therapist)—especially those that seem confusing and shameful or that were previously suppressed or forbidden in abusive or unsupportive relationships.

A stance of artificial neutrality or passive and intellectualized detachment on the part of the therapist is largely ineffective and potentially harmful to clients with major attachment injuries. These run the risk of creating iatrogenic reenactments of clients' traumatic relational experiences of neglect, abandonment, and rejection—what Linehan (1993) aptly termed "invalidating environments." In contrast, a therapist's ability to tolerate questioning or conflict without defensiveness, retaliation, or criticism and a stance of interest, receptivity, and humility can create conditions for personal expression and emotional and relational growth, even in clients who have suffered the most severe traumatization and resultant developmental deficits (Kinsler et al., 2009).

Another way to manage the various therapeutic challenges is to clearly establish the rights and responsibilities of both members of the therapeutic dyad, the topic of the next section.

RIGHTS AND RESPONSIBILITIES OF CLIENTS AND THERAPISTS

Psychotherapy for clients with complex trauma histories is explicitly based on established ethical codes and standards of professional practice that are at the core of training across all behavioral health and medical professions. In a landmark article more than 30 years ago, Hare-Mustin, Marecek, Kaplan, and Liss-Levinson (1979) described how the "responsibilities of therapists" are inextricably related to "rights of clients." A number of versions of a "Clients' Bill of Rights" have been developed in the past 25 years, including a consensus document outlining patient rights created in 1997 and approved or supported by organizations representing more than 600,000 mental and behavioral health professionals and major advocacy groups for people with mental and behavioral health disorders in the United States (see Tables 3.1 and 3.2). See Tables 3.3 and 3.4 for sample codes of ethics.

Commitment to Professional Competence and Accountability

Knowledge and Professional Expertise

Psychotherapy is a professional endeavor that is based on a course of training and the attainment of qualifications and licensing following the demonstration of achieved knowledge and competence. In terms of the treatment of complex traumatic stress disorders, the therapist needs training beyond the basics of the generic psychotherapy curriculum. Unfortunately, organized training in the competencies needed to treat traumatized clients (much less those with complex trauma histories) has rarely been available or provided in organized professional training (Courtois, 2003; Courtois & Gold, 2009; DePrince & Newman, 2011). With the increasing availability of preprofessional (Ford, 2009b) and continuing professional education training materials (see, e.g., *www.nctsnet.org*, *www.istss.org*, *www.apa-traumadivision.org*, *www.isstd.org*, or *www.ncptsd.org*), this situation is improving gradually. Until preprofessional and professional training curricula systematically address trauma, PTSD, dissociation, and complex traumatic stress disorders and their assessment and treatment, therapists must find other ways to gain the necessary knowledge and to develop competence in treating these posttraumatic conditions through ongoing specialized courses of study (including continuing education), focused self-study and reading (including developing familiarity with best-practices statements and treatment guidelines published by professional organizations; Forbes et al., 2010), and consultation and supervision.

Self-study and periodic continuing education seminars are not optimal ways to develop needed knowledge and skills. In recognition of this deficit and the percentage of mental health clients with a history of trauma, several

TABLE 3.1. An Outline of Patient Rights

Commitment

Our commitment must be to provide quality mental health and substance abuse services to all individuals without regard to race, color, religion, national origin, gender, age, sexual orientation, or disabilities.

The Right to Know Benefits

Individuals have the right to be provided information from the purchasing entity (such as employer or union or public purchaser) and the insurance/third party payer describing the nature and extent of their mental health and substance abuse treatment benefits. This information should include details on procedures to obtain access to services, on utilization management procedures, and on appeal rights. The information should be presented clearly in writing with language that the individual can understand.

Professional Expertise

Individuals have the right to receive full information from the potential treating professional about that professional's knowledge, skills, preparation, experience, and credentials. Individuals have the right to be informed about the options available for treatment interventions and the effectiveness of the recommended treatment.

Contractual Limitations

Individuals have the right to be informed by the treating professional of any arrangements, restrictions, and/or covenants established between third party payer and the treating professional that could interfere with or influence treatment recommendations. Individuals have the right to be informed of the nature of information that may be disclosed for the purposes of paying benefits.

Appeals and Grievances

Individuals have the right to receive information about the methods they can use to submit complaints or grievances regarding provision of care by the treating professional to that profession's regulatory board and to the professional association.

Individuals have the right to be provided information about the procedures they can use to appeal benefit utilization decisions to the third party payer systems, to the employer or purchasing entity, and to external regulatory entities.

Confidentiality

Individuals have the right to be guaranteed the protection of the confidentiality of their relationship with their mental health and substance abuse professional, except when laws or ethics dictate otherwise. Any disclosure to another party will be time limited and made with the full written, informed consent of the individuals. Individuals shall not be required to disclose confidential, privileged or other information other than: diagnosis, prognosis, type of treatment, time and length of treatment, and cost.

Entities receiving information for the purposes of benefits determination, public agencies receiving information for health care planning, or any other organization with legitimate right to information will maintain clinical information in confidence with the same rigor and be subject to the same penalties for violation as is the direct provider of care.

Information technology will be used for transmission, storage, or data management only with methodologies that remove individual identifying information and assure the protection of the individual's privacy. Information should not be transferred, sold or otherwise utilized.

TABLE 3.1. *(continued)*

Choice

Individuals have the right to choose any duly licensed/certified professional for mental health and substance abuse services. Individuals have the right to receive full information regarding the education and training of professionals, treatment options (including risks and benefits), and cost implications to make an informed choice regarding the selection of care deemed appropriate by individual and professional.

Determination of Treatment

Recommendations regarding mental health and substance abuse treatment shall be made only by a duly licensed/certified professional in conjunction with the individual and his or her family as appropriate. Treatment decisions should not be made by third party payers. The individual has the right to make final decisions regarding treatment.

Parity

Individuals have the right to receive benefits for mental health and substance abuse treatment on the same basis as they do for any other illnesses, with the same provisions, co-payments, lifetime benefits, and catastrophic coverage in both insurance and self-funded/self-insured health plans.

Discrimination

Individuals who use mental health and substance abuse benefits shall not be penalized when seeking other health insurance or disability, life or any other insurance benefit.

Benefit Usage

The individual is entitled to the entire scope of the benefits within the benefit plan that will address his or her clinical needs.

Benefit Design

Whenever both federal and state law and/or regulations are applicable, the professional and all payers shall use whichever affords the individual the greatest level of protection and access.

Treatment Review

To assure that treatment review processes are fair and valid, individuals have the right to be guaranteed that any review of their mental health and substance abuse treatment shall involve a professional having the training, credentials and licensure required to provide the treatment in the jurisdiction in which it will be provided. The reviewer should have no financial interest in the decision and is subject to the section on confidentiality.

Accountability

Treating professionals may be held accountable and liable to individuals for any injury caused by gross incompetence or negligence on the part of the professional. The treating professional has the obligation to advocate for and document necessity of care and to advise the individual of options if payment authorization is denied.

Payers and other third parties may be held accountable and liable to individuals for any injury caused by gross incompetence or negligence or by their clinically unjustified decisions.

(continued)

TABLE 3.1. *(continued)*

Approving Organizations
American Association for Marriage and Family Therapy (membership: 25,000) Anthony Jurich, Ph.D., President
American Counseling Association (membership: 56,000) Gail Robinson, Ph.D., President
American Family Therapy Academy (membership 1,000) Evan Imber-Black, Ph.D., President
American Nurses Association (membership: 180,000) Beverly L. Malone, Ph.D., RN, President
American Psychological Association (membership: 142,000) Dorothy W. Cantor, PsyD, President
American Psychiatric Association (membership: 42,000) Harold I. Eist, M.D., President; American Psychiatric Nurses Association (membership: 3,000) Nancy M. Valentine, President
National Association of Social Workers (membership: 155,000) Jay J. Cayner, ACSW, LCSW, President
National Federation of Societies for Clinical Social Work (membership: 11,000) Elizabeth Phillips, Ph.D., President
Supporting Organizations
National Mental Health Association
National Depressive and Manic–Depressive Association
American Group Psychotherapy Association
American Psychoanalytic Association
National Association of Drug and Alcohol Abuse Counselors

Note. Retrieved October 26, 2010, from *www.oregoncounseling.org/LawsRights/PatientRights.htm#The%20Right%20to%20Quality%20Mental%20Health%20Care.*

professional organizations are calling for the inclusion of courses addressing theory, research, assessment, and treatment of traumatic stress disorders in professional curricula across all major medical and mental health professions, as well as in allied professions (Courtois, 2003; Courtois & Gold, 2009). At least five professional organizations—the American Psychological Association, Division 56; the International Society for the Study of Trauma and Dissociation (ISSTD); the International Society for Traumatic Stress Studies (ISTSS); the National Child Traumatic Stress Network (NCTSN); and the National Association of Social Workers (NASW)—have developed lists of professional competencies that are required to treat traumatized individuals and have work groups whose members (including both authors) are currently tasked with the development of guidelines for the assessment and treatment of complex traumatic stress disorders.

TABLE 3.2. The Layperson's Guide to Counselor Ethics: What You Should Know about the Ethical Practice of Professional Counselors

Approved by the ACA Governing Council, October 1999
Logistics update, May 2009

As clients make decisions concerning the professional counselor from whom they will seek services, they should realize that there are standard practices and procedures that they can expect. Many of these practices and procedures are driven by the code of ethics that your professional counselor is bound to follow, the American Counseling Association's (ACA's) 2005 Code of Ethics. This document offers some highlights specifically relevant to you as consumer. You have the right to ask your professional counselor for a complete copy of the ACA 2005 Code of Ethics. The following will highlight some of these practices and procedures that you should expect from your professional counselor.

What to Expect

- Your professional counselor will describe her or his qualifications and areas of expertise.
- Your professional counselor will treat you with respect and dignity, especially in regard to age, color, culture, disability, ethnic group, gender, race, religion, sexual orientation, marital status, or socioeconomic status.
- Your professional counselor will inform you of the purposes, goals, techniques, procedures, limitations, potential risks, and benefits of all counseling services that you will receive. You may request this information in writing.
- Your professional counselor will inform you of and give you the opportunity to discuss matters of confidentiality, privacy, and disclosure of information. She or he will also inform you of the limitations to confidentiality.
- Your professional counselor will inform you of all financial arrangements related to service prior to entering the counseling relationship. You may request this information in writing.
- Your professional counselor will, when necessary, assist in making appropriate alternative service arrangements. Such arrangements may be necessary following termination, at follow-up, and for referral.
- When questions or concerns arise regarding services requested or services received, please discuss them immediately with your professional counselor. If such questions cannot be answered or a resolution reached, please call or contact ACA for advice and/or counsel at 1-800-347-6647, X314, or at ethics@counseling.org.

Note. Retrieved October 26, 2010, from *www.counseling.org/Resources/CodeOfEthics/TP/Home/CT2.aspx.*

Therapist Emotional Health and Self-Regulation

In addition, every therapist must develop enough personal maturity, clinical wisdom, and capacity for good judgment to effectively and safely conduct psychotherapy, an imperative that is especially important in the treatment of this population. The emotion dysregulation and insecure and disorganized attachment of complex trauma clients elicit strong emotional reactions from others, even those in their support network, including therapists. Reactions can range from sympathy, sorrow, fear, and guilt to frustration, impatience, anger/rage, hostility, and disgust or contempt. Related actions

TABLE 3.3. Excerpts from the American Association for Marriage and Family Therapy Code of Ethics

Principle I
Responsibility to Clients

Marriage and family therapists advance the welfare of families and individuals. They respect the rights of those persons seeking their assistance, and make reasonable efforts to ensure that their services are used appropriately.

1.1. Marriage and family therapists provide professional assistance to persons without discrimination on the basis of race, age, ethnicity, socioeconomic status, disability, gender, health status, religion, national origin, or sexual orientation.

1.2 Marriage and family therapists obtain appropriate informed consent to therapy or related procedures as early as feasible in the therapeutic relationship, and use language that is reasonably understandable to clients. The content of informed consent may vary depending upon the client and treatment plan; however, informed consent generally necessitates that the client: (a) has the capacity to consent; (b) has been adequately informed of significant information concerning treatment processes and procedures; (c) has been adequately informed of potential risks and benefits of treatments for which generally recognized standards do not yet exist; (d) has freely and without undue influence expressed consent; and (e) has provided consent that is appropriately documented. When persons, due to age or mental status, are legally incapable of giving informed consent, marriage and family therapists obtain informed permission from a legally authorized person, if such substitute consent is legally permissible.

1.3 Marriage and family therapists are aware of their influential positions with respect to clients, and they avoid exploiting the trust and dependency of such persons. Therapists, therefore, make every effort to avoid conditions and multiple relationships with clients that could impair professional judgment or increase the risk of exploitation. Such relationships include, but are not limited to, business or close personal relationships with a client or the client's immediate family. When the risk of impairment or exploitation exists due to conditions or multiple roles, therapists take appropriate precautions.

1.4 Sexual intimacy with clients is prohibited.

1.5 Sexual intimacy with former clients is likely to be harmful and is therefore prohibited for two years following the termination of therapy or last professional contact. In an effort to avoid exploiting the trust and dependency of clients, marriage and family therapists should not engage in sexual intimacy with former clients after the two years following termination or last professional contact. Should therapists engage in sexual intimacy with former clients following two years after termination or last professional contact, the burden shifts to the therapist to demonstrate that there has been no exploitation or injury to the former client or to the client's immediate family.

1.6 Marriage and family therapists comply with applicable laws regarding the reporting of alleged unethical conduct.

1.7 Marriage and family therapists do not use their professional relationships with clients to further their own interests.

1.8 Marriage and family therapists respect the rights of clients to make decisions and help them to understand the consequences of these decisions. Therapists clearly advise the clients that they have the responsibility to make decisions regarding relationships such as cohabitation, marriage, divorce, separation, reconciliation, custody, and visitation.

TABLE 3.3. *(continued)*

1.9 Marriage and family therapists continue therapeutic relationships only so long as it is reasonably clear that clients are benefiting from the relationship.

1.10 Marriage and family therapists assist persons in obtaining other therapeutic services if the therapist is unable or unwilling, for appropriate reasons, to provide professional help.

1.11 Marriage and family therapists do not abandon or neglect clients in treatment without making reasonable arrangements for the continuation of such treatment.

1.12 Marriage and family therapists obtain written informed consent from clients before videotaping, audio recording, or permitting third-party observation.

1.13 Marriage and family therapists, upon agreeing to provide services to a person or entity at the request of a third party, clarify, to the extent feasible and at the outset of the service, the nature of the relationship with each party and the limits of confidentiality.

Principle II
Confidentiality

Marriage and family therapists have unique confidentiality concerns because the client in a therapeutic relationship may be more than one person. Therapists respect and guard the confidences of each individual client.

2.1 Marriage and family therapists disclose to clients and other interested parties, as early as feasible in their professional contacts, the nature of confidentiality and possible limitations of the clients' right to confidentiality. Therapists review with clients the circumstances where confidential information may be requested and where disclosure of confidential information may be legally required. Circumstances may necessitate repeated disclosures.

2.2 Marriage and family therapists do not disclose client confidences except by written authorization or waiver, or where mandated or permitted by law. Verbal authorization will not be sufficient except in emergency situations, unless prohibited by law. When providing couple, family or group treatment, the therapist does not disclose information outside the treatment context without a written authorization from each individual competent to execute a waiver. In the context of couple, family or group treatment, the therapist may not reveal any individual's confidences to others in the client unit without the prior written permission of that individual.

2.3 Marriage and family therapists use client and/or clinical materials in teaching, writing, consulting, research, and public presentations only if a written waiver has been obtained in accordance with Sub-principle 2.2, or when appropriate steps have been taken to protect client identity and confidentiality.

2.4 Marriage and family therapists store, safeguard, and dispose of client records in ways that maintain confidentiality and in accord with applicable laws and professional standards.

2.5 Subsequent to the therapist moving from the area, closing the practice, or upon the death of the therapist, a marriage and family therapist arranges for the storage, transfer, or disposal of client records in ways that maintain confidentiality and safeguard the welfare of clients.

2.6 Marriage and family therapists, when consulting with colleagues or referral sources, do not share confidential information that could reasonably lead to the identification of a client, research participant, supervisee, or other person with whom they have a confidential relationship unless they have obtained the prior written

(continued)

TABLE 3.3. (*continued*)

consent of the client, research participant, supervisee, or other person with whom they have a confidential relationship. Information may be shared only to the extent necessary to achieve the purposes of the consultation.

Principle III
Professional Competence and Integrity

Marriage and family therapists maintain high standards of professional competence and integrity.

3.1 Marriage and family therapists pursue knowledge of new developments and maintain competence in marriage and family therapy through education, training, or supervised experience.

3.2 Marriage and family therapists maintain adequate knowledge of and adhere to applicable laws, ethics, and professional standards.

3.3 Marriage and family therapists seek appropriate professional assistance for their personal problems or conflicts that may impair work performance or clinical judgment.

3.4 Marriage and family therapists do not provide services that create a conflict of interest that may impair work performance or clinical judgment.

3.5 Marriage and family therapists, as presenters, teachers, supervisors, consultants and researchers, are dedicated to high standards of scholarship, present accurate information, and disclose potential conflicts of interest.

3.6 Marriage and family therapists maintain accurate and adequate clinical and financial records.

3.7 While developing new skills in specialty areas, marriage and family therapists take steps to ensure the competence of their work and to protect clients from possible harm. Marriage and family therapists practice in specialty areas new to them only after appropriate education, training, or supervised experience.

3.8 Marriage and family therapists do not engage in sexual or other forms of harassment of clients, students, trainees, supervisees, employees, colleagues, or research subjects.

3.9 Marriage and family therapists do not engage in the exploitation of clients, students, trainees, supervisees, employees, colleagues, or research subjects.

3.10 Marriage and family therapists do not give to or receive from clients (a) gifts of substantial value or (b) gifts that impair the integrity or efficacy of the therapeutic relationship.

3.11 Marriage and family therapists do not diagnose, treat, or advise on problems outside the recognized boundaries of their competencies.

3.12 Marriage and family therapists make efforts to prevent the distortion or misuse of their clinical and research findings.

3.13 Marriage and family therapists, because of their ability to influence and alter the lives of others, exercise special care when making public their professional recommendations and opinions through testimony or other public statements.

3.14 To avoid a conflict of interests, marriage and family therapists who treat minors or adults involved in custody or visitation actions may not also perform forensic evaluations for custody, residence, or visitation of the minor. The marriage and family therapist who treats the minor may provide the court or mental health professional performing the evaluation with information about the minor from the marriage and family therapist's perspective as a treating marriage and family therapist, so long as the marriage and family therapist does not violate confidentiality.

TABLE 3.3. *(continued)*

3.15 Marriage and family therapists are in violation of this Code and subject to termination of membership or other appropriate action if they: (a) are convicted of any felony; (b) are convicted of a misdemeanor related to their qualifications or functions; (c) engage in conduct which could lead to conviction of a felony, or a misdemeanor related to their qualifications or functions; (d) are expelled from or disciplined by other professional organizations; (e) have their licenses or certificates suspended or revoked or are otherwise disciplined by regulatory bodies; (f) continue to practice marriage and family therapy while no longer competent to do so because they are impaired by physical or mental causes or the abuse of alcohol or other substances; or (g) fail to cooperate with the Association at any point from the inception of an ethical complaint through the completion of all proceedings regarding that complaint.

Principle VII
Financial Arrangements

Marriage and family therapists make financial arrangements with clients, third-party payors, and supervisees that are reasonably understandable and conform to accepted professional practices.

7.1 Marriage and family therapists do not offer or accept kickbacks, rebates, bonuses, or other remuneration for referrals; fee-for-service arrangements are not prohibited.

7.2 Prior to entering into the therapeutic or supervisory relationship, marriage and family therapists clearly disclose and explain to clients and supervisees: (a) all financial arrangements and fees related to professional services, including charges for canceled or missed appointments; (b) the use of collection agencies or legal measures for nonpayment; and (c) the procedure for obtaining payment from the client, to the extent allowed by law, if payment is denied by the third-party payor. Once services have begun, therapists provide reasonable notice of any changes in fees or other charges.

7.3 Marriage and family therapists give reasonable notice to clients with unpaid balances of their intent to seek collection by agency or legal recourse. When such action is taken, therapists will not disclose clinical information.

7.4 Marriage and family therapists represent facts truthfully to clients, third-party payors, and supervisees regarding services rendered.

7.5 Marriage and family therapists ordinarily refrain from accepting goods and services from clients in return for services rendered. Bartering for professional services may be conducted only if: (a) the supervisee or client requests it, (b) the relationship is not exploitative, (c) the professional relationship is not distorted, and (d) a clear written contract is established.

7.6 Marriage and family therapists may not withhold records under their immediate control that are requested and needed for a client's treatment solely because payment has not been received for past services, except as otherwise provided by law.

Principle VIII
Advertising

Marriage and family therapists engage in appropriate informational activities, including those that enable the public, referral sources, or others to choose professional services on an informed basis.

8.1 Marriage and family therapists accurately represent their competencies, education, training, and experience relevant to their practice of marriage and family therapy.

(continued)

TABLE 3.3. (*continued*)

8.2 Marriage and family therapists ensure that advertisements and publications in any media (such as directories, announcements, business cards, newspapers, radio, television, Internet, and facsimiles) convey information that is necessary for the public to make an appropriate selection of professional services. Information could include: (a) office information, such as name, address, telephone number, credit card acceptability, fees, languages spoken, and office hours; (b) qualifying clinical degree (see sub-principle 8.5); (c) other earned degrees (see sub-principle 8.5) and state or provincial licensures and/or certifications; (d) AAMFT clinical member status; and (e) description of practice.

8.3 Marriage and family therapists do not use names that could mislead the public concerning the identity, responsibility, source, and status of those practicing under that name, and do not hold themselves out as being partners or associates of a firm if they are not.

8.4 Marriage and family therapists do not use any professional identification (such as a business card, office sign, letterhead, Internet, or telephone or association directory listing) if it includes a statement or claim that is false, fraudulent, misleading, or deceptive.

8.5 In representing their educational qualifications, marriage and family therapists list and claim as evidence only those earned degrees: (a) from institutions accredited by regional accreditation sources recognized by the United States Department of Education, (b) from institutions recognized by states or provinces that license or certify marriage and family therapists, or (c) from equivalent foreign institutions.

8.6 Marriage and family therapists correct, wherever possible, false, misleading, or inaccurate information and representations made by others concerning the therapist's qualifications, services, or products.

8.7 Marriage and family therapists make certain that the qualifications of their employees or supervisees are represented in a manner that is not false, misleading, or deceptive.

8.8 Marriage and family therapists do not represent themselves as providing specialized services unless they have the appropriate education, training, or supervised experience.

Note. Retrieved October 26, 2010, from *www.aamft.org/resources/lrm_plan/ethics/ethicscode2001.asp*.

can range from overinvolvement on the one hand to withdrawal and abandonment on the other. As well, therapists are not immune to "secondary" or "vicarious" traumatization or countertransference reactions. Indeed, therapists may be particularly affected because of their commitment not to just be tolerant and offer generic moral support (e.g., the Hippocratic oath to "first do no harm") but to be emotionally engaged, responsive, and attuned to the client. Although empathy and attunement do *not* equate with becoming emotionally distraught and overinvolved, therapists with even the best instincts, training, and consultation often find themselves emotionally flooded or drained (or both) when meeting regularly with a client (or more than one) who has had major experiences of trauma, especially those that are interpersonal, premeditated, and deliberately cruel or demeaning (Wilson & Lindy, 1994).

In order to fulfill the professional commitment to provide "*quality* mental health and substance abuse services to *all* individuals without regard to race, color, religion, national origin, gender, age, sexual orientation, or *disabilities*" (italics added; see Table 3.1), "therapist's expertise in emotional self-regulation (Ford, 2012), emotional health, and mature judgment are just as important as technical and clinical expertise (Pope & Keith-Spiegel, 2008). The importance of therapist self-care to the provision of competent psychotherapy has been increasingly recognized in recent years. A variety of continuing education seminars and courses are now available that address self-care issues and provide guidance to the novice or experienced therapist (see Resources for Therapist Self-Care in the online supplement to this book). In addition, therapists must be well informed about the ethical standards, principles, and guidelines of their professional discipline (e.g., see Tables 3.4 and 3.5).

The three key words italicized in the preceding paragraph—*quality, all, disabilities*—are directly related to therapist self-care because an impaired or destabilized therapist cannot provide services without gaps in quality. Therapists who are preoccupied with personal stresses may be highly skilled, knowledgeable, and caring, but cannot bring their full therapeutic abilities to bear without inevitable skips in attention, empathy, or technical precision. No therapist is free from competing personal and professional agendas (some of which may involve life transitions or life crises and may be of sudden onset), but therapeutic quality suffers when personal concerns that result in physical or emotional exhaustion, stress or worry, or irritation or frustration occupy the foreground rather than the background of the therapist's attention and emotional and cognitive focus. Under those conditions, it is natural for anyone, even experienced and well-trained therapists, to either avoid or to be overly drawn to clients whose personal characteristics or symptoms are "triggers" for their own personal issues. The problem for the therapist, which unfortunately can transfer to and become an even bigger problem for the client, is of being so caught up in unfinished personal business that the therapy is essentially overtaken and compromised.

So, although no therapist is immune to personal stresses and issues, and to countertransference reactions, the heart of therapist self-care is developing and following through on a personal commitment to emotional health and *emotion self-regulation*, starting with balance between professional and personal life domains. Based on the complex trauma perspective—but switching the perspective from one of trauma to the dialectical opposite of healthy personal growth and development—emotion self-regulation involves reliable access to (and accessing of) relationships that are grounded in secure mutual emotional attachment. In order to provide, as well as receive, attachment security, the therapist must be able to recognize, contain the intensity of, and recover from distressing emotion states. It is for this reason that self-care involves the therapist developing a personal life that includes engagement in emotionally restorative and

TABLE 3.4. Excerpts from the American Psychological Association Ethical Principles of Psychologists and Code of Conduct: 2010 Amendments

General Principles

This section consists of General Principles. General Principles, as opposed to Ethical Standards, are aspirational in nature. Their intent is to guide and inspire psychologists toward the very highest ethical ideals of the profession.

Principle A: Beneficence and Non-maleficence

Psychologists strive to benefit those with whom they work and take care to do no harm. In their professional actions, psychologists seek to safeguard the welfare and rights of those with whom they interact professionally and other affected persons, and the welfare of animal subjects of research. When conflicts occur among psychologists' obligations or concerns, they attempt to resolve these conflicts in a responsible fashion that avoids or minimizes harm. Because psychologists' scientific and professional judgments and actions may affect the lives of others, they are alert to and guard against personal, financial, social, organizational, or political factors that might lead to misuse of their influence. Psychologists strive to be aware of the possible effect of their own physical and mental health on their ability to help those with whom they work.

Principle B: Fidelity and Responsibility

Psychologists establish relationships of trust with those with whom they work. They are aware of their professional and scientific responsibilities to society and to the specific communities in which they work. Psychologists uphold professional standards of conduct, clarify their professional roles and obligations, accept appropriate responsibility for their behavior, and seek to manage conflicts of interest that could lead to exploitation or harm. Psychologists consult with, refer to, or cooperate with other professionals and institutions to the extent needed to serve the best interests of those with whom they work. They are concerned about the ethical compliance of their colleagues' scientific and professional conduct. Psychologists strive to contribute a portion of their professional time for little or no compensation or personal advantage.

Principle C: Integrity

Psychologists seek to promote accuracy, honesty, and truthfulness in the science, teaching, and practice of psychology. In these activities psychologists do not steal, cheat, or engage in fraud, subterfuge, or intentional misrepresentation of fact. Psychologists strive to keep their promises and to avoid unwise or unclear commitments. In situations in which deception may be ethically justifiable to maximize benefits and minimize harm, psychologists have a serious obligation to consider the need for, the possible consequences of, and their responsibility to correct any resulting mistrust or other harmful effects that arise from the use of such techniques.

Principle D: Justice

Psychologists recognize that fairness and justice entitle all persons to access to and benefit from the contributions of psychology and to equal quality in the processes, procedures, and services being conducted by psychologists. Psychologists exercise reasonable judgment and take precautions to ensure that their potential biases, the boundaries of their competence, and the limitations of their expertise do not lead to or condone unjust practices.

(*continued*)

TABLE 3.4. *(continued)*

Principle E: Respect for People's Rights and Dignity
Psychologists respect the dignity and worth of all people, and the rights of individuals to privacy, confidentiality, and self-determination. Psychologists are aware that special safeguards may be necessary to protect the rights and welfare of persons or communities whose vulnerabilities impair autonomous decision making. Psychologists are aware of and respect cultural, individual, and role differences, including those based on age, gender, gender identity, race, ethnicity, culture, national origin, religion, sexual orientation, disability, language, and socioeconomic status and consider these factors when working with members of such groups. Psychologists try to eliminate the effect on their work of biases based on those factors, and they do not knowingly participate in or condone activities of others based upon such prejudices.

Note. Retrieved October 26, 2010, from *www.apa.org/ethics/code/index.aspx?item=3*.

rejuvenating relationships and a professional life that also involves supportive connections with others. Relationships provide for physical and emotional nurturance—including intimacy, sustained friendship and family ties, recreation, socializing, and civic participation. The key to effective involvement in the provision of responsive therapeutic practice is that these activities are based, in part, on the therapist's mental health and emotional self-regulation. (More on this topic in Chapters 9 and 10.)

Consistent with an emotion self-regulation perspective, therapists do well to carefully prepare their clients with emotion regulation skills before they assist them in recalling past traumatic experiences. Such preparation involves helping clients enhance or more reliably access skills and resources (particularly secure and timely contact with key people in their support system) to maintain or regain emotional balance and hope even when confronted with feelings of severe distress and related cognitions and behaviors (e.g., dissociation or impulses to self-harm; see Chapters 8 and 9).

Therapists, no matter how well prepared they are technically, are likely to have a full range of emotional reactions when hearing what a client has experienced. Even when the details of a client's trauma history are not known or only partly disclosed, the client's suffering is almost always palpable—although sometimes not immediately (as in the case of Doris's initial session, in which she appeared to be only mildly distressed and high functioning) and at other times only indirectly (as in the case of Hector's intense disavowal of emotional needs or distress) or by inference (as was the case with both Doris and Hector when they felt emotionally numb and empty, including episodes of severe dissociative detachment).

It is worth noting that thinly veiled or disavowed emotional distress and a detached/dismissive relational style can be at least as evocative as the most intense forms of direct emoting—and at times even more so, because the undercurrent of wordless terror, rage, grief, self-loathing, shame, or guilt that is expressed nonverbally is much harder to understand than verbal expressions. In addition, the silent client may be experienced as

TABLE 3.5. Excerpts from the Code of Ethics of the National Association of Social Workers

Approved by the 1996 NASW Delegate Assembly
and revised by the 2008 NASW Delegate Assembly

Social workers promote social justice and social change with and on behalf of clients. "Clients" is used inclusively to refer to individuals, families, groups, organizations, and communities. Social workers are sensitive to cultural and ethnic diversity and strive to end discrimination, oppression, poverty, and other forms of social injustice. These activities may be in the form of direct practice, community organizing, supervision, consultation administration, advocacy, social and political action, policy development and implementation, education, and research and evaluation. Social workers seek to enhance the capacity of people to address their own needs. Social workers also seek to promote the responsiveness of organizations, communities, and other social institutions to individuals' needs and social problems.

The mission of the social work profession is rooted in a set of core values. These core values, embraced by social workers throughout the profession's history, are the foundation of social work's unique purpose and perspective.

The following broad ethical principles are based on social work's core values of service, social justice, dignity and worth of the person, importance of human relationships, integrity, and competence. These principles set forth ideals to which all social workers should aspire.

Value: *Service*

Ethical Principle: *Social workers' primary goal is to help people in need and to address social problems.*

Social workers elevate service to others above self-interest. Social workers draw on their knowledge, values, and skills to help people in need and to address social problems. Social workers are encouraged to volunteer some portion of their professional skills with no expectation of significant financial return (pro bono service).

Value: *Social Justice*

Ethical Principle: *Social workers challenge social injustice.*

Social workers pursue social change, particularly with and on behalf of vulnerable and oppressed individuals and groups of people. Social workers' social change efforts are focused primarily on issues of poverty, unemployment, discrimination, and other forms of social injustice. These activities seek to promote sensitivity to and knowledge about oppression and cultural and ethnic diversity. Social workers strive to ensure access to needed information, services, and resources; equality of opportunity; and meaningful participation in decision making for all people.

Value: *Dignity and Worth of the Person*

Ethical Principle: *Social workers respect the inherent dignity and worth of the person.*

Social workers treat each person in a caring and respectful fashion, mindful of individual differences and cultural and ethnic diversity. Social workers promote clients' socially responsible self-determination. Social workers seek to enhance clients' capacity and opportunity to change and to address their own needs. Social workers are cognizant of their dual responsibility to clients and to the broader society. They seek to resolve conflicts between clients' interests and the broader society's interests in a socially responsible manner consistent with the values, ethical principles, and ethical standards of the profession.

(continued)

TABLE 3.5. *(continued)*

Value: *Importance of Human Relationships*

Ethical Principle: *Social workers recognize the central importance of human relationships.*

Social workers understand that relationships between and among people are an important vehicle for change. Social workers engage people as partners in the helping process. Social workers seek to strengthen relationships among people in a purposeful effort to promote, restore, maintain, and enhance the wellbeing of individuals, families, social groups, organizations, and communities.

Value: *Integrity*

Ethical Principle: *Social workers behave in a trustworthy manner.*

Social workers are continually aware of the profession's mission, values, ethical principles, and ethical standards and practice in a manner consistent with them. Social workers act honestly and responsibly and promote ethical practices on the part of the organizations with which they are affiliated.

Value: *Competence*

Ethical Principle: *Social workers practice within their areas of competence and develop and enhance their professional expertise.*

Social workers continually strive to increase their professional knowledge and skills and to apply them in practice. Social workers should aspire to contribute to the knowledge base of the profession.

Note Retrieved October 26, 2010, from *www.naswdc.org/pubs/code/code.asp.*

withholding, oppositional, and sulking or as holding the therapist "hostage" in ways that elicit resentment and other negative responses. Because it is not unusual that relational and other forms of traumatization began when the client was preverbal, he or she may not have words. The lack of access to emotions or to words to describe them is known as *alexithymia* and is a common response to trauma. What the client is likely to have instead is somatosensory, behavioral, dissociative, and relational manifestations that therapists must seek to understand and translate into words, a process that involves hard work and intense focus.

In this way, this psychotherapy can be understood as a process of translating wordless (implicit, somatosensory, unconscious, or dissociated) affective distress and states into the more bounded and manageable form of words and conscious thoughts, a function of the left brain. The treatment of complex developmental trauma requires a therapist who has the ability to stay emotionally present and available while simultaneously being able to process her or his own internal emotional reactions without allowing them to discharge unfiltered onto the client (Pearlman & Courtois, 2005). The current treatment may be further compounded if the client has a long-standing history of marginally effective or ineffective treatment. Therapists must have sufficient emotional maturity and compassion to deal with the painful material and the relational difficulties that attend these clients.

Therapists who have not had training to anticipate these issues may have great difficulty managing transference, countertransference, enactments and reenactments, and their own vicarious trauma reactions, leading them to make therapeutic errors they might not make otherwise (Pearlman & Caringi, 2009). Furthermore, it is not unusual for the ill-equipped or inadequately trained or immature therapist to become overly personally involved or invested or to do too much for the client (a process labeled "vicarious indulgence" by Turkus [personal communication, 2008]). Behaviors such as these frequently backfire and, if untended or unmanaged, can lead therapists to become resentful, frustrated, disappointed, discouraged, and angry with the client or to continue to overgratify and merge with the client in other ways that unfortunately lead to retraumatization rather than to resolution of issues from the past. Such a response is often at root of crossed boundaries, including sexual transgressions.

Another classic dictum, "physician, heal thyself," is also implicated in the therapist's mental health and emotional regulation. In this case, the "healing" is not necessarily a completed course of personal therapy, although many therapists find this to be professionally as well as personally useful. Personal therapy provides a first-person experience "on the receiving end" to work on personal issues that can also heighten the ability to empathize. Of course, it is essential not to overgeneralize issues and reactions from the therapist's personal therapy to that of any client; however, it can provide the lived (rather than merely textbook, or vicariously observed) experience of facing, struggling with, and coming to terms with (however imperfectly) emotions that—even for the highest functioning or most enlightened therapist—can be confusing, complicated, unruly, and unpleasant. In this way, personal therapy can be a way of directly experiencing the challenge of learning how to emotionally self-regulate; that is, how to be aware of and proactively deal with and recover from (rather than avoid or defer) one's own troubling unfinished emotional business.

Personal therapy is not the only way for therapists to enhance or elaborate their emotional self-regulation skills. At present, numerous training resources covering a wide variety of topics are available. Web-based training programs and supervision that have increased exponentially in recent years are broadening the range of options. Therapeutic training and supervision or consultation based on an emotion-regulation approach to psychotherapy (see e.g., Ford, 2012; Fisher & Ogden, 2009; Ogden & Fisher, 2013; Fosha, Paivio, Gleiser, & Ford, 2009; Johnson, 2002; Paivio & Pascual-Leone, 2010) can provide the opportunity not only to learn but also to get feedback and guidance while putting into practice emotion regulation strategies with clients.

Therapist Wisdom and Judgment

Therapists treating complex trauma clients are frequently required to make decisions and judgment calls not needed when working with other populations. They will find themselves questioning when they should hold firm to boundaries and when to take a more problem-solving and flexible approach. As with other issues, there is no one right answer and no "one size fits all." Therapists gain maturity and skill over time and with ongoing or episodic supervision and consultation recommended as a support system for exploration and perspective. Wisdom is not something that is necessarily taught but instead develops from experience and from having to deal repeatedly with different variations of similar situations. A recent survey of therapists identified as being wise by their peers (Levitt, 2011) identified a common theme among these therapists: striving to achieve empathy by pushing themselves to understand their clients' experiences and frames of reference. Drawing on research on the psychobiology of wisdom (Meeks & Jeste, 2009), Ford (2012) suggests that psychotherapeutic wisdom results from a dual commitment to (1) enable the client to empathically observe and understand his or her own mental processes ("mentalization"; Allen, Fonagy, & Bateman, 2008) and (2) use the same framework and skills to regulate their own affect. Thus therapeutic wisdom includes characteristics such as curiosity, determination, respect, humility, and integrity—truly "walking the walk" (i.e., taking responsibility for one's own affect regulation and active engagement and pushing to understand the client's experience, both past and present) rather than simply "talking the talk" (i.e., preaching, lecturing, or cheerleading from the sidelines while the client does all the work).

Informed (and Empowered) Consent and Refusal

Clients have the right to know what will be required of them and provided to them in therapy—including fees for treatment and whether and how they will be able to utilize their insurance or other health care benefits (see the Right to Know Benefits, Contractual Limitations, Appeals and Grievances, Parity, Discrimination, Benefit Usage, and Benefit Design sections of Table 3.1). They also should be informed about the choices they have for treatment and treatment providers and the rights they and their supporters have in determining treatment choices (see Table 3.1, sections on Choice, Determination of Treatment, and Treatment Review). At the start of treatment and throughout its course, clients and therapists engage in collaborative treatment planning, with clients being advised about the approaches and strategies used, the parameters of the treatment relationship, and how they can bring any concerns about therapy to the attention of the therapist or to external sources of help. For example, Table 3.2 provides a sample informational handout created by the American Counseling Association to explain to new clients what they can expect from the therapist and from the professional relationship.

Information about clients' rights and what they can expect helps to make therapy more "transparent" and assists clients in giving a truly informed consent or refusal to various aspects of the treatment to make it a collaborative endeavor. This offsets the fear, belief, or expectation of "being done to" by an authority figure and having to defer to or comply with his or her requirements. Clients have the right to accept or refuse aspects of the treatment, to question its course or its effectiveness, to seek outside consultation, and to end treatment without penalty (although with responsibility to pay any outstanding balance). They should also be advised quite specifically about confidentiality and how, as well as when and to whom, private information may be released. Many therapists create a contract regarding the terms of treatment and rights and responsibilities of both parties that client and therapist sign, a strategy recommended by all professional mental health organizations, many of which have developed templates for such contracts based on their ethical principles (see Figure 7.1), that gives clients this information, along with the basic ground rules of the treatment relationship, including financial and business elements. In addition, specialized informed consent forms are advisable in the event that any out-of-the ordinary or experimental treatment procedure is proposed, giving clients the right to knowledgeably accept or refuse it.

As part of the contract, therapists are advised to explain treatment parameters, including how it is organized (e.g., frequency and length of meetings, duration, special requirements) and therapist responsibilities, roles, boundaries, availability, and limitations, for example, how he or she will communicate with the client outside of treatment sessions, when and how the therapist is available between sessions and during a crisis, times of unavailability, boundaries and limitations on availability, vacations and other absences, backup coverage by other professionals during absences, whether e-mails or other means will be used to communicate (now ever changing due to developments in electronic and social media, new means of communication, and telehealth options and strategies). This document lays out the "rules of the road" and is what the therapist returns to when and if problems or miscommunication arise.

Clients should also be advised that, although personal empowerment and collaboration are encouraged and informed consent or refusal is in effect, the therapist has rights and responsibilities as well. Therapy is not laissez-faire, and the client does not run the therapy; the therapist maintains the responsibility for its course and strategy and for the client's welfare (and, by extension, the general welfare of others in relationship with the client; Courtois, 1999). Clients are advised about specific issues that might require the breaking of their confidentiality, such as an imminent threat of suicide or homicide, the client's report of the probable abuse of children or the legal requirements of the jurisdiction. They are further informed of behaviors that are problematic and that could cause a termination of the treatment. These might include lack of motivation or cooperation with the agreed-to treatment plan; impulsive and unplanned disclosures to and confrontations of alleged abusers or the mounting of lawsuits (or other actions) against them that are not discussed with the therapist beforehand (with the therapist maintaining the right to advise for or against such a course of action and to assist the client in weighing its pros and cons and further to determine whether the client is emotionally prepared for such an action and its possible repercussions); threatening behavior toward the therapist, including physical stalking or cyberstalking; engaging in dual therapies without letting the therapist know of a concurrent treatment; excessive lateness for sessions or absences and "no shows"; unwillingness to sign a release of information so the therapist can coordinate treatment with other providers or the retraction of a signed release during times of crisis, when it might be most needed; and other "therapy-interfering behaviors" (Linehan, 1993).

As discussed previously, although a certain amount of client resistance and mistrust is to be expected and worked with, when these issues prove to be intractable over time, the therapist may need to advise the client to "shape up" or to face the possible end of the treatment. Linehan (1993) has been explicit in her recommendation that the therapist must "reinforce the right thing," that is, to hold the line on what is acceptable and what is not and to withdraw from the treatment contract if the client is not sufficiently motivated or is in a position of constantly being at odds with the therapist and the agreed-upon goals of treatment and demarcated therapeutic boundaries. Nevertheless, this does not mean that the therapist needs to be harsh and judgmental in setting limits or can simply abandon the client; rather, he or she has the right to insist on certain standards and to be matter-of-fact in applying them.

Duration of Treatment

On average, treatment for complex traumatic stress disorders (including its co-occurring conditions and disorders) is longer term than treatment for less complicated presentations. For some clients, treatment can literally last for decades or may even be lifelong, whether provided continuously or episodically. For others, treatment duration is delimited and occurs on an episodic and as-needed basis. Some of the newer treatment models (described in following chapters), designed to be implemented in anywhere from 10 to 20 sessions, can be considered to be very short term; each developer of these modalities notes that more sessions are often required. Obviously, goals and duration of treatment should be paired to the client's ability to benefit, willingness to engage, and resources (personal and social, as well as financial/insurance, agency limitation, etc.), and the therapist should limit goals when length of time, resources, and client motivation are in short supply and when the therapist's time is delimited in some way (e.g., an intern or extern year, the therapist's pending retirement). In such cases, intervention may be directed toward education, safety, support, stabilization, limited skill building, and what has come to be known as resourcing (i.e., helping the client to develop practical and interpersonal resources to support his or her functioning).

Frequency of Sessions

Most therapy occurs on a once- or twice-a-week basis (50- to 75-minute individual sessions; 75- to 120-minute group sessions); however, when multiple modalities are needed (e.g., substance abuse treatment in addition to psychotherapy, couple and/or family work in addition to individual therapy, partial hospitalization in addition to or instead of individual therapy, an occasional inpatient stay), more sessions per week are obviously in order. The therapist should be careful to exceed this usual standard of no more than two individual sessions per week and should hold more frequent weekly sessions or contacts (1) when symptom severity or crisis level is such that it is required; (2) if mandated by his or her theoretical orientation (e.g., psychoanalysis three to four times per week); and/or (3) in the event of an ongoing emergency especially if the client is unable to gain timely admission to an inpatient or partial hospital unit. Too-frequent sessions, especially if oriented toward rescuing the client or toward trauma processing without adequate skill building and careful preparation (Chapters 5 and 6), may emotionally flood the client, causing destabilization. For others, too-frequent sessions and unlimited therapist availability between sessions may set up unrealistic expectations, while conveying that the client is not responsible for his or her own behavior or capable of recovery. This can lead to client overdependence that, over time, is exhausting and frustrating, in some cases leading to acting-out behavior (including abrupt termination and abandonment) by an angry, resentful, overextended therapist. It is for reasons such as these that therapists are advised to carefully set and maintain treatment boundaries that are reasonable and that are ultimately protective of the therapy and its continuance.

Corollary Treatment and Alternatives

A number of treatments in addition to psychotherapy might be necessary or beneficial. These should be explained to the client beforehand, either in the treatment contract or verbally. Hospitalization might be required due to clear and present danger to self or others or to inability to function. It is recommended that hospitalization occur on a voluntary basis (in collaboration with the therapist and as part of the overall treatment) rather than on an involuntary basis that involves the courts, police, and the use of physical and/or chemical restraints. Most of this therapy occurs in an outpatient setting and hospitalization might be rarely used, at times due to restrictions placed on admission by insurance companies. We have found that the treatment sequence and process, as described in the next chapters, often work against the need for hospitalization. Nevertheless, hospital admission must be maintained as an option in the event that the client deteriorates, is unable to function, or is in danger. It is advisable that the therapist never take the option of hospitalization off the table, although some clients may ask that the therapist promise never to hospitalize them, as they were previously hospitalized against their will or threatened with admission to or incarceration in a psychiatric facility. Unfortunately, some have had negative experiences with psychiatric stays, such as misunderstanding and stigmatization of their symptoms, along with substandard care involving but not limited to misdiagnosis, mistreatment, neglect, and exposure to further abuse, including sexual or physical abuse by staff members or other patients and excessive use of restraints, medications, and seclusion. The therapist can empathize with these unfortunate (and at times, unethical) situations but still should not trade off the option of an inpatient stay in the event that it is needed. It is quite helpful for the therapist to have an ongoing association with or attending privileges at a hospital and to be knowledgeable about specialized units that have a trauma-informed orientation to treatment. Sadly, only a few of these are in operation at the present time.

Similarly, medication is a recommended adjunctive treatment for the traumatized, but it may be highly adverse to some complex trauma clients, especially those whose abuse involved the use of drugs or those with addictions. Although medication is often helpful in managing severe symptoms (e.g., of PTSD, depression, anxiety, mood disorders, attention disorders, or psychotic symptoms), clients have the right to agree to or refuse their use (informed consent or refusal). Therapists should be prepared to offer alternative techniques and strategies and to discuss natural substances (such as St. John's wort for depression, melatonin for sleep) that might be more acceptable and more in keeping with the client's beliefs or preferences—or resources, when clients are unable to afford the high cost of psychotropic medications (see Self-Help Resources and Workbooks [in the online supplement to this book] with suggested strategies and exercises that may be relevant for clients with complex trauma histories). When psychotropic medications are suggested, it benefits both client and therapist to have a collaborative working relationship with the prescribing professional, optimally someone experienced in treating posttraumatic conditions as a specialty (see Friedman & Davidson, 2007, and Opler, Grennan, & Ford, 2009, for discussion of medication choices along with recommendations for area management of issues that might arise).

Alternative care approaches are ever more standard as adjuncts to psychotherapy and should be clearly described, within the limits of their evidence base, as well as the reasons why they might be helpful. For example, mindfulness or yoga practices or acupuncture or massage were rarely considered to be psychotherapy techniques, and a focus on spirituality was not seen as within the domain of psychotherapy until relatively recently. These and a wide variety of other mind–body approaches are now used routinely and add significantly to the therapist's armamentarium of approaches in treating clients with histories of complex trauma especially regarding somatic concerns and physical regulation (see Chapters 5–7).

Clients' Responsibilities

Clients have responsibilities that should be articulated in the treatment contract and the initial discussions regarding the psychotherapy. These include attending scheduled therapy sessions (or providing reasonable notice of cancellation if unable to attend), paying the therapist's or agency's fees (or arranging for third-party payment and making the copayment), respecting the privacy of other clients in the therapist's practice or agency, being honest, and engaging in therapy in good faith (e.g., not using therapy only as a way to obtain legal assistance or financial advantage or as a means of obtaining compensation or other financial gain). It is standard practice to ask the client to attend one final session should he or she decide to stop therapy. This strategy helps to ensure that the ending is without misunderstandings or erroneous communications, some of which might be harmful to the client or be a cause for him or her to later take legal, licensing, or ethics action against the therapist. It also provides for an ending and a good-bye along with the expression of associated emotions, something the client might seek to avoid by leaving abruptly and without notice. As part of the treatment contract that the client signs, it is standard for her or him to agree in general not to leave treatment impulsively or without first discussing her or his reasons for doing so in a final face-to-face session.

Client responsibilities should be stated up front, clearly, and without hesitation or coercion. If a client feels desperate to get help, the therapist should carefully evaluate and discuss whether he or she is able to freely agree to fulfill the expected responsibilities. Clients with complex trauma histories often are very unsure of their ability to tolerate disappointment and to follow through and complete what they have started, so it is reasonable to expect some ambivalence or uncertainty in this regard at the outset of treatment. What is important is that clients genuinely understand what is expected and have sufficient internal (psychological) and external (physical health, financial, transportation, child care) resources to be able to make an honest effort at achieving those expectations. As with therapists, perfection is neither expected nor required, and this is one of the hallmark "corrective emotional experiences" of successful therapy. Therapists must expect some failures on the part of clients in these practical areas while remaining calmly consistent in reinforcing the importance of good faith effort and the reasonable likelihood of success by the client. Also, anticipating and planning for potential relapses—meaning a return to old symptomatic states of mind, coping and other behavior patterns, and reengagement in dangerous relationships—is recommended because posttraumatic adaptations have been overlearned (Foa & Kozak, 1986) and therefore are likely to reoccur despite the best efforts of clients or therapists. To be able to honestly buy into, rather than simply acquiesce to, and achieve expectations that originate from another person is an invaluable opportunity for complex trauma clients to learn by experience that cooperation and shared expectations (along with support and reinforcement) can be helpful and enriching rather than critical or exploitive.

CONCLUSION

Preparing to undertake psychotherapy with a complex trauma survivor is paradoxically no different and entirely different from preparing to work with any troubled individual. The therapist's personal and professional boundaries and readiness to provide consistent, reliable, empathic, evidence-based attention and interventions is no different with these clients than with any others. However, because the extreme stressors to which complex trauma survivors have had to adapt tend to lead to correspondingly extreme states of emotion (both in intensity and shutdown), cognition (including black-and-white thinking, severe hopelessness, and distrust), physical response and distress (including unremitting pain, breakdown in bodily functions, and other symptoms), and behavior (including avoidance, defiance, rejection, and dependency), additional preparation and anticipation on the part of the therapist is recommended (Ford, 2012). The material provided in this chapter is intended, therefore, to alert clinicians to the crucial issues they face with regard to this treatment and to inform them about strategies, tools, and resources available to meet some of its singular challenges. We turn next, in Chapter 4, to a discussion of goals of treatment based on an initial comprehensive assessment. Strategies and instruments for the assessment and reassessment of complex trauma clients over the course of treatment are presented.

CHAPTER 4

Treatment Goals and Assessment

Survivors of complex trauma often experience symptoms of both PTSD and complex traumatic stress disorders, along with their associated features and co-occurring disorders (Ford & Kidd, 1998; Lanius et al., 2010). Therefore, at the outset, the therapist must assess and identify the specific symptoms that are most troubling and cause the greatest degree of personal and interpersonal impairment. We first summarize goals related to PTSD treatment and then discuss necessary goals for addressing the additional symptoms of complex traumatic stress disorders. For each goal, we provide an illustrative but not exhaustive summary of potential assessment tools in Table 4.1. Additionally, we discuss assessment issues and strategies.

GOALS FOR PTSD TREATMENT

Marmar, Foy, Kagan, and Pynoos (1994, p. 127) described the following goals for the treatment of PTSD that are representative of those proposed by other trauma treatment models. They include:

1. To increase the capacity to respond to threat with realistic appraisal rather than exaggerated or minimized/minimizing responses.
2. To maintain normal levels of arousal rather than hypervigilance or psychic numbing.
3. To facilitate the return to normal development, adaptive coping, and improved functioning in work and interpersonal relations.
4. To restore personal integrity and normalize traumatic stress response by validating the universality of stress symptomatology and by establishing a frame of meaning.
5. To conduct treatment in an atmosphere of safety and security in order to ensure that the threat of retraumatization is minimized.

6. To regulate the level of intensity of traumatic aspects to facilitate cognitive reappraisal.
7. To increase capacity to differentiate remembering from reliving of past traumas, for both external reminders and internal cues.
8. Neither to eradicate the memories of the trauma nor to avoid and overreact rigidly to reminders; rather, to place trauma in perspective and regain control over life experiences.
9. To attend to biological and social learning risk factors that shape the trauma response.
10. To intervene actively to address secondary adversities and prevent future complications, including the risk for spreading comorbidities.
11. To facilitate a transformation in self-concept from a victim to an individual with a sense of constructive engagement in daily life and future goals.
12. To enhance personal courage in approaching the memories and reminders of the traumas.

Numerous treatment models for PTSD are currently available and many can be found in the online resource list that accompanies this text.

ADDITIONAL GOALS FOR THE TREATMENT OF COMPLEX TRAUMATIC STRESS DISORDERS

As discussed in Chapters 1 and 2, clients with complex trauma histories tend to have self-, relational, developmental, and life/social skill deficits beyond those of PTSD. Additional goals that build on the twelve listed above are needed to address developmental deficits and the seven symptom categories of complex PTSD/DESNOS:

13. To face, rather than avoid, the trauma memory and its associated feelings, cognitions, beliefs and schema about self and others.
14. To experience the relational safety and attunement in the treatment relationship as a "secure base" from which to develop or regain secure inner working models.
15. To develop and/or restore emotion regulation, that is, the ability to access and identify emotions (especially core emotions and affective schemas such as shame, horror, self-loathing, exploitation, and betrayal) and increase the capacity for and tolerance of emotional expression (emotion regulation) as a means of self-development.
16. To shift self-concept from permanently damaged to resilient and recovered from injury.
17. To shift self-concept from helpless/ineffective to autonomous self-determination.

18. To acquire or regain capacities for bodily self-awareness and arousal regulation that have been split off or compartmentalized in the form of somatoform dissociation.
19. To develop or regain self-regulatory capacities to recognize and reduce the severity and frequency of dissociation, addiction, self-harm, impulsivity, compulsion, and aggression toward self and others.
20. To identify reenactments of traumatic events and develop self-protection and self-enhancement skills to prevent revictimization and retraumatization.

METAGOALS FOR PSYCHOTHERAPY WITH COMPLEX TRAUMA SURVIVORS

This listing contains so many multifaceted goals that it is difficult for most therapists to attend to all of them while simultaneously getting to know the client. In consequence, we suggest that therapists refer to the complete list of goals periodically throughout treatment, while using the following list of "metagoals" as ongoing reference points.

Challenge Avoidance through Attachment Security and Skill Development

Avoidance in the service of self-protection is a hallmark of traumatic stress disorders because it keeps the individual from reexperiencing painful memories and emotions; however, it has the simultaneous negative side effect of overgeneralizing to similar situations and of preventing the processing of traumatic memories and emotions that is necessary for resolution. The first two goals of psychotherapy with complex trauma survivors address both the core injuries that lead these individuals to overrely on a myriad of avoidance strategies—these injuries being deprivation of security in primary relationships and of the opportunity, the consistent role modeling, and the coaching to develop the ability to regulate emotions (Courtois & Ford, 2009). Whereas the fear of the repetition of traumatic events or of the negative affect states associated with trauma memories (e.g., fear, anxiety, shame) hypothesized to be at the core of PTSD (Dalgleish, 2004) is fairly straightforward, avoidance in the aftermath of complex trauma is more convoluted. It involves fear of experiencing intolerable and unmanageable internal physical and affective states of diffuse emotional distress and fear of the very people who are also the sources of emotional security. In the past, this has involved the irresolvable separation from needed relational and social support, especially when most needed. The problematic states of hypo- and hyperarousal, dissociation, alienation, deactivation of attachment, resignation, terror, horror, and loathing of self or others that characterize complex traumatic stress disorders thus can be understood as largely unconscious forms of avoidance in the face of dysregulated emotions and of attachment insecurity and disorganization. Although often driven by a healthy motivation to survive overwhelming experiences, avoidance (especially when overlearned and habitual) exacts a high price.

The resultant loss of emotional, cognitive, behavioral, and interpersonal functioning tends to overgeneralize, affecting many, if not most, domains of the individual's life. Additionally, and perhaps most importantly, pervasive avoidance prevents emotional and cognitive processing that might allow resolution of posttraumatic reactions. The reversal of avoidance and the mastery of skills required to face painful events or memories and emotions are viewed as essential to the treatment of PTSD, particularly the processing of trauma-related emotional distress, which is the focus of cognitive-behavior therapies for traumatized individuals (Foa, Keane, Friedman, & Cohen, 2009; Resick, Nishith, Wearer, Astin, & Feuer, 2002). Attachment-based therapies (Muller, 2010; Wallin, 2007), experiential and emotion-focused therapies (Fosha, Siegel, & Solomon, 2009), and somatosensory awareness-focused therapies (Ogden et al., 2006) are also important interventions for avoidant clients.

Complex trauma clients first and foremost require assistance with their attachment insecurity and emotion dysregulation in order to progressively learn to recognize and modify the ways in which they use avoidance to cope with actual or anticipated danger or distress. Attachment security and emotion regulation provide a basis for clients to identify other ways to modulate distress and develop more effective coping tactics. With this therapeutic foundation, clients can be assisted in achieving several other crucial goals.

Enhance Self-Determination and Autonomy

Attachment security and emotion regulation are important not only for therapeutic healing and recovery, but also for achieving the cornerstone goal of treatment of enhanced self-determination and autonomy. In general, autonomy refers to the client's right to freedom of action and choice without being placed in a position of dependency (on the therapist or others) or of undue external control or coercion (by the therapist or others). With regard to complex trauma survivors, self-determination and autonomy require that the therapist treat each client as the "authority" in determining the meaning and interpretation of his or her personal life history, including (but not limited to) traumatic experiences (Harvey, 1996). Therapists can inadvertently misappropriate the client's authority over the meaning and significance of her or his memories (and associated symptoms, such as intrusive reexperiencing or dissociative flashbacks) by suggesting specific "expert" interpretations of the memories or symptoms. Clients who feel profoundly abandoned by key caregivers may appear deeply grateful for such interpretations and pronouncements by their therapists, because they can fulfill a deep longing for a substitute parent who makes sense of the world or takes care of them. However, this delegation of authority to the therapist can backfire if the client cannot, or does not, take ownership of her or his own memories or life story by determining their personal meaning. Moreover, the client can be trapped in a stance of avoidance because trauma memories are never experienced, processed, and put to rest. Helping the client to develop a core sense of relational security and the capacity to regulate (and recover from) extreme hyper- or hypoarousal is essential if the client is to achieve a self-determined and autonomous approach to defining the meaning and impact of trauma memories, a crucial goal of posttraumatic therapy.

Many chronically traumatized clients have learned to "read" and respond to the signals of others—especially abusers or anyone else in a position of power—in an attempt to stay safe and avoid further mistreatment or due to their learned caretaking. Some become experts at "making themselves invisible" or "blending into the woodwork," others at "responding in kind"—essentially becoming chameleons who change according to the whims or needs of others and not due to their own feelings or agency. Briere (1996) identified this process as "other-directedness," the development of an external locus of control, undertaken at the behest of dominant/abusive others or otherwise in the interest of safety and hypervigilance. Freyd (1994) furthered this line of reasoning and posited that maintaining an attachment with the perpetrator or other primary caregivers is at root of the complex trauma client's loss of self-awareness and, at times, memory.

The focus on autonomy and self-determination does not mean, however, that clients cannot or should not develop healthy dependence on the therapist (or on significant others in their lives). In fact, because attachment insecurity was the norm in the families of many, their healthy dependence needs were likely frustrated, forcing them instead to meet the needs of others (i.e., becoming "caretakers" or "enablers") even from a very young age. Steele and Van der Hart (2009) noted that the dependence that complex trauma clients exhibit over the course of the treatment should not be rebuffed, stigmatized, or disregarded, nor should it be overindulged. Rather, the therapist should assess the client's attachment style and dependence needs and balance his of her emotional support accordingly. Some clients (preoccupied attachment style) are more dependent and require more closeness, whereas others (dismissive/detached attachment style) require more distance at least initially. The disorganized/disoriented style involves a confusing blend of closeness and detachment. For clients with this style, being close to someone is contradictory: It feels dangerous instead of comfortable, causing them to detach rather than attach. Many iterations of this pattern play out in the treatment and the therapist must learn about their origins and not take the distancing personally (even when it is personalized and aggressive, as was illustrated earlier in the example of Doris). Rather, the therapist can notice the pattern and encourage reflection by the client as to its meaning and purpose. Over time and with repeated nondefensive notice and discussion, the client experiences enough security to lessen the detachment defense. In all attachment styles, but especially the disorganized/disoriented one, the therapist's attunement, predictability, and consistency are all essential.

Enhance Ability to Manage Extreme Arousal States

Psychotherapy with complex trauma survivors is geared toward the identification of the extreme arousal states, which include the physiological hyperarousal characteristic of PTSD and also states of insufficient arousal, numbing, and dissociation. Heightening of arousal may take the form of intense and unremitting states of anxiety/agitation, dysphoria, impulsivity, aggression (toward self as well as toward others), confusion, anguish, and the somatic (somatoform) variant of dissociation (such as persistent distress due to physical pain, discomfort, or disability that is not readily diagnosed medically). States of extreme depletion (hypoarousal) make up the opposite end of the PTSD spectrum. It may take the form of dissociation—which is primarily psychoform (psychological) but also can be somatoform (physical), such as analgesia or conversion symptoms—or variants of PTSD's emotional numbing that include avoidance, a profound sense of estrangement or alienation from self or others, and self-loathing and self-disregard. Many clients are desperate to lessen these opposing states of arousal and "nothingness" and describe wanting to do anything to be "out of their skin." Attempts to feel or to stop feeling something are at root of many clients' often maladaptive self-soothing attempts. Once these states and the usual coping strategies have been identified, clients can learn to monitor them through specific instruction in emotional identification, involving awareness of body state and the visceral processes at the core of emotions and the labeling of these feeling states by the therapist, and skills training in more adaptive and healthy self-management (discussed in detail in upcoming chapters). In this way, as clients learn to identify their emotions and self-regulate their states of hyper- and hypoarousal, they are no longer at the mercy of them, nor are they reliant on the therapist or someone or something outside of themselves to help them self-regulate.

Enhance Sense of Self and Personal Identity

The most significant consequence of pervasive developmental trauma is its effect on the child's core sense of self and identity. As discussed earlier, the self-concept of most abused children is highly negative, as they routinely incorporate the blame for their mistreatment and neglect. The compromised self must therefore be an essential focus of treatment. A primary goal is to provide conditions that allow and encourage self-exploration (in all senses of the word), a process that was largely interrupted by abuse, neglect, and other forms of insecure attachment, hopefully to allow a more positive sense of self to develop. These conditions include acceptance and reflection of the client back to him- or herself through the therapist's empathy and emotional and physical synchrony. Schore (2001, 2003b) described the significance of such "right brain to right brain" attunement of therapist and client as the foundation of creating new neuronal pathways that contribute to actual development of the brain and of heretofore implicit self. Siegel (2001) also compellingly discussed the need for and the significance of a reflective or mirroring other (a relationship of acceptance and attunement rather than disregard and criticism) to the healthy development of the mind of the child and later the adult. Siegel's triangular model of self-development includes the brain, the mind, and the relationship.

Enhance Sense of Personal Control and Self-Efficacy

Developmentally adverse interpersonal trauma, in particular, fundamentally disrupts the acquisition of personal control and self-efficacy (Solomon & Siegel, 2003). Particular attention needs to be paid to assisting clients in recognizing ways that they are (or can be) personally and interpersonally effective and able to feel a sense of pride and confidence without being overwhelmed by negative emotions such as fear, alienation, self-hatred, and shame (Phases 1 and 3; see Chapters 5 and 6). Trauma memory and symptom processing (Phase 2; see Chapter 6) must be timed and structured to support the client's ability not only to tolerate trauma memories and emotional responses but also to gain a sense of self-efficacy along with a life story that encompasses success and growth. Quoting Courtois and colleagues (2009):

> At no point should therapy substitute for living life, or be a direct precipitant of—or tacit collusion with—a view of the client as permanently damaged. Empathizing with the client's struggle with altered self-control facilitate growth rather than a sense of disability. Helping the client to experience and work through painful emotions, traumatic memories, and altered beliefs about self, others, and life meaning bolsters the client's positive self-esteem and internal and external resources. (p. 95)

Maintain Functioning and Overcome Co-Occurring Difficulties and Disorders

It should be recognized, however, that unfortunately some clients' functioning is permanently compromised in that it never matches or returns to their original potential. As well, clients' functioning may be reduced temporarily at critical junctures in therapy when they experience symptomatic relapses related to personal safety, trauma memory reminders and reactions, and problems in relationships and life pursuits. These clients often are steeped in helplessness due to their having been repeatedly disempowered; consequently, some are prone to co-occurring (or comorbid) symptoms and disorders such as anxiety, depression, and dissociation. Often, the disempowerment causes them to feel unable to cope with, manage, or overcome symptoms such as these and life in general. Chronic helplessness and disempowerment are best addressed by teaching specific skills such as assertiveness, goal setting, decision making, problem solving, and boundary management. As noted by Gold (2000), it is the lack of these very basic life skills that were not taught which cause clients to feel unequipped to manage effectively in the world and to not feel "normal".

Recognize and Prevent Traumatic Reenactments

Goals are also developed for highly individualized concerns based on clients' specific and subjective trauma histories and the ways in which these are reenacted in relationships with others and, more generally, in life. Such reenactments tend to be replays of themes and dilemmas that were part of the original trauma and, although they are not *intrinsically* traumatic, they can be (and often are) retraumatizing, as well as stressful and dangerous. Reenactments involve an impairment or loss of functioning in an area in which clients would ordinarily (based on their core physical, intellectual, and interpersonal capacities) be able to function adequately or better, if not for the compensatory coping used to deal with traumatic stress reactions or the ways past methods of coping are replayed. When they involve actual danger, life threat, risk, or other traumatic and abusive acts or circumstances involving self and others, immediate action, crisis management, problem solving, and safety planning are required. As an example, traumatic reenactments may be dealt with over the course of the treatment process through a hierarchy of interventions (developed by phase of treatment). These interventions might include (1) other strategies for coping or for improving function; (2) an overarching safety plan that includes specific attention to reenactments; (3) a strategy for safety in interactions with formerly or currently abusive others; (4) a plan for parent skill training (as needed); (5) a workplace plan to counter harassment or prevent underperforming; (6) a letter of confrontation or reconciliation in a primary relationship—which may actually be sent or not; or (7) a family intervention or other therapeutic approach to addressing safety concerns or family dynamics. A case example illustrates how posttraumatic reenactments can be identified and reduced in frequency and intensity even early in treatment. This, in turn, helps reduce the automaticity and severity of posttraumatic reenactments before the trauma processing and completion phases of therapy.

Doris

After the therapist's initial surprise at Doris's unexpected hostility in session 2, she quickly realized that the incident provided an almost textbook example of an unconscious posttraumatic reenactment that warranted examination with Doris later in therapy. The therapist was able to avoid several potential missteps by not "taking the bait" and engaging Doris in a debate or attempting to "instruct" Doris about her behavior. Instead, she made a mental (and written) note to be vigilant in watching and listening for examples in Doris's life in which she was unintentionally reenacting a "script" of (1) feeling and acting perfectly competent and secure when interacting with a person from whom she is seeking help (or some form of approval or attachment security), followed by (2) reacting as if the same individual has betrayed, abandoned, exploited, and abused her. The therapist did not explicitly discuss this with Doris as a reenactment until several such examples had occurred, been identified, and worked through. These included incidents with Doris's friends and family members, whom she alternately described in effusive and idealized terms ("She's my best friend, the only person whom I can really trust because she knows exactly how I feel") or in a highly derogatory, suspicious, and contemptuous manner ("She is a snake in the grass, a liar who will say or do anything to get even with me and pull me down to her level"). Similar shifts between idealization and subsequent devaluation of the therapist were also given consideration.

Rather than viewing this pattern as reflective of a personality disorder—Doris had been diagnosed with both borderline and narcissistic personality disorders previously—the therapist focused on how it could be a reenactment of early attachment failures with the additional emotional imprinting of traumatic threats to Doris or her caregivers. Indeed, as additional history was gathered in Phase 1, it became clear that Doris had experienced a similar scenario as a child with her mother. She described her mother as at times telling her that Doris was her best and only friend, only to turn around and berate her for being a "monster" who "should never have been born" and "didn't deserve to be loved by anyone as loving as I am," as well as describing Doris as a "compulsive liar" who "would always be unhappy and make everyone around her unhappy." It was not clear exactly what part of this diatribe was actually spoken by her mother (who apparently had multiple inpatient hospitalizations for major mood instability associated with bipolar disorder) and what part was the result of the emotional confusion and helplessness that Doris experienced from having been physically and sexually abused by a father who also was violent toward Doris's mother. Doris tended to describe the abuse and witnessed domestic violence in a matter-of-fact manner that defended against experiencing emotions associated with the violation and life-threatening danger to which she and her mother had been subjected, which could then make her vulnerable to unconsciously reenacting the less traumatically dangerous but more emotionally painful dilemma of emotional abuse.

In Phase 1, while consolidating the therapeutic relationship and helping Doris to build a foundation of emotional security, the therapist did not refer to this scenario directly but commented obliquely on how much of a loss it must be to Doris when she felt betrayed by someone whom she'd looked up to or befriended and trusted—and how it might be a loss for those people also if Doris was angry with them, emphasizing that Doris's positive regard might be highly valued. The therapist also pointed out that she herself had to step back and remember that the relationship between therapist and client was strained but need not be permanently damaged or lost when Doris felt angry and believed the therapist had betrayed her. The therapist "talked through" the emotions she personally experienced when Doris was angry with her as a way to model experiencing and recovering from manageable distress. Only later in therapy, when helping Doris to therapeutically process memories of abuse and family violence, did the therapist begin to point out the parallel between Doris's experience with her mother (and how that was amplified by the abuse and violence) and Doris's reactions when she felt vulnerable.

Repair the Mind–Body Split

Posttraumatic dissociation and detachment occur in both mind and body. Van der Kolk (1996) famously coined the phrase "the body keeps the score" to emphasize the connection between body and mind in the trauma response. Physical and emotional trauma engenders major physiologically based coping or defensive responses (e.g., fight, flight, freeze, or collapse). Such responses are involuntary, encoded implicitly, and, when they are repeated and of sufficient intensity, they result in a physiological condition known as *allostatis* (a chronic stress response of unremitting arousal that occurs even in the absence of current danger and even when the individual is in a relaxed physical state or circumstance; Friedman & McEwen, 2004), the physiological basis of PTSD. Even when the client is not conscious of her or his own physical state, somatoform dissociation might nevertheless be the body's attempt to split off both the trauma and its reaction.

Treatments for PTSD, especially those directed toward somatosensory experiencing, encourage mind–body integration on the level of arousal management and regarding unfinished or incomplete physical actions and emotional responses. For example, progressive muscle relaxation often is taught early in treatment, and awareness of bodily sensations during traumatic memory processing is encouraged. Recently developed sensorimotor therapy interventions (i.e., Ogden et al., 2006; Ogden & Fisher, 2012) involve experiential exercises designed to increase the client's awareness of physical sensations and to address symptoms of somatoform dissociation. Although such interventions have not been as extensively tested in scientific studies as emotion regulation and attachment-focused interventions (e.g., Cloitre et al., 2010; Ford, Steinberg, Hawke, Levine, & Zhang, 2012; Ford, Steinberg, & Zhang, 2011), they currently have a broad clinical consensus and are widely recognized by clinicians as critical in working with this population (Adults Surviving Child Abuse, 2012; Cloitre et al., 2011). Moreover, they draw on the substantial research base of biofeedback (Clum, 2008) and mindfulness or meditative approaches (Follette & Vijay, 2009; Waelde, Silvern, Carlson, Fairbank, & Kletter, 2009).

GENERAL ASSESSMENT ISSUES AND APPROACHES

The specific nature and form of treatment goals change according to phase and focus of treatment and to the emergence of individualized concerns, as well as crisis circumstances. The development of the preliminary treatment goals follows the initial psychosocial assessment. Ongoing evaluation across the domains of symptoms and functioning is essential to the tracking of progress (or lack thereof) and to the reformulation of the original goals and the identification of additional ones as treatment progresses. It is now well recognized by therapists who specialize in this population that the achievement of a goal and/or the resolution of an issue might lead to the emergence of other concerns that were previously dormant (including the use of dissociative processes), unavailable to conscious awareness, or otherwise not in evidence.

As is the case in more general forms of psychotherapy, a psychosocial assessment occurs before treatment; yet such an assessment with clients with complex trauma may present issues that differ from those of the nontraumatized. These individuals can be difficult to engage due to mistrust and suspicion of the therapist's motive, a tendency toward reflexive self-protection, resistance to discussing information that is a painful reminder of what has been avoided, generalized fear and terror, fear of losing control and actual loss of control or decompensation due to emotional flooding or numbing. Assessment, therefore, is best not approached as a one-time event but rather as a process that occurs over time, with additional assessments built on the original to evaluate progress and keep the treatment planning updated. Moreover, repeat assessments are needed if and when new symptoms and problems emerge, something that is rather routine in complex trauma (e.g., dissociative symptoms are likely to emerge and to become more prominent as enough safety develops and as the client's defenses begin to give way). In the following sections, we present strategic considerations for successful assessment, whether by clinical interview, formal psychological testing, or both. We discuss approaches to the assessment of the previously traumatized individual and special issues that can arise with suggestions for their management.

Assessment as Providing Baseline Information

Assessment begins with an intake interview and a comprehensive psychosocial evaluation (that may include medical examinations or other evaluations as needed, to rule out physical illness or other conditions). Notes from the intake assessment provide a baseline of information about the individual's status at the time and so are quite important, especially when memory is unclear or otherwise at issue (Courtois, 1999); it is not unusual for clients to defensively "forget" something they previously reported. Most therapists begin by conducting at least a limited mental status examination (expanded on when indicated) and recording their observations, including appearance, behavior, personality traits, and general cognitive functioning. A clinical interview is usually the basis of the more broad-based assessment, parts of which might be in writing or completed via computer. The interview includes a wide range of issues, beginning with basic demographic information; the individual's chief complaint/presenting concern (or reasons for seeking treatment); a review of principal symptoms, including their onset, sequence, course and duration; previous episodes and treatment if any; past and current life stressors, including lack of personal safety; and any current medication.

A second major area for discussion involves personal and social histories. These include the achievement of developmental milestones and major events; family history, status, functioning, and crises; parental relationship and its quality, along with parental functioning and relationship between parents; stepparents, substitute parents, adoption, or foster placements; past family and individual medical history (including gynecological/obstetrical history for women, genitourinary history for men) and major illnesses or injury; and any past or present involvement in the legal/criminal justice system. Other contextual issues, such as cultural background, social class, religion, ethnicity, gender, sexual identity and orientation, refugee or immigrant status, country or culture of origin (and whether repressive or not), or other issues that might shape or the individual's presentation or perspective merit inquiry.

A third area of attention involves the individual's personal strengths and resources, including ego strength and self-capacities, as well as personal support network. The therapist seeks to capitalize right from the start on available strengths and resources. This section also specifically involves assessment of clinical signs, symptoms, and personality and diagnostic indicators (e.g., mood disturbances; reality testing and psychosis; predominant defensive operations and characterological structure; substance use and abuse; personal, relational, sexual, and social/vocational problems; depression, anxiety, and associated problems; suicidality and other forms of self-harm; risk of interpersonal violence) and their respective onset, duration, intensity, degree of disruption, and subjective level of distress, including a history of suicide attempts (the number of previous attempts and their severity), and any prior psychiatric hospitalizations. A general risk assessment is part of the overall assessment and includes questions about past or current trauma, current safety and risk of violence to or from others, domestic violence and other important family dysfunction, such as substance abuse and history of major mental illness, and additional crises, trauma, and major losses during the individual's lifetime (e.g., significant deaths or separations, accidents or disasters, traumatic brain injuries, major illnesses and associated treatment, and medical emergencies).

Such detailed inquiry as well as queries about abuse, violence, and trauma, although essential, can be quite evocative for the traumatized, and so they must be made neutrally, using descriptive, behavioral questions that are open ended (e.g., "Did you ever experience such and such?"; "Did such and such ever happen to you?"; "Please tell me about it"; "Can you tell me anything more about it?") Disclosure of past abuse and trauma has been shown to be influenced by the terminology used, how questions are phrased, and the attitude and openness of the assessor. Open-ended questions prompt free recall; the interviewee describes the situation in his or her own words, in writing or recorded verbatim by the therapist. The assessor must be prepared to ask for details in follow-up questioning and to be open to the responses given without minimizing them or downplaying their significance or without amplifying them (or correcting or judging them). Particularly in response to open questions such as these, the therapist should pay attention to *how* the individual describes his or her experience. Discourse that is digressive and incoherent or disjunctive is most often indicative of a background involving disorganized attachment (Crittenden & Landini, 2011; Main, Goldwyn, & Hesse, 2002), an important consideration in the assessment.

The therapist should inquire about any earlier treatment and the reason(s) for it, whether it was helpful or not, conditions of its ending, previous diagnoses, and why the individual currently is seeking treatment with a different therapist or one using a different approach. A request for the release of information or records from prior treatment should be made so the therapist can seek to ascertain its quality and effectiveness.

Another area of inquiry has to do with the client's living situation and economic status, including housing, personal support network, financial and job security, and health care funding, if any. A treatment plan must be in line with available resources and should start with deficits that must be remediated or addressed for treatment to proceed (e.g., building up a personal support system, finding stable and safe housing, finding steady employment, getting health insurance or disability coverage, getting additional case management or social services). It is clearly unhelpful to propose a treatment that exceeds the individual's ability to pay for it or that further destabilizes an already precarious living situation.

In the assessment phase and throughout the treatment process, adjunctive consultations and testing for corollary medical, psychiatric, substance abuse, or neurological conditions and adjunctive services, such as career development, vocational rehabilitation, substance abuse services, or testing for learning difficulties and disorders may be in order. A second opinion might prove useful even after a comprehensive workup, especially in cases that are unclear, complicated, or perplexing and when the therapist has residual concerns about the scope of the symptom picture, the diagnostic formulation, and treatment recommendations. Assessment of the individual's suggestibility and hypnotizability is sometimes justified, as the therapist needs to be especially cautious and circumspect when treating an individual who is suggestible.

One final and nonstandard area of inquiry deserves mention: determining whether the individual has undertaken, is currently involved in, or is contemplating a lawsuit or other legal action for any reason, but particularly for past abuse and trauma (especially if it was incestuous abuse, alleged on the basis of recovered memory). The therapist needs to know whether, at some point, litigation would call for his or her involvement in the forensic setting, something that might affect the decision to treat the client in the first place. For example, some therapists, if they do agree to treat, clarify at the outset that they are not willing to testify in a legal case, or they make clear that any testimony that would be required of them must concern their role as the treating therapist/fact witness and *not* as an expert witness—two different roles that require different stances toward the litigant client. The client may be asked to sign an additional consent form agreeing with this stipulation.

The Need for "Supportive Neutrality"

By definition, trauma victims (of severe and/or repeated interpersonal victimization, whether past or present or both) have experienced intrusion and damage at the hands of others and are therefore highly suspicious of the motives and intentions of anyone wanting to know about them, even though they sought out the treatment. Being asked to discuss highly personal events and reactions may feel intrusive and like "ripping off the bandage," resulting in an overly skittish, noncooperative, shut down, or even antagonistic stance. To the degree possible, the therapist should have a very calm and respectful demeanor that is encouraging but not pressuring. A stance of "supportive neutrality" is recommended, as the individual may be unable to disclose traumatic events and circumstances unless supported in doing so through direct yet sensitive questioning.

ct of Assessment on the Traumatized Individual Therapist

In any event, and no matter how gently or sensitively conducted, the assessment process is likely to be stressful. It is therefore crucial to create an environment and conditions that are safe and to develop a degree of rapport by explaining the inquiry procedure and being open to questions. The therapist should indicate that he or she is not expecting particular responses, there are no right or wrong answers and, although assessment is not intended to be hurtful, it is likely to cause some discomfort and upset because it focuses attention on painful episodes and experiences that may previously have been avoided. The individual is encouraged to maintain as much control as possible, to communicate whether he or she is beginning to feel overwhelmed or numb, to ask for clarification if uncertain about a question or its meaning, to choose to answer or not, to choose to give details or not, and to take breaks as needed in order to make the process as much a joint venture as possible.

At times, it is necessary to adjust the pacing of the assessment or to suspend it altogether if it is overly unsettling or causes decompensation (Briere, 2004). A high level of unmanageable and unmodulated distress is counterproductive as it can negatively influence and even contaminate the entire assessment. If, despite the therapist's best efforts, destabilization occurs during or afterward (as suggested by flashbacks, numbing/dissociation, regressive behavior, anger, anxiety, panic, suicidal ideation or action, attempts at self-harm), the process must be halted and the individual restabilized. Conducting a trauma assessment can create conditions of personal and professional stress to the therapist due to traumatic transference or vicarious traumatization (discussed further in Chapters 10 and 11). The therapist can be profoundly affected by the difficult and stressful interpersonal context of the assessment, which involves hearing about atrocities (especially when committed by family members or others who are related to or known to the victim or when the details are especially graphic or horrific and are of the sort that can cause shock and strain credibility) and hearing about their painful and damaging consequences.

Under- and Overreporting

Traumatized individuals may under- or overreport their experiences and symptoms, especially when questions are indirect, imprecise, or misunderstood. It is necessary for questions to be phrased precisely but neutrally, using behavioral descriptions (i.e., "Did you, as a child, ever have a sexual experience with an adult? . . . a family member? . . . another child?" "Have you ever been exposed to or witnessed violence or sexual abuse between members of your family, or in the community?" "Have you ever been pressured into unwanted sexual contact of any sort?"

"Have you ever been physically injured by a member of your family or by someone else?").

Gelinas (1983) described common characteristics and manifestations of what she termed the *disguised presentation* that include a constellation of symptoms consisting of "a characterological depression with complications and atypical compulsive and dissociative elements" (p. 326). Further, she noted the particular presentation made by "parentified" clients who come across as competent, responsible, confident, and mature. Their social and professional accomplishments are in fact genuine, but they are expert at masking difficulties and concerns and at taking care of others and can often be described as pseudomature. The overly responsible client closely resembles the apparently normal personality (ANP) described by Van der Hart et al. (2006) in their structural model of dissociation. The traumatic reactions and emotions (and even memory) are sequestered from awareness in one or more emotional personalities (EPs) from the time of the trauma and later. As a result, the emotional material is not available in the pretreatment assessment and may be accessible only over the course of treatment with deliberate elicitation by the therapist and as enough trust and relational security develop for its emergence.

In addition to dissociation, some of the most common reasons for the disguised presentation (or underreporting) include but are not limited to, the following: lack of awareness about past abuse/victimization; naivete or ignorance about it (it was the norm in its context); gender (with males on average being more reluctant to disclose, although this seems to be gradually changing with more reporting of clergy and coach abuse, and more recognition that boys can be abused); age and life-stage issues (with adolescents and older clients possibly more reluctant to disclose); and the chronic nature of the symptoms; trauma bonding, attachment, and loyalty to the abuser or others in a family, organization, or group setting; threat, terror, or silence used against the victim (these may be ongoing, up to the time of assessment and treatment); previous negative experience with disclosure; feelings of stigma and shame; use of silence as protection (of oneself or others); mistrust of others; and any past history of treatment, whether it was helpful or not and whether or not it identified or addressed the trauma history. Other reasons may be highly idiosyncratic (e.g., parent was a member of a gang involved in the production and sale of child pornography who threatened reprisal; abuser was a clergy member who threatened the victim with fire and brimstone in the afterlife; etc.; Courtois, 2010).

Underreporting can also result from memory difficulties, due to dissociative (out of consciousness) amnesia or due to more conscious motivated suppression or forgetting. Clients might say such things as "I never remembered, but I never forgot. Who would want to remember this anyway?" or "Now that you ask me, I remember that." Underreporting additionally may be due to shame, avoidance, and emotional pain associated with the trauma story or may be a way to protect the assessor from having to hear it, especially if the client perceives or is given indications of aversion, judgment, or personal distress (one of us [CAC] recently heard of a case in which a *therapist* ended up in a fetal position during an assessment interview with a complex trauma client, a circumstance that prompted the client to take care of the therapist and to be concerned that she had damaged her with her story—certainly an untherapeutic contact for the client!).

Overreporting is also possible, for one or more of the following reasons: secondary gain (such as gaining sympathy, attention, friendship, compensation, or other financial benefit); retribution or vindictiveness; an explanation for life's problems; social inclusion; memory errors, misunderstandings and misperceptions; delusions due to psychosis or other severe personality disturbance; psychopathy; and personal traits of suggestibility or fantasy-proneness that increase compliance with suggestions from an authority figure. When these characteristics are noted, is it advisable for the therapist to conduct specialized personality assessment, as well as assessment of malingering and psychopathy. At the present time, it is unknown how often past trauma is over- or underreported or reported in error and how much is due to false memory, false belief, or other factors, but all are possible (Courtois, 1999).

The Crisis Presentation

A full-blown crisis can develop with the unplanned and spontaneous emergence of delayed aftereffects and symptoms associated with the original trauma that are stirred up by events or other stimuli that serve as reminders. The symptoms, depending on their severity, can bring on acute states of anxiety, depression, or dissociation, explosive or impulsive behavior (including acting out or violence toward oneself or others), and decompensation involving reactive psychosis or vegetative and even states of dissociation and catatonia. The reemergence of the trauma and its symptoms would be highly distressing to anyone; however, it is most distressing to past victims who have no conscious memory of having been abused or otherwise traumatized (i.e., those whose experience is highly dissociated and for which they are amnestic). Crisis intervention involves emotional support and stabilization, assurances of and planning for safety, normalization of reactions, and a calm and nonjudgmental stance regarding the symptoms and the shock that accompanies their sudden emergence. In the most severe cases involving decompensation (up to and including total inability to function and suicidal or homicidal urges), sedation and hospitalization may be needed. Needless to say, the therapist can be taken aback by the intensity of such a response or presentation and may need to use others as backup (professional colleagues, client's spouse or partner or friends) or call on other resources (e.g., police, EMTs, ambulance) for assistance.

For complex trauma survivors, various life events, whether they are distressing and *decremental* (e.g., involving illness, miscarriage/stillbirth, other deaths or losses, anniversary dates, abuse scandals in the community or media, relationship separation and divorce, loss of status or functioning, job and economic loss, legal charges) or, paradoxically, are happy and *incremental* (e.g., development of an intimate relationship, marriage or other relationship commitment, pregnancy, the birth of a child) can trigger symptoms that meet criteria for ASD or delayed-onset PTSD. Quite paradoxically, these incremental events and transitions can cause crisis reactions when they provide enough security for defenses to lessen, resulting in the emergence of memories, symptoms, or negative emotions such as fear, anxiety, and guilt. Negative events may allow emotionally numb clients to suddenly have intense feelings or to close down even more. The loss or death of a perpetrator or any other significant person, for example, can disrupt dormant emotions and memories or, alternatively, create a major numbing of response or a swing between the two. Some types of events are especially evocative, including those that either directly or more indirectly symbolize or resemble the original trauma (e.g., reexposure to the original circumstance, especially after having been apart from it for a period of time; revictimization; additional betrayal, including the discovery of other abuse in a family or community; and media coverage, especially when sensationalized and of the saturated and pervasive sort; Courtois, 1988; 2010). The Penn State scandal serves as a recent example.

The case of **Hector**—and the triggering that occurred from his war zone activities and exposure, the sexual assault perpetrated on him by other soldiers, and the media reports of ongoing scandal in the Catholic Church, possibly implicating the pope—is illustrative of a complex trauma client who was triggered by present events into flashbacks and intrusions of past abuses. He was also triggered when his mother mentioned to him almost in passing that she had heard that his perpetrator priest had been arrested on child molestation charges that she adamantly refused to believe.

When Trauma and Abuse Victimization Are Disclosed

When trauma and abuse victimization are disclosed during the course of an assessment, the therapist should inquire about both the *objective* factors (who, what, when, where, how long, severity, progression, use of force, any physical injury, the individual's role, actions taken or not) and the *subjective* thoughts, beliefs, and feelings about its occurrence and its effects and should *record responses factually*. The therapist must ask questions regarding these issues in direct but supportive fashion, all the while staying attuned to the toll the questioning might be taking and either modifying its pace accordingly or stopping the process (Briere, 2004). Some traumatized individuals (due to their ability to separate or dissociate thoughts from feelings and to present "just the facts" without the emotions) have the capacity to respond to such detailed questions without much discomfort, but others experience strong reactions and need to respond slowly over a more extended period of time. Still others show no outward reactions (i.e., keep a well-practiced "poker face") but report delayed or "boomerang" responses that occur later, and some dissociate all or part of the assessment and later deny or are confused about their responses to the questions.

The therapist should also attempt to discern the meaning of disclosure of past trauma and learn about any childhood messages or beliefs about divulging information. Then the therapist should monitor how the client is reacting to the questioning and disclosure. It is good policy for the therapist to inform the client regarding possible postassessment reactions and the normalcy of delayed reactions and to offer suggestions for managing them. Most significantly, the therapist must make explicit that the client is supported and safe and that what was reported is confidential (except under the exceptions described in Chapter 3). Where there is difficulty in describing or remembering specific details or conflicting details and memories, the therapist does not press for certainty but instead indicate and model a tolerance for uncertainty.

When past abuse and trauma is disclosed, the therapist must further evaluate for possible posttraumatic reactions and associated conditions of dissociation, substance abuse and other addictive and compulsive behaviors, intense emotional states, learning difficulties, memory disturbances, medical problems and psychosomatic reactions, attachment status and interpersonal difficulties (for which a variety of assessment instruments are now available; see listing in Table 4.1), criminal justice or legal difficulties or history, or contemplated or pending litigation. As the formal evaluation wraps up, it must be made explicit that *disclosure does not mean resolution but rather signifies the beginning of the treatment process of which resolution is a major goal.* Confidentiality of the material disclosed should again be emphasized.

Despite all, it is definitely the case that some individuals are immediately and obviously relieved to be asked about their trauma history and experience (Courtois, 1988). The assessment may be the first time anyone has indicated interest in their experiences, and they may find the interview (especially one that is well paced and conducted with sensitivity and interest) to be immediately cathartic and therapeutic for them.

When Trauma and Abuse Victimization Are Not Disclosed

As discussed earlier in this section, trauma and victimization that are explicitly known may not be divulged even when questions are direct and unambiguous and asked with sensitivity. In other circumstances, traumatic experiences are not disclosed because they are not known but are suspected (or they might not even be suspected). Another possibility is that they did not occur; therefore, there is nothing to disclose (See Courtois, 1999 for detailed discussion). When the fact of occurrence is unclear, the individual's expectations and motivations for treatment must be ascertained. In some cases, they may need to be reworked or even challenged. For example, some expectations are eminently reasonable (e.g., "I want help to determine whether there is any basis to my suspicions," or "I want to determine whether something I'm not sure about is causing my symptoms"), but others are not and might even pose potential hazards to the individual or the therapist (e.g., I want *you to tell me that I was abused* so that I can sue my parents, or the Catholic Church" [or whoever]; "I want you *to find my incest memories* for me and tell me what happened"; "My friends/support group tell me *I act and look like I was abused* but I don't remember, so I might as well find out. I don't remember, but I'm sure I was"; "I want to find out if I was really abused so I can legitimately kill myself").

As a general rule, the therapist should not assume the meaning of a lack of disclosure. However, when the symptom picture is acute and/or has a strong resemblance to the co-occurring disturbances of the complex PTSD formulation, or when the therapist observes certain behavioral and response patterns commonly associated with trauma and victimization, its possibility should be contemplated. The therapist might develop a degree of suspicion or develop a hypothesis that is optimally kept private in order not to be suggestive, but he or she must also concede the patient's not knowing and/or not disclosing. In some of the most traumatized individuals, especially those who are highly dissociative, the story might surface only in a disguised, highly fragmented and incoherent manner. Possibly, memories might become available only when the client has developed enough trust and made enough advances (developed sufficient ego resources and self-capacities, resolved substance abuse or other addictions) for memories to emerge.

The therapist must be especially cautious when trauma and abuse are not known to the client but are suspected, even when the basis for suspicion is quite compelling (e.g., when dream content is replete with victimization scenarios; when behavioral reenactments within or outside of the therapy seem to point to it; or when the client has posttraumatic symptoms). It is necessary to inquire about how suspicions of abuse came about in the absence of specific memory and to assess possible personal and interpersonal motivations. As mentioned previously, these can include secondary gain or loss, malingering, the desire for a particular diagnosis or explanation for symptoms, compensation, and/or for revenge, or any sources of suggestion and misinformation (e.g., social influences, media reports, books, previous suggestive therapeutic activities).

When specific memory is absent, the therapist should not speculate about, fill in, or try to confirm suspicions. Both therapist and client in such a circumstance need to tolerate uncertainty, with the therapist urging an open-ended exploratory stance over time. He or she should also correct any misinformation about the impact of trauma on memory processes and clarify appropriate goals of treatment (explicitly charting both the misinformation and the correction).

On a final but related matter, psychosis does not automatically rule out the occurrence of trauma. In fact, positive symptoms of psychosis have been documented in samples of PTSD patients (Butler, Mueser, Sprock, & Braff, 1996), and trauma and abuse victimization have been documented as common occurrences in the background of a subset of psychotic patients (Read, 1997) that can cause psychosis. Psychotic and posttraumatic symptoms can co-occur, and psychotic symptoms might, in reality, be the posttraumatic and dissociative hallucinatory intrusion and reexperiencing of real traumatic events and circumstances. Many posttraumatic and dissociative patients have been misdiagnosed as schizophrenic or bipolar and the reality and possibility of past trauma discounted, downplayed, or ignored (Ellason & Ross, 1995).

ASSESSMENT USING STANDARD AND TRAUMA-SPECIFIC PSYCHOLOGICAL INSTRUMENTS

A number of trauma-specific psychological instruments are available to supplement the psychosocial interview. More accurate assessment of both traumatic experiences and trauma-related symptoms can be made with psychometrically sound instruments constructed specifically for such assessment that are neutral and precise. Particularly in forensic evaluations, in which accuracy and neutrality are so crucial, the assessment should include the use of the instruments with the best quality of standardization. Trauma-specific assessment instruments and strategies are presented here, with attention to those that are the most commonly used and the most methodologically sound. Table 4.1 includes a listing of instruments and inventories that are paired with associated treatment goals. Not all are included in the following discussion, but the table contains a listing of authors and developers.

Five types are discussed: (1) generic psychological inventories with specialized subscales for traumatic response and symptoms and structured clinical interviews; (2) dedicated measures of traumatic events, experiences, and symptoms; (3) structured interviews to elicit detailed information about the traumatic event(s) or for the purposes of diagnosis; (4) assessments of attachment status; and (5) psychophysiological, biological, and neurological/neuropsychological instruments and approaches. Trauma-specific instruments can be supplemented with those that are more generic (e.g., for depression and anxiety), with specialized assessments (of beliefs, intentions, locus of control, health status, substance abuse, eating disorders, self-harm, suicidality, level of functioning, quality of life, hypnotizability

TABLE 4.1. Sample Evidence-Informed Assessment Instruments for Complex Trauma Cases

Domain: Posttraumatic appraisals/cognitions
Goals 1, 6, 11, 12, 15, and 16

- Post-Traumatic Cognitions Inventory (Foa, Ehlers, Clark, Tolin, & Orsillo, 1999)
- World Assumptions Scale (Janoff-Bulman, 1992)
- TSI Belief Scale (McCann & Pearlman, 1992)
- Trauma and Attachment Belief Scale (Pearlman, 2003)
- Trauma-Related Guilt Scale (Kubany, Abueg, Kilauano, Manke, & Kaplan, 1997)
- Centrality of Event Scale (Berntsen & Rubin, 2006)
- Trauma Symptom Inventory Impaired Self-Reference Scale (Briere & Elliott, 2003; Elliott, Mok, & Briere, 2004)
- Cognition Distortion Scales (Briere, 2000a)
- Young Schema Questionnaire–3 (Young & Brown, 2001)
- Initial Trauma Review for Adolescents (Briere & Lanktree, 2012)

Domain: Psychic numbing and hyperarousal/hypervigilance
Goal 2

- Clinician-Administered PTSD Scale (Weathers, Keane, & Davidson, 2001)
- PTSD Checklist (McDonald & Calhoun, 2010)
- Posttraumatic Symptom Scale (Foa, Johnson, Feeny, & Treadwell, 2001; Foa & Tolin, 2000)
- Trauma Symptom Inventory (Briere & Elliott, 2003; Elliott et al., 2004)

Domain: Work and interpersonal functioning
Goal 3

- Social Adjustment Survey—Self-Report (Weissman, Olfson, Gameroff, Feder, & Fuentes, 2001)
- Inventory of Interpersonal Problems Short Form (Barkham, Hardy, & Startup, 1996)
- Trauma Symptom Inventory–2: Sexual Concerns and Dysfunctional Sexual Behavior Scales (Briere, 2011)
- Relationship Questionnaire (Bartholomew & Horowitz, 1991)
- Experiences in Close Relationships (Brennan, Clark, & Shaver, 1998)

Domain: Intrusive reexperiencing and avoidance
Goals 4, 7, and 12

- Trauma Memory Questionnaire (Halligan, Michael, Clark, & Ehlers, 2003)
- Interpretation of PTSD Symptoms Scale (Halligan et al., 2003)
- Personal Beliefs About Memory Inventory (Lineweaver & Hertzog, 1998)
- Trauma Symptom Inventory Intrusive Experiences and Avoidance Scales (Bennett & Wells, 2010)
- Clinician-Administered PTSD Scale (Weathers et al., 2001)
- PTSD Checklist (McDonald & Calhoun, 2010)
- Posttraumatic Symptom Scale (Foa et al., 2001; Foa & Tolin, 2000)

(continued)

TABLE 4.1. *(continued)*

Domain: Retraumatization

Goals 5, 10, and 13

- Traumatic Events Screening Instrument (Daviss et al., 2000; Ford et al., 2000; Ford & Smith, 2008)
- Conflict Tactics Scale (Straus & Douglas, 2004; Straus, Hamby, Finkelhor, Moore, & Runyan, 1998)

Domain: Self-efficacy and sense of personal control

Goals 8 and 12

- Hope Scale (Snyder et al., 1996, 1997)
- World Assumptions Scale (Janoff-Bulman, 1992)
- TSI Belief Scale (McCann & Pearlman, 1992)

Domain: Biological and familial risk factors

Goal 9

- Anxiety Sensitivity Index (Osman et al., 2010; Taylor et al., 2007)
- Event-Related Rumination Inventory (Cann et al., 2011)
- Conflict Tactics Scale (Straus & Douglas, 2004; Straus, Hamby, Finkelhor, Moore, & Runyan, 1998)
- Childhood Trauma Questionnaire (Bernstein et al., 1994)

Domain: Comorbidities/co-occurring disorders

Goal 10

- Beck Depression Inventory (Steer, Ball, Ranieri, & Beck, 1997, 1999)
- Beck Anxiety Inventory (Kohn, Kantor, DeCicco, & Beck, 2008; Leyfer, Ruberg, & Woodruff-Borden, 2006)
- Trauma Symptom Inventory–2; Anxious Arousal and Depression Scales; Dysfunctional Behaviors Scale (Briere, 2011)
- State–Trait Anxiety Inventory (Spielberger & Vagg, 1984)
- K6 and K10 (Kessler et al., 2002, 2010)
- Brief Symptom Inventory (Derogatis & Melisaratos, 1983)
- Personal Health Questionnaire (PHQ) (Spitzer et al., 1999)
- Eating Attitudes Test (Garner & Garfinkel, 1979)

Domain: Attachment working models

Goal 13

- Revised Adult Attachment Scale (Collins, Ford, Guichard, & Allard, 2006; Ravitz, Maunder, Hunter, Sthankiya, & Lancee, 2010)
- Relationship Scales Questionnaire (Bartholomew, 1997; Ravitz et al., 2010)
- Parental Bonding Instrument (Parker, 1989; Ravitz et al., 2010)
- Adult Attachment Inventory (Main et al.,2002)
- Trauma Symptom Inventory–2; Insecure Attachment Styles Scale (Briere, 2011)

(continued)

TABLE 4.1. *(continued)*

Domain: Emotion regulation

Goal 14

- Expectancies for Negative Mood Regulation (Catanzaro & Mearns, 1990; Catanzaro, Wasch, Kirsch, & Mearns, 2000)
- Difficulty with Emotion Regulation Scale (Tull, Barrett, McMillan, & Roemer, 2007; Tull, Jakupcak, McFadden, & Roemer, 2007)
- Test of Self-Conscious Affect Scale (Shame) (Tangney, Wagner, Fletcher, & Gramzow, 1992)

Domain: Dissociation

Goals 17 and 18

- Psychoform Dissociation Questionnaire—Peritraumatric (Nijenhuis, Van Engen, Kusters, & Van der Hart, 2001)
- Somatoform Dissociation Scale (Nijenhuis et al., 2001)
- Trauma Symptom Inventory–2; Dissociation Scale (Briere & Elliott, 2003; Elliott et al., 2004)
- Multidimensional Inventory of Dissociation (Dell, 2006)
- Multiscale Dissociation Inventory (Briere, Weathers, & Runtz, 2005)
- Dissociative Experiences Scale–2 (Carlson & Putnam, 1993; Merritt & You, 2008; Modestin & Erni, 2004)
- Dissociative Disorders Interview Schedule (uses DSM-III diagnostic criteria) (Ross et al., 1989, 1990)
- Structured Clinical Interview for DSM-IV Dissociative Disorders, Revised (Steinberg, 1994)
- Office Mental Status Examination for Complex Dissociative Symptoms and Multiple Personality Disorder (Loewenstein, 1991)

Domain: Anger/aggression

Goals 18 and 19

- State–Trait Anger Expression Inventory (Forgays, Forgays, & Spielberger, 1997; Spielberger, Reheiser, & Sydeman, 1995)
- Buss–Durkee Hostility Inventory (Buss & Durkee, 1957; Riley & Treiber, 1989)
- Trauma Symptom Inventory–2; Anger Scale (Briere, 2011)

Domain: Self-harm and suicide

Goals 18 and 19

- Risk Taking and Self-Harm Inventory (Vrouva, Fonagy, Fearon, & Roussow, 2010)
- Suicide Concerns for Offenders in Prison Environment (Perry & Gilbody, 2009)
- Adult Suicidal Ideation Questionnaire (Reynolds, 1991)
- Beck Scale for Suicidal Ideation (Beck, Brown, & Steer, 1997)
- Self-Injury Questionnaire (Santa Mina et al., 2006)

(continued)

TABLE 4.1. *(continued)*

Domain: Addiction
Goals 18 and 19

- Alcohol, Smoking and Substance Involvement Screening Test (Humeniuk et al., 2008)
- Global Assessment of Individual Needs (Dennis, Chan, & Funk, 2006; Dennis, Funk, Godley, Godley, & Waldron, 2004)
- Trauma Symptom Inventory Tension Reduction Scale (Briere & Elliott, 2003; Elliott et al., 2004)
- Michigan Alcoholism Screening Test (Selzer, 1971)
- Substance Abuse Subtle Screening Inventory–3

and suggestibility, psychopathy, traumatic bereavement, and malingering, to name but a few), and with information from collateral sources.

Generic Psychological Inventories and Structured Clinical Interviews

The therapist can start by assessing symptoms and personality variables using generic and widely accepted psychological self-report inventories, such as the Minnesota Multiphasic Personality Inventory (MMPI-2; Hathaway & McKinley, 1989), the Millon Clinical Multiaxial Inventory (MCMI-III; Millon, 1987), the Personality Assessment Inventory (PAI) (Morey, 1991, 2007), the Symptom Checklist-90—Revised (SCL-90-R; Derogatis, 1977; Derogatis & Unger, 2010), and the Rorschach (Rorschach, 1981). The Structured Clinical Interview for DSM-IV Disorders (SCID-I; First, Gibbon, Spitzer, Williams, & Benjamin, 1997) covers DSM-IV diagnostic categories, but is weak as concerns PTSD and somatoform disorders. The SCID-II covers criteria of the 11 DSM personality disorders (First et al., 1997). Because these will change as the DSM revision becomes finalized, new versions of the SCID are likely to develop.

For the most part, these measures were not designed to assess symptoms associated with posttraumatic or dissociative response and symptoms and are not trauma specific; however, subscales have been developed and specialized interpretations that take trauma into consideration have appeared for some. On average, trauma survivors have tended to have highly elevated scales, yielding a symptom profile that, until relatively recently, suggested other serious psychopathology, especially personality disorders and schizophrenia, or suggested that the responses were invalid. This stance has now been modified. An elevated profile might well be an accurate report of acute and pervasive symptomatology often of the sort associated with complex traumatic stress, and that high item endorsement might further signify a cry for help. It is now recommended that profile interpretation take into account reports or suspicions of traumatization to avoid misinterpretation of symptoms and resultant misdiagnosis.

Measures of Posttraumatic and Dissociative Symptoms and Disorders

Other instruments and structured diagnostic interviews are now available that include scales that go beyond the usual symptoms of depression, anxiety, and personality disturbance to assess the symptoms of PTSD (traditional and complex), dissociation, somatization, enduring personality characteristics, attachment style, and relational and sexual difficulties. Discussion of trauma symptom scales now in use in assessing dimensions of complex trauma can be found in Briere (2004), Briere and Lanktree (2012), Briere and Spinazzola (2005, 2009), D. Brown (2009), and Keane and Wilson (2004).

A large number of instruments have been developed to directly assess posttraumatic symptoms and disorders. The following are among the most well known and most used: the Clinician-Administered PTSD Scale (CAPS; Blake et al., 1995), the Posttraumatic Stress Diagnostic Scale (PDS; Foa, 1995), the Detailed Assessment of Posttraumatic Stress (DAPS; Briere, 2001), the Inventory of Altered Self Capacities (IASC; Briere, 2000a), and the Cognitive Distortions Scale (CDS; Briere, 2000b). Additionally, the Structured Interview for Disorders of Extreme Stress (SIDES; Pelcovitz, Van der Kolk, Roth, Mandel, Kaplan, et al., 1997) and the Trauma Symptom Inventory 1 and 2 (TSI-1, Briere, 1995; TSI-2; Briere, 2011), with their focus on trauma symptoms associated with classic PTSD and the criteria for complex PTSD/DESNOS, are clinically useful with the population under discussion.

Measures for the assessment of dissociative symptoms and disorders have been developed in the past several decades: the Dissociative Experiences Scale (DES), Carlson and Putnam (1993), the Dissociative Disorders Interview Schedule (DDIS; uses DSM-III diagnostic criteria; Ross et al., 1989, 1990), the Multiscale Dissociation Inventory (MDI; Briere, 2002), the Multidimensional Inventory of Dissociation (MID; Dell, 2006), the Somatoform Dissociation Questionnaire–20 (SDQ-20; Nijenhuis, Spinhoven, Van Dycke, Van der Hart, & Vanderlinden, 1996), and the Structured Clinical Interview for DSM-IV Dissociative Disorders, Revised (SCID-D, Rev.; Steinberg, 1994). The Office Mental Status Examination for Complex Dissociative Symptoms and Multiple Personality Disorder (Loewenstein, 1991) is an organized set of questions found to have great clinical utility about types of dissociative experiences and symptoms and for the diagnosis of dissociative disorders (but the interview has no psychometric properties). Where the therapist needs a psychometrically sound instrument for the diagnosis of the dissociative disorders (especially for a forensic evaluation), Steinberg's SCID-D, Rev. is the instrument of choice.

Measures of Traumatic Events and Experiences

Instruments that explore details of specific types of traumatic events and experiences have been developed and are accessible in different formats, usually as structured sets of questions posed by the interviewer, who records responses verbatim, or as paper-and-pencil or computerized self-report measures. They elicit specific information about the experience(s) and event(s) when a trauma history has been disclosed and a more detailed description is sought. The Courtois Incest History Questionnaire (IHQ; Courtois, 1988, 2010) is an example.

Assessment of Attachment Style

In a recent chapter, D. Brown (2009) described a theory-driven strategy for multi-instrument assessment of attachment style, complex trauma history, and resultant complex traumatic stress and impairments. He wrote: "Given the extent to which early attachment status predicts a significant portion of the variance of adult psychopathology, independent of or in combination with traumatic events, it is imperative to measure attachment status as part of a comprehensive assessment of complex trauma" (p. 129). The Adult Attachment Inventory (AAI; Main et al., 2002) is perhaps the most used instrument for determining attachment style, the degree to which loss and/or trauma are unresolved, and the assessment of metacognitive reflection or mentalization, an important component of psychological recovery (Bateman & Fonagy, 2004a, 2004b). Crittenden and Landini (2011) have recently published a book on the assessment of adult attachment.

Psychophysiological, Biological, Neurological, and Medical Assessment

As discussed in Chapter 2, substantial research on the psychobiological and psychophysiological responses to trauma and resulting PTSD has provided a consistent picture of greater physiological reactivity, including startle response and biological alterations in individuals who develop PTSD versus those who do not. Psychophysiological and biological measures of PTSD are increasingly under development and currently include those for heart rate, blood pressure, muscle tension, skin conductance level and response, and peripheral temperature, as well as physiological challenge tests in response to standardized or personalized challenges or scripts of actual or potentially traumatic experiences (Orr, Metzger, Miller, & Kaloupek, 2004). Neuropsychological assessment provides another means of evaluating the possible neurocognitive aspects of PTSD symptoms including and apart from traumatic brain injuries (TBI) and of making differential diagnoses (Knight & Taft, 2004). Neurological conditions may be related to past and present physical abuse or battering (e.g., head or brain trauma and TBI resulting from childhood or adult physical abuse or repeated choking or suffocation to the point of unconsciousness during episodes of abuse, particularly common in intimate partner abuse). Medical examinations, general and specialized, might also be necessary when medical illness or injury is evident or a medical condition needs to be ruled in or out. The therapist should consider a generic or more specialized medical workup and psychophysiological, biological, and/or neurological assessments as independent means of evaluation that supplement or clarify psychological data. Additional discussion of assessment of psychological trauma and PTSD can be found in Briere (2004), Briere and Lanktree (2012), Carlson (1997), and Wilson and Keane (2004) and of the dissociative disorders in Dell and O'Neil (2009).

Other Common Issues for Assessment

Because substance abuse disorders are so common (along with the other addictive/compulsive problems, such as eating disorders, sex or pornography addictions) among those with PTSD, specialized assessment is often warranted. Screening questions can provide a starting point, with detailed assessment to follow as indicated. Additionally, specialized assessment of such issues as health status, sleep, lifestyle and quality of life, stress management and level of functioning, risk of violence to and from others, risk of suicide and lethality, hypnotizability and suggestibility, psychopathy, traumatic bereavement, and malingering might be indicated.

Collateral Assessment: Interviews and Information Gathering

Collateral assessments (e.g., with spouses or partners, family members, friends, teachers, employers and coworkers, former therapists) can at times be warranted to obtain more objective observational information or to provide information about events for which the client has little or no recollection. In addition, collateral reports can help the therapist assess or understand the impact the client has on others and the ways he or she interacts and interprets personal experiences and symptoms, providing supplementary data not otherwise available. Seeking collateral information from sources external to the treatment is best decided and undertaken collaboratively; yet, even so, the suggestion to include information from outside sources must be judicious and have a clear rationale (and can only be obtained with the client's explicit permission and release of information, except in emergency situations) because it can be counterproductive and even damaging to the client, the assessment, or the therapy (Carlson, 1997). It may cause the client to feel disbelieved and out of control, reinforcing his or her alienation from and mistrust of others. An additional caution needs mention: Although the strategy of seeking collateral information seems reasonable, experts in the dynamics of interpersonal trauma (especially involving a family or other group) point out some major shortcomings, particularly that perpetrators and others (bystanders or those in positions of authority in organizations) deny and minimize their behavior and that of other members. Consequently, if collateral information is sought, the therapist must not automatically take the family or organization's word over that of the client. Such collateral sources sometimes provide substantiation for a report of trauma (e.g., a sibling who witnessed incestuous abuse by a parent, a neighbor who witnessed beatings, a teacher who noticed and reported bruises); however, others provide nothing so conclusive or provide misinformation. As with other aspects of the assessment, the information must be weighed in aggregate, with conclusions drawn over time.

Records (medical, school, police, legal, child protective services, psychotherapy, employment, and military records, as well as information from other sources, such as diaries, pictures, photo albums, and media accounts and newspaper reports) can provide other sources of supplemental information that elaborate on and possibly corroborate the client's disclosure and reports of past symptoms and functioning. Clients may seek out the information themselves, or it may be sought by the therapist, obviously with the client's permission and with the recognition that such information can have serious implications. For example, when a client seeks (or otherwise gains) outside corroboration that supports memories or triggers recall, the information can be validating but highly upsetting. This was the case with **Hector**, when his mother told him that his abuser priest had been arrested on charges of molesting other boys in the parish. Hector was validated but shocked and upset; this information was not sought and felt "out of the blue" for Hector when it was disclosed to him while he was in the war zone. On the other hand, inquiries and research that does not result in any confirmatory information can be an outcome that is upsetting, leading to additional self-doubt or to further mistrust of others, or it may be relieving if it helps resolve ongoing uncertainty.

Prognostic Indicators

Richard Kluft pioneered early treatment for complex developmental dissociative forms of PTSD, particularly DID (Kluft, 1984, 1985, 1999). In 1994, he documented different "treatment trajectories" that had to do with the unique circumstance of each client and his or her strengths/resources and liabilities and other factors related to a client's capacity to make use of the treatment and to result in positive outcomes. He posited three main trajectories. Clients in the *low trajectory* typically had conditions of chronic trauma and chronic mental illness, chaotic lives and unstable families, multiple crises, self-injury and suicidality, addictions, limited support and motivation, and difficulty agreeing to and abiding by the therapeutic agenda. Many had long histories of unsuccessful treatment and their prognosis for recovery was generally poor. *Middle trajectory* clients were in better shape overall, that is, they had more stability in their lives and greater resources at their disposal, yet still required years of treatment in order to achieve a stable recovery. They had more personal resources to call upon, but emotional regulation was a major treatment task. They also had a general mistrust of therapy and therapists but not to the degree of their low trajectory peers and they were more likely to develop a treatment alliance over time and to agree to and abide by the treatment goals. *High trajectory* clients, as the name implies, have the most personal and interpersonal capacities to apply—their treatment is likely to be the least crisis-prone and the most efficient and to take the least amount of time. Based on observations of the trajectories of clients in his own caseload and in his inpatient treatment population, Kluft developed a preliminary tool for assessment of the client's prognosis, The Dimensions of Therapeutic Movement Instrument (DTMI). He was able to show that a number of individual and contextual factors could be associated with therapeutic capacity and progress (Kluft, 1994a). This model is helpful to therapists in determining possible prognosis but also in understanding that not all clients heal from trauma and certainly that not all heal in the same way or to the same degree of emotional resolution and life enhancement.

Recently, Baars et al. (2011) extended this work in predicting stabilizing treatment outcomes based on an expertise-based prognostic model for the treatment of complex PTSD and DID. Based on two waves of expert therapist surveys, the researchers developed a prognostic model for the treatment of complex trauma that contained 51 factors clustered into 8 main categories: lack of motivation; lack of healthy relationships; lack of healthy therapeutic relationships; lack of other internal and external resources; serious Axis I comorbidity; serious Axis II comorbidity; poor attachment; and self-destruction. An additional 5 DID-specific items were constructed. The model they developed supports the current sequenced treatment model described in this book and elsewhere (Chu, 2011; Courtois, 1999, 2010; Courtois & Ford, 2009; Ford, Courtois, Steele, Van der Hart, & Nijenhuis, 2005; Herman, 1992b; Steele, Van der Hart, & Nijenhuis, 2001, and others). At the present stage of the development of this model, therapists can use the factors and clusters as a checklist that assists them in determining their clients' relative strengths and weaknesses and likely prognoses and trajectory. This information can assist in the assessment and treatment planning aspects of the treatment. Quoting the study's authors: "Therapists can use the results of the checklist to focus their therapeutic attention toward specific treatment goals related to the prognostic categories (e.g., improving treatment motivation), or, in the case of a low total score, they can be aware that treatment goals might be limited to the stabilization phase only" (Baars et al., 2011, pp. 84–85).

PULLING IT ALL TOGETHER: COMPREHENSIVE AND DESCRIPTIVE DIAGNOSIS

As discussed in the first two chapters, arriving at a postassessment diagnostic formulation for a complex trauma client is complicated by the number of symptoms and developmental consequences that span more than one diagnostic category (or axis in the DSM system) and the co-occurring symptoms that are in evidence or that emerge over the course of treatment. Research has found that among patients with PTSD, 80% have at least one associated disorder (Brady, 1997) and that traumatic or dissociative symptoms are frequently misdiagnosed, most often as bipolar, schizoaffective, or psychotic (Read, 1997; Ross, 1996). Difficulties in differential diagnosis occur because traumatic stress symptoms can resemble and mimic those of other mental disturbances and because some DSM diagnostic formulations lack clarity and rigor. As specifically suggested in DSM-IV-TR (American Psychiatric Association, 2000), multiple diagnoses (listed in descending order of priority) within each axis can and should be given when necessary to describe the current condition.

The conceptualization of complex PTSD/DESNOS is a more parsimonious way of organizing multiple symptoms and associated diagnoses (including symptoms not included in the current PTSD diagnosis) across different axes in the DSM system, as is the diagnosis of "enduring personality change after catastrophic events" included in ICD-10 (World Health Organization, 2005). Both of these match what therapists usually see in clients with complex trauma, and they offer a way of organizing and explaining complex symptoms and prioritizing the treatment. We recently offered the following inclusive formulation to account for these elements: "*Complex traumatic sequelae* are the changes in mind, emotions, body, and relationships experienced following complex psychological trauma, including severe problems with dissociation, emotion dysregulation, somatic distress, or relational or spiritual alienation, hereafter referred to as *complex traumatic stress disorders*" (Courtois & Ford, 2009, p. 13; italics in original). The therapist who utilizes one of these formulations will likely find them highly applicable and useful but must be aware that *complex PTSD or complex traumatic stress disorders are not freestanding diagnoses in the DSM and should not be assigned as such* (nor can they be used for insurance purposes, except as an associated feature of PTSD).

CONCLUSION

Goals for the treatment of complex trauma that include but extend beyond those developed for the symptoms of more standard forms of PTSD were outlined and discussed in this chapter. Assessment before goal setting and treatment is a necessity and an ethical imperative. Issues surrounding assessment and assessment instruments tied into particular goals were discussed, as were challenges and pitfalls of assessment of which the evaluator must be aware. The latter part of the chapter reviewed how the conceptualization of complex PTSD helps to pull the various assessment and treatment strands together to assist in the planning and implementation of an organized and systematic treatment. We now turn to the next two chapters in which we describe the three phases of the recommended sequenced treatment model and their associated goals and tasks.

CHAPTER 5

Phase 1

Safety, Stabilization, and Engagement— Measured in Skills, Not Time

This chapter begins with a brief review of the sequenced three-phase treatment model for complex trauma that follows the assessment pretreatment described in the previous chapter. The first phase, the focus of this chapter, has as its primary emphasis personal and environmental safety and safety planning as needed. The aftereffects of trauma cannot be treated successfully if the client is still in danger from others. In such a circumstance, he or she needs to continue to use survival defenses. Additionally, if a client is a danger to him- or herself in any way and/or is involved in compulsive activities or has active addictions, these require early intervention (however some degree of trauma processing might need to occur before a client is truly free from self-harming behavior or before he or she can give up addictions or compulsions). While safety is being addressed, other tasks such as educating the client about trauma and posttraumatic reactions and laying the foundation of the therapy relationship can take place. As well, the client must be assisted in the development of specific skills, especially emotion identification and methods to achieve emotional regulation.

Once a relative degree of safety and self-regulation have been achieved, these skills can be further developed and others that increase self-control and establish ongoing life stabilization introduced. This phase involves "resourcing" the client and building on his or her available strengths and resilience. It might also involve the introduction of skills in stress management and self-care that begin to address posttraumatic symptoms and those of associated anxiety and mood disorders. Assessment for medication and treatment of illnesses or medical conditions might also be indicated. Some clients (typically those with lower trajectory prognosis) are unable to move beyond Phase 1 and some are satisfied with the gains made in Phase 1 and choose not to go further in the process.

The second phase of the sequenced model is designed to help the client face and process the trauma and its attendant emotions, beliefs, and cognitions in enough detail to achieve mastery over its memory and the emotion states associated with traumatic stress symptoms and those of co-occuring disorders. The client uses the self- and emotion-regulation skills learned in the previous phase and applies them to the emotions associated with the trauma. In this phase, the triad of symptoms of PTSD (i.e., intrusive reexperiencing, avoidance, and hypervigilance) is treated directly through a variety of exposure, adaptive resolution, and emotion-based techniques while further strengthening and expanding the capacity for emotion tolerance and regulation. The exposure to the trauma must be carefully balanced so as not to overwhelm the client's capacity. If the client is challenged beyond his or her emotional tolerance, a return to previous maladaptive coping skills often results in relapse and is a major issue for the therapist to attend to. Clients must be encouraged to return to the skills first introduced in Phase 1 in order to reestablish safety and stability before proceeding with the processing. Again, safety is the foundation, and the ability to modulate emotions is the skill essential to the processing and resolution of past trauma.

Phase 2 requires a high degree of motivation on the part of the client and ongoing support and encouragement from the therapist. The emergence of long-suppressed feelings and details of the trauma can be daunting for both. Processing involves facing and accepting the victimization and its associated personal and life toll. When processing is successful, the client is more in control of his or her reactions and not as subject to posttraumatic emotional hijacking. The ability to successfully resolve past trauma leads to greater personal control, a sense of empowerment and hope rather than helplessness and hopelessness. Moreover, once a client understands more and can put the pieces of the story together into a more coherent narrative, he or she has increased self-understanding and self-compassion, resulting in improved self-esteem, along with more capacity for self-determination and assertiveness.

Phase 3 involves applying the skills, knowledge, and increased self-worth and self-confidence acquired in the first two phases to all facets of current (and future) daily life. This crucial consolidation of therapeutic gains serves as a new lease on life for many. Issues that were previously unaddressed or unmanageable are usually undertaken during this phase. Many involve relationships with others (e.g., friendships, intimate relationships, parenting of one's own children, relationships with abusive others from the past or in the present) and the client's changed attachment style to one of "earned secure" is applied in these other relationships.

Although systemic therapy modalities (group, couple, and family therapy) can be introduced at any treatment phase, they are more likely to occur in the latter phases after clients have a more developed sense of self, greater capacity for emotional regulation, and more realistic expectations of relationships based on increased attachment security. The specifics of Phases 2 and 3 are presented in Chapter 6 and systemic treatments in Chapter 7. We now return to the detailed discussion of Phase 1, the focus of the current chapter.

PHASE 1

The first phase of psychotherapy with clients with complex trauma histories builds on the pretreatment assessment and is specifically directed toward "resourcing" the client. It resembles more general forms of psychotherapy and models developed for PTSD treatment more specifically. It focuses on further identification of client strength and resilience (including survival skills and adaptations) on which to build; continued assessment of client attachment style in order to tailor approaches and strategies; continued assessment of risk and danger (and the active teaching of skills for the maintenance of whatever safety is possible); ongoing education on victimization and trauma, including symptoms and secondary elaborations, and on complex trauma and its developmental impacts; engagement of the client in treatment and the development of the treatment alliance; and skills training for emotion regulation, life enhancement, and stabilization. As we have shown, these goals do not occur spontaneously, but instead require careful planning, deliberate education, and directed action by the therapist.

Some clients with secure attachment histories and more personal and interpersonal resources (i.e., high trajectory clients) may have many of the tasks and skills of this phase mastered and so will spend little or no time on safety, alliance building, skill development, and life stabilization before moving to directed work on the trauma. On the other hand, clients with insecure attachment styles, and especially those whose styles are disorganized or unresolved, may need to spend large amounts of time mastering the tasks and skills of this phase, and some never move beyond this phase. This does not imply failure, as clients who achieve the goals of this phase benefit directly. As discussed in Chapter 2, clients are individuals, with idiosyncratic needs and resources and differing prognoses and treatment trajectories (Baers et al., 2012; Kluft, 1994).

We now turn our attention to the essential tasks of safety assessment and planning, stabilization, enhancing readiness for change and motivation, and building a therapeutic working relationship. The final section of this chapter is devoted to the elements of the therapeutic setting and therapist style that play a role in assisting the client in establishing safety, stability, and engaging in this foundational treatment phase.

Ensuring Safety

A key initial task is to help the client to establish sufficient safety and stability to diminish exposure to any current stress, life instability, and imminent danger. Only with a decrease in danger or its ongoing threat can the client begin to disengage the "survival brain" in order to engage the "learning brain" (Ford, 2009b, 2009c) in the therapy and in outside life.

By definition, individuals who have been traumatized have been made unsafe. The individual who is still in danger, whether from self or others, will be hard-pressed to lower emotional defenses and to process posttraumatic symptoms sufficiently to heal. The *treatment must be geared towards the development of safety in the client's life*, something that might be both a short- and long-term goal and an ongoing process that can take a long time to achieve. In some cases, quite realistically, it might not be very achievable (i.e., for those who live in violent communities or cultures and who have no option to move). It might also be built on the achievement or resolution of some other treatment issues (e.g., leaving an abusive relationship, becoming clean and sober, finding a safe place to live, achieving financial or other life stability, and, in some cases, processing traumatic events sufficiently to foster safety).

As discussed in Chapter 3, the therapist's initial emphasis on physical and psychological safety can be very surprising and disconcerting to those who have rarely (or never) had anyone concerned about their safety. Therapists certainly cannot change the objective circumstances of a client's life, nor is it their function to serve as case manager to organize the client's life or to get the resources needed for safety and stability (although in some settings the two roles overlap). The major way that therapists *can* uniquely contribute to clients' safety and stability is by helping them to do a personal assessment of safety issues, to educate them, and to develop a realistic and detailed plan for dealing with—rather than being unaware or avoidant of—threats to safety or psychosocial stability or of being repeatedly revictimized.

Addressing safety (as discussed in the last chapter) involves assessment of the presence and severity of potentially dangerous conditions in the environment (e.g., abusive others, domestic or community violence, abuse, drugs, weapons) and symptoms (e.g., suicidality, self-harm, aggression, impulsivity, addiction, dissociative fugue). Although it is essential to assess these critical indicators of danger from the outset of treatment and to monitor them throughout, it is not realistic for the therapist to assume responsibility for eradicating danger from the client's life. It is entirely understandable that for both altruistic and self-serving reasons—a combination of the desire to preserve the client's welfare and save them from further harm and to contain personal anxiety and sense of powerlessness—therapists feel a strong urge to rescue their clients. When a client's transference includes the wish to be protected or saved, the therapist may experience a strong countertransference reaction as the client's rescuer.

However, from a developmental and strengths-based perspective, safety is most likely to be attained not when the therapist rescues but when he or she assists the client in developing a realistic awareness and appraisal of potential dangers and a sense of both responsibility and options for maintaining personal safety. The way that therapy can best enhance client safety is—with rare exceptions—not by attempting to eliminate danger from the client's life nor by exhorting the client to do so. In fact, when therapists pressure their clients to take obvious steps to eliminate or confront sources of physical danger, this can backfire—in some cases tragically. Simplistic solutions to chronic or complex dangers (e.g., "Just stand up to that aggressor"; "Just leave that abusive relationship") can lead to severe backlash in the client's relationships and community that may cause more harm than good. Furthermore, a "quick fix" approach communicates a distrust in the client's own judgment and ability to determine when and how best to deal with danger, and such distrust can undermine both the client's self-efficacy and the therapeutic alliance. Although objective danger should never be ignored or taken lightly, therapy can best help reduce the client's vulnerability by increasing awareness either of the danger itself or of ways to proactively separate from and escape it. Alternatively, the client can be taught to deescalate and transform it into a manageable challenge that results in safety from further harm.

Ensuring safety also includes careful attention to the objective set of conditions that make up the client's life circumstances, including place of residence, neighborhood/community, and workplace or school, recreation, self-improvement, relationships and their quality, and socioeconomic resources and barriers. It is quite usual for these clients to underestimate the degree of actual or potential danger they face on an ongoing basis, as it may be the norm for them and all they know. They may use their "tried and true" coping skills, such as dissociation or drugs, to manage their fears, strategies that paradoxically render them more vulnerable. Although it is not totally in the therapist's purview to determine what is or is not acceptable in terms of objective safety, it is clinically and ethically warranted for therapists to carefully assess and evaluate the nature and extent of actual or potential threats to safety and to raise concerns directly in the context of discussion of realistic options and constraints for its maintenance. It is important not to become so caught up in the client's emotional distress on the one hand or in the client's apparent indifference, detachment, powerlessness, or hopelessness on the other that objective threats to the client's safety go unnoticed are not thoughtfully discussed. Moreover, it is important to follow jurisdictional reporting requirements, where warranted.

A second area to be assessed regarding safety is how the client subjectively makes sense of and deals with these life circumstances, including his or her degree of awareness and appraisal. Because the objective conditions of the client's life generally are beyond the therapist's ability to change, it is these subjective appraisals and perspectives that undergird the client's behavioral responses that the therapist should seek to influence. When the therapist demonstrates sincere interest in understanding both the client's objective circumstances and the subjective meaning assigned to them, he or she can help the client consider not only how to change perspective but also how to change behaviors. This can be a way to regain hope, as well as to improve actual life circumstances, especially important for clients who profoundly devalue themselves, who are self-defeating, or who have become resigned to being victimized. It also provides a model for how therapy can help the client recognize, plan ways to address, and actually achieve goals that are of personal importance. As therapy progresses, the therapeutic "field of vision" can expand to include other goals of importance to the client, such as being able to enjoy rather than dread life challenges and opportunities. However, *safety is the focus in early treatment, as it lays the groundwork for other goals directed toward life stabilization and enhancement—that is, for a life without ongoing danger, abuse, victimization, and other forms of trauma.*

Two examples illustrate the importance of dealing with safety right from the start. The first involves the external danger faced when an individual is in a primary relationship with a violent and emotionally abusive partner. Engaging in therapy can actually intensify the danger because it might threaten a controlling and insecure partner (e.g., fearing exposure of the "secret" battering, losing control of the abused partner, having a third party influence the partner, or facing the risk that the partner might feel sufficiently strong and supported to actually leave the relationship). It is crucial in the first phase of treatment to educate the client concerning known patterns of violence and abuse and to develop a shared understanding of the full extent of actual and potential danger and how she or he has remained in the relationship and has handled the danger. Rather than insisting that the client must leave the relationship in order to remain in treatment, it is preferable to brainstorm the pros and cons. If undertaking therapy is judged to pose overly great risks, then the therapist can assist the client in getting other sources of immediate help (e.g., from domestic violence shelters or legal advocates) while leaving the door open for a return to therapy once safety from immediate danger is established.

The other major threat to personal safety may be internal and self-generated rather than due to external factors. It usually results from a combination of risk taking, danger seeking, disinhibition, impulsivity, emotional lability, self-injury, and suicidality and feelings of fear, anxiety, depression, and dissociation, not infrequently supported by substance abuse. Clients with these problems may be in real danger (as the case of **Hector** demonstrates). Indeed, they may have previously been refused treatment for being too dangerous and out of control. Treatment is oriented toward helping the client to understand the possible motivations and reasons behind self-endangerment in order to begin planning ways to gain control over impulses. This may take a great deal of time and effort. The initial screening or assessment is a first opportunity to provide a prospective client with education about the role of traumatic stress reactions in contributing to the vicious cycle of emotional dysregulation (e.g., feelings and thoughts of hopelessness, helplessness, or worthlessness), resignation and isolation, and the use of suicide, self-harm, self-disregard, or addiction to escape from or control the emotional pain and entrapment (or as a reenactment of feelings associated with being abused and abandoned). This education is then continued in the safety-oriented work of Phase 1.

The focus on personal safety does not mean that the client must defer treatment for traumatic stress problems until she or he has achieved control of all high-risk symptoms. Therapy should not be framed as "all or nothing," with the client pressured into making a commitment to personal safety that is not possible to keep as a condition of remaining in treatment; however, the client must develop motivation to change and must make an honest effort to develop a personal safety plan (rather than a safety contract, as described later in this book) and to work its various steps. Safety planning is an ongoing process that involves building a hierarchy of practical steps (optimally suggested by the client, who determines what is feasible and doable) that the client agrees to implement when he or she begins to identify risk of danger from self or others. The client's achievement of a sufficient degree of safety to be able to engage productively in therapy without unacceptable and avoidable risk (and related liability for the therapist) is the first step on which to base additional treatment goals and tasks. Shapiro noted that some clients are paradoxically unable to achieve safety until they have processed traumatic material sufficiently to allow them to be safe (Francine Shapiro, personal communication, 2011).

Stabilization

In other cases, symptoms may not be so imminent a threat to a client's safety but nevertheless compromise the ability to function in daily life and to engage productively in therapy. As discussed in previous chapters, symptoms are debilitating and severely affect the life quality of clients with complex trauma. Fortunately, a variety of therapeutic approaches, including cognitive-behavioral and interpersonal psychotherapies (some evidence-based) have shown promise in stabilizing and reducing anxiety (Meichenbaum, 1985; Stangier, Von Consbruch, Schramm, & Heidenreich, 2010) or depressive symptoms. Dialectical behavior therapy (DBT; Linehan, 1993) and mindfulness models of psychotherapy such as acceptance and commitment therapy (ACT; Hayes, Luoma, Bond, Masuda, & Lillis, 2006) help clients tolerate and regulate extreme emotional reactivity and even psychotic symptoms. Clinical reports have described the application of these treatments, which were originally developed for clients with borderline personality disorder, to clients with complex trauma (Follette, La Bash, & Sewell, 2010; Harned, Jackson, Comtois, & Linehan, 2010; Vujanovic, Youngwirth, Johnson, & Zvolensky, 2009; Wagner, Rizvi, & Harned, 2007). Several pharmacotherapy agents also contribute to reducing the severity of these symptoms (Laddis, 2011; Opler et al., 2009). Gold (2000) has discussed the significance of teaching basic life skills such as assertiveness, decision-making, home organizing, and so on to enhance life stability.

The stabilization of even one, let alone several, chronic and persistent symptoms can seem an overwhelming problem—especially if little progress, or at most transient partial remission, has been accomplished in any previous episodes of treatment. Yet it is essential to stabilize symptoms and life circumstances that are causing emotional distress (these often meet criteria of chronic stress and are in addition to the traumatic stress) in order to increase the client's ability to think clearly and to maintain and increase functioning. These skills are also needed for the client to address the posttraumatic legacy. A recent study demonstrated that the trauma-memory-processing component of therapy for women with childhood abuse histories and PTSD was better tolerated (i.e., 50% fewer dropouts) and more effective when preceded by therapy sessions designed to enhance skill in emotion regulation and interpersonal effectiveness (Skills Training for Affect and Interpersonal Regulation [STAIR]; Cloitre et al., 2010). Elements of that therapy model, and other similar interventions designed to enhance emotion regulation, attachment security, and personal agency—for example, Trauma Affect Regulation: Guide for Education and Therapy (TARGET; Ford et al., in press-a, in press-b); Seeking Safety (Najavits, 2002a); and emotion-focused therapy (EFT; Paivio, Jarry, Chagigiorgis, Hall, & Ralston, 2010; Paivio & Nieuwenhuis, 2001)—provide strategies that can be adapted by therapists for symptom and life stabilization with complex trauma survivors. A number of books for therapists and workbooks for clients on skill building and symptom and emotional regulation are now available. (See Self-Help Resources and Workbooks in the online supplement to this book.)

Focusing

A first step in symptom stabilization is gaining or regaining the presence of mind necessary to observe life problems or symptoms and to be able to discuss them rather than being flooded by or habitually repeating them without control or relief. The sophisticated self-reflection or "mentalizing" (Allen et al., 2008, 2012) required to therapeutically process trauma memories or traumatic stress symptoms begins with the simpler but still difficult mental act of reorienting attention to the present moment. This has been described variously as "grounding" (Horowitz, 1997), mentalization (Allen, 2012), mindfulness (Hayes et al., 2006; Linehan, 1993) and experiential (Gendlin, 1982) or mental focusing (Ford & Russo, 2006).

Experiential (Fosha, Siegel, & Solomon, 2009; Paivio & Pascual-Leone, 2010) and sensorimotor (Fisher & Ogden, 2009; Ogden & Fisher, 2013) treatments provide a variety of techniques for therapists to use in modeling and guiding clients in the practice of directing their attention to the present moment and to "stilling" or quieting. A widely used basic approach is to help the client to do a mental scan of physical sensations (e.g., tension, tightness, pain, warmth, and strength).

Meditative approaches to attentional reorienting engage clients in nonjudgmental self-observation of spontaneous thoughts or in the breathing or in a selected thought or image as a focal point on which to concentrate. Cognitive-behavioral models teach clients to use body awareness or simple body movements (e.g., tensing and relaxing muscle groups) or visual images (e.g., visualizing a place that is associated with feeling peaceful and safe) to enhance physical and mental relaxation. Such focusing interventions have the dual benefit of shifting attention temporarily away from symptoms and associated distress while teaching clients experientially and behaviorally to change or distract from their ruminative thoughts rather than passively being preoccupied or overwhelmed by them. Thus a preliminary step in symptom stabilization is helping the client to understand through experiential learning that thoughts and feelings need not control his or her mind, thinking, or actions; rather, they can be observed and selectively focused on, to increase personal control. For many clients, this is a major revelation and forms the basis for increased self-control and behavioral change.

Behavior-Analytic Interventions to Enhance Mindful Awareness

The second step in symptom reduction is increased rather than decreased awareness of both the symptom and its precursors. From a behavioral-analytic perspective (Follette, Iverson, & Ford, 2009), every symptom (or feeling, thought, or behavior) is a part of a "chain" that includes antecedents (i.e., precursor events or stimuli), the symptom itself, and consequences (i.e., subsequent events or stimuli that increase or decrease the likelihood of the symptom recurring), sometimes abbreviated as the A–B–C (antecedents–behavior–consequences) chain. Symptoms tend to be more manageable if they are consciously recognized, rather than actively avoided, dissociated, or otherwise not noticed and if their antecedents and consequences also are recognized. Self-monitoring of symptoms can, without any other intervention, lead to a reduction in their frequency and severity.

This process is fundamentally different from the alternating pattern of first avoiding awareness and then ruminating obsessively, typical of PTSD. The act of consciously and purposefully paying attention to symptoms and their antecedents and consequences makes the symptoms more an objective target for thoughtful observation than an intolerable source of subjective anxiety, dysphoria, and frustration. In ACT, the act of accepting symptoms as an expectable feature of a disorder or illness, has been shown to be associated with relief rather than increased distress (Hayes et al., 2006). From a traumatic stress perspective, any symptom can be reframed as an understandable, albeit unpleasant and difficult to cope with, reaction or survival skill (Ford, 2009b, 2009c). In this way, monitoring symptoms and their environmental or experiential/body state "triggers" can enhance client's willingness and ability to reflectively observe them without feeling overwhelmed, terrified, or powerless. This is not only beneficial for personal and life stabilization but is also essential to the successful processing of traumatic events and reactions that occur in the next phase of therapy (Ford & Russo, 2006).

Cognitive-Behavioral Interventions to Enhance Self-Management Skills

Therapeutic interventions designed originally for the treatment of fears and phobias (e.g., systematic desensitization, flooding), anxiety (e.g., relaxation training, biofeedback, cognitive therapy), and obsessive–compulsive disorder (e.g., exposure and response prevention) are very helpful in stabilization and skill building. These interventions offer education and practical self-management skills that have been described as "stress inoculation training" (SIT; Meichenbaum, 1985; Meichenbaum & Novaco, 1985; Saunders, Driskell, Johnston, & Salas, 1996) or "anxiety management training" (AMT; Hembree, 2008). SIT and AMT involve instructing patients about why and how to use cognitive and behavioral skills to recognize and intentionally reduce anxious feelings (e.g., cognitive restructuring: reevaluating and replacing anxiety-evoking beliefs) and physiological arousal (e.g., progressive muscle relaxation, guided imagery, autogenics). When these skills were repeatedly practiced and honed, substantial improvement in the hyperarousal symptom cluster was achieved by a number of participants in small studies. Clinically, SIT and AMT make sense for clients who have had little helpful guidance or role modeling in how to cope with stress reactions. However, with adults who are suffering from PTSD or ASD in the wake of a traumatic event, SIT and AMT have not been shown to consistently provide relief from the intrusive reexperiencing of unwanted memories and reminders of traumatic events (Cahill, Rothbaum, Resick, & Follette, 2009), necessitating the use of other interventions.

Not surprisingly, even when arousal can be reduced using SIT or AMT skills, the continuing struggle with unwanted memories and reliving of traumatic dilemmas in otherwise innocuous current experiences can cause sufficient distress to evoke conscious and involuntary forms of avoidance, thus perpetuating rather than breaking the vicious cycle of intrusion–avoidance–hyperarousal in PTSD. Trauma memory processing therapies therefore were developed to assist trauma survivors in therapeutically recalling, rather than avoiding, intrusive memories of traumatic experiences (see Phase 2 in Chapter 6, this volume).

Enhancing Readiness for Change through Education

Client education is an integral component of Phase 1 and optimally begins right from the start of treatment. As many traumatized individuals know little or nothing about trauma and posttraumatic reactions, they have limited understanding that their symptoms may be related to their past experiences, making education about trauma and its impact extremely important. It may effectively help a client to understand reactions and to develop increased personal perspective and compassion, and may even result in a lessening of prominent symptoms such as depression and self-blame (Allen, 2005; Jehu, 1988). Additionally, it can demystify the process of psychotherapy, an endeavor that might be terrifying to these clients. Education is also the foundation for teaching specific skills that cover a number of domains: the identification and regulation of emotional states and the development of assertiveness, coping, problem solving, decision making, personal mindfulness, self-care, and social functioning. Affect identification, regulation, and modulation are perhaps the most important self-regulatory skills to develop.

Relationships and a personal support network are also crucial to address in this treatment phase. Therapy must help clients to acquire more interpersonal skills, including the ability to negotiate relationships and to develop a reasonable degree of trust in others. Optimally, the treatment relationship starts the process by providing the client a new model of attachment, a "secure base" from which to explore different ways to be in relationship with trustworthy and reciprocal others. Group therapy can also assist in this regard (see Chapter 7).

Individuals in treatment progress through a number of "stages of change" (Prochaska & DiClemente, 1992). At the start, most clients are either in the precontemplation or contemplation stage, either not viewing change as desirable or necessary or just beginning to consider that change may be possible and worth attempting. A primary goal in the first phase of therapy is therefore for the client to move from precontemplation or contemplation into the next stage, preparation for change. It is important to bear in mind, however, that being (or even feeling) ready and prepared to change can feel alien and be anxiety provoking, no matter how well the preparation has gone, because these clients may have phobias about changing and even about being prepared to do so. Traumatic stressors, by definition, do not permit a person to be more than partially prepared. Even when these events or experiences occur repeatedly and somewhat predictably (e.g., for military or emergency response personnel or for victims of chronic childhood abuse or domestic violence), there is no way to be fully ready for the next exposure (even with hypervigilance and anticipatory anxiety) because its exact timing and nature are uncertain. The victim learns to try not to be a target and to be continuously on alert for the inevitable, whenever it comes. As a result, being or feeling prepared without the accompanying anxiety can seem like a luxury that simply is not possible.

What is more, many of these clients have had their core expectations for the future—whether it is possible, realistic, or safe to prepare for one—challenged, diminished, or destroyed. Like other survivors of more delimited types of trauma, they have a sense of a foreshortened future and hopelessness about any possibility of having a happy and satisfying life. They may have learned that any attempt is doomed to fail and that preparation and anticipation are simply futile, a trap that causes false hopes to develop (e.g., that being prepared can reduce exposure to further trauma or enable them not to be as overwhelmed when the next traumatic shock occurs) or that it will result in a false sense of confidence against the inevitability of the next traumatic experience. The discouragement associated with failure makes it easier to be passively resigned to being a victim and hopeless regarding the possibility of change.

Related perspectives and beliefs are often at play when clients are encouraged to actively engage in therapy. They may revert to a stance of passivity, to having it "done to them" rather than carrying it out. Collaboration may be quite at odds with what they have experienced previously, and they may resist any active involvement in goal setting and in working on agreed-upon therapy goals and associated tasks. Even when clients recognize that therapy is an active rather than a reactive or passive endeavor, they may be hampered by the inertia created by many years or even a lifetime of habitual avoidance. Chu (2011) discussed such "chronic disempowerment" and advised therapists to challenge clients to do what they have agreed to do, *even if they do not want to*, from a position of empathic rather than direct confrontation. Gold (2009) gave a compelling example of a therapist challenging a recalcitrant client who actively avoided doing agreed-upon therapeutic tasks and who resisted his efforts while complaining that expected change was not happening.

Another potential trauma-related reaction against therapeutic engagement involves the typical "fight–flight–freeze" defensive reactions to danger. When trauma is ongoing, entrapping, and inescapable, one further reaction has been noted to occur in humans as it does in animals, namely, collapse or "tonic immobility" (Marx, Forsyth, Gallup, Fuse, & Lexington, 2008), a state of involuntary biological shutdown (Porges, 2011, 2013). This immobility is a form of dissociation and involves both psychic shutdown (e.g., catatonia, loss of ability to maintain consciousness) and somatoform symptoms (e.g., physical collapse and paralysis, inability to respond to stimuli, blindness, deafness, analgesia, anesthesia; Nijenhuis et al., 2001; Porges, 2011, 2013). Tonic immobility is now recognized as a response to traumatic victimization that is more common than previously recognized and that might be lifesaving in that it keeps the victim from struggling (and possibly being more injured or even killed) and provides relief from physical sensations through analgesia and anesthesia.

This state of immobility may actually occur during the course of treatment, both in and out of sessions. Its occurrence should be treated as an indication that the individual is totally overwhelmed (often due to multiple life crises or to triggers in and out of the treatment, the pace and pressure of the treatment, insufficient stabilization and emotion regulation, and possibly to ongoing abuse and having been recently revictimized) to the point of not being able to maintain consciousness and personal awareness. If it occurs in the session (e.g., the client stills, collapses, or "faints," closes his or her eyes, takes shallow breaths, is unresponsive but still conscious), the best practice is to first attempt to "ground" the client using the least restrictive approaches (such as encouraging him or her to open closed eyes, to breathe, to pay attention to the surroundings, to focus on colors or objects in the room, to the therapist and his or her voice, to physical grounding through sensory stimulation and engagement, including the therapist's touch—but only with permission—and mindfulness interventions such as those discussed earlier). If these are not successful after an extended period of time and the client is not able to restabilize safely in the "here-and-now," more intensive or longer term interventions become necessary. In cases in which clients cannot be "brought back," psychiatric evaluation in the emergency room and/or hospitalization is usually indicated.

Beginning in the pretreatment phase, a combination of motivational enhancement (Miller & Rollnick, 2009, 2012) and paradoxical prescription (Selvini, Boscolo, Cecchin, & Prata, 1980) may be used to prepare clients for therapy. Motivational enhancement involves helping them to carefully consider the pros and cons of change, including: (1) what they view as important to change in their lives and their own personal reasons for wanting to change, particularly based on discrepancies between their goals and values and their actual outcomes and actions in their lives; and (2) what they do not want to change or view as lower priorities for change and the reasons why they do not want to change in these areas, as well as in areas in which they *do* want to change, particularly identifying perceived costs of attempting or achieving change. With an examination of both sides, clients can make an informed choice and feel more in control about what they are willing and able to work on in therapy and what they are not.

Personal control and the ability to choose involve a fundamental paradigm shift for many of these clients, as they are not just permitted but actually encouraged and assisted in articulating their fears, reservations, and limitations and in making personal choices without criticism, judgment, or negative consequence. This therapeutic dialogue offers the opportunity to experience the freedom to identify and express goals, values, aspirations, and intentions with empathic validation and thoughtful reflection on their views and preferences. Although this type of preparatory motivational enhancement is important in any psychotherapy, it is crucially important with complex trauma clients, as coercion, exploitation, stigma, and disempowerment have made up their template for how relationships work and do not work.

Motivational enhancement also involves "rolling with the resistance" (Miller & Rollnick, 2009), that is, finding ways to nonjudgmentally acknowledge and redirect clients' subtle and obvious attempts to avoid either engagement in the therapeutic dialogue or the practicing of new skills (or their application outside of the treatment setting). Clients may be reluctant to explicitly state their feelings, especially when they feel pressured, overwhelmed, or in disagreement with the therapist's suggestions and observations due to patterns of learned and superficial compliance. A key way to prevent or reduce the likelihood or intensity of client pushback or avoidance is for the therapist to be very circumspect and cautious about making suggestions until the client feels that the therapist has enough knowledge to (1) have his or her best interests at heart; (2) anticipate areas of particular sensitivity, posttraumatic reactivity, and hypervigilance; (3) gauge the client's emotional capacity and tolerance; and (4) phrase suggestions as natural logical extensions of what the client already is saying or thinking. When a client avoids or takes an opposing stance, the therapist can then "roll with the resistance" by empathically validating the core concerns and goals that underlie this "resistance." This process communicates that the therapist and client are not in opposition but in fact are fundamentally on the same side.

Even if the therapist fully intends to "roll with the resistance," when clients hold beliefs, state intentions, or engage in behaviors that have substantial downsides, it can be difficult for him or her not to get caught in a knee-jerk reaction of overprotecting, rescuing, teaching, or correcting the client (not to mention such other reactions as criticizing, judging, chastising, or feeling and communicating disgust). At the start of treatment, such client beliefs or incidents are quite common and might lessen only with considerable therapeutic focus and engagement. Clients may be acting on what they know or have learned from their past exposure to negative role modeling that has made risky or harmful behavior acceptable or even desirable. Alternately, these beliefs and behaviors can result in reenactments and repetition compulsions designed to gain a sense of mastery (i.e., by being the one to engage in and control the behavior rather than being the victim). The "prescription" is not a tacit or explicit statement of permission or endorsement of any specific choice about how to think or act but a shift in focus to validate the client's right to give opinions and to give due consideration to each choice. The paradox is not that the therapist prescribes any specific choice but that he or she supports the client in considering the pros and cons of any important decision. Complex trauma usually involves exactly the opposite prescription, namely, that the client must do what a victimizer requires with neither the right nor the ability to rethink, challenge, or change that choice. It often takes many sessions and repeated therapeutic interaction and encouragement for the client to acquire a new set of emotionally significant experiences that are fundamentally different from those involved in victimization.

Building a Therapeutic Working Alliance

The development of a working alliance is crucial because it addresses a psychic phobia associated with relationships that is common in complex trauma clients. As we discussed, when primary relationships are sources of profound disillusionment, betrayal, and emotional pain, any subsequent relationship with an authority figure who offers an emotional bond or other assistance might be met with a range of emotions, such as fear, suspicion, anger, or hopelessness on the negative end of the continuum and idealization, hope, overdependence, and entitlement on the positive. Therapy offers a compensatory relationship, albeit within a professional framework, that has differences from and restrictions not found in other relationships. On the one hand, the therapist works within professional and ethical boundaries and limitations in a role of higher status and education and is therefore somewhat unattainable for the client. On the other, the therapist's ethical and professional mandate is the welfare of the client, creating the perception of an obligation to meet the client's needs and solve his or her problems. Furthermore, the therapist is expected to both respect the client's privacy and accept emotional and behavioral difficulties without judgment, while simultaneously being entitled to ask the client about his or her most personal and distressing feelings, thoughts, and experiences. Developing a sense of trust in the therapist, therefore, is both expected and fraught with inherent difficulties that are amplified by each client's unique history of betrayal trauma, loss, and relational distress.

Despite these difficulties, building a working alliance is an essential component in the development of personal safety and stabilization and a precursor to further therapeutic work. As well, the therapeutic relationship provides a crucial opportunity for clients to have a different relational experience involving trust and security from which to decrease their isolation and improve their relationship skills and expectations. Much has been written about the nature and essential function of the therapeutic relationship and working alliance in psychotherapy (see more discussion in the Part III of this book), so we focus here on how therapists can establish a collaborative alliance, given the difficulties and dilemmas a history of interpersonal trauma creates.

A core strategy is to explicitly acknowledge and reframe the threatening aspects of the relationship. Betrayal trauma results in the mistrust of others (particularly authority figures perceived as stand-ins for parents and others) or a paradoxical overreliance on them (Freyd, 1994). Therapists can clearly acknowledge and empathically validate clients' deep fear of being deceived and betrayed yet again, and their simultaneous longing for a trustworthy relationship. The therapist can convey that trust is not expected to be automatically given but that it needs to be earned over time through consistency, reliability, and honesty in the therapist's words and actions. Clients can be encouraged to expect that the therapist's actions are in accordance with what he or she has communicated verbally. They can further be encouraged to trust conditionally as they get to know the therapist while they continue to assess whether their trust is warranted. Yet they should also anticipate that the therapist is human and should not be held to an unrealistic standard of perfection. The therapist will make various mistakes and missteps but strive to rectify them in consultation with the client. It is this ability to discuss mistakes and to repair them that differs significantly from relationships in which lack of communication and punitive responses including emotional shutdown prevail.

The second alliance threat is fear of abandonment. In this case, it is important for the therapist to acknowledge the fear associated with being rejected or left. As noted in the previous paragraph, the reality of imperfection and the inevitability of empathic failures are realities. The therapist can discuss with the client up front that there will be times when he or she will not fully understand or pay sufficient attention to thoughts, feelings, or events that are of vital importance to the client. There will be other times when the therapist will not be fully available to or present with the client, including times when regular appointments cannot occur due to travel or vacation, when after-hours calls cannot be returned right away, or when not having had enough sleep or having competing professional or personal agendas lessens the ability to keep adequate focus in a session. These issues, too, can be noted and discussed by therapist and client, and the therapist must be able to acknowledge such lapses and discuss how to rectify them nondefensively and without retaliation. The counterbalancing message is that the therapist is striving to earn the client's trust despite being imperfect. Like caregivers, therapists can at best be "good enough" (Winnicott, 1971)—not perfect—in their responsiveness and availability.

A third threat to the alliance is the fear that the therapist might use her or his authority and expertise to intimidate, coerce, belittle, or otherwise usurp or violate the client. Clients who have experienced victimization, exploitation, devaluation, or retaliation by those in positions of authority are understandably prone to fear and to expect similar behavior from others. This expectation is heightened if the therapist presents as a detached and mysterious observer/evaluator, as the "authority on high," or as an overly indulgent and available purveyor of care and salvation. However, it is possible for even the best-intentioned therapist to feel an internal or external pressure to take a stance of hyperneutrality in order to maintain appropriate professional boundaries or to err in the opposite direction and try too hard to provide the client with remoralizing reassurance and hope. The challenge is for the therapist to maintain a stance of supportive openness and empathic attunement with limits and boundaries, the distance determined by the client's needs, personal resources, and the respective attachment styles of therapist and client. For example, clients with a preoccupied style may need a more engaged and available therapist, whereas the detached/avoidant client may need more distance, at least initially. The disorganized/dissociated client has difficulty regulating distance and is likely to behave in ways that are contradictory and confusing. The therapist needs awareness of his/her own attachment style and to modify his or her stance according to the client's requirements. (See Chapters 9 and 10 in this volume for in-depth discussion of these issues.)

A fourth alliance threat occurs with the client who has become resigned to, or even ambivalently comfortable with, the "sick" role. The therapist and the therapeutic process can threaten clients' dysfunctional but familiar and apparently manageable equilibrium by producing relief from symptoms and greater functionality. Whereas "neurotic" clients have been described as prone to avoid change by making a "flight into health" (i.e., claiming to have remarkably rapid symptom relief and resolution in order to avoid facing anxiety-provoking inner conflicts in therapy), some clients with complex trauma are more likely to flee in the opposite direction and report symptom worsening as a kind of rebound effect if their symptoms begin to diminish. For some, maintaining the "patient" role can be a way of maintaining the therapist's attention (this may be the most nurturing and important relationship the clients have ever experienced and thus not something they want to give up), and getting better runs the risk of losing the therapist.

The client's dependency needs must be accepted and understood rather than criticized (Steele et al., 2001). It is helpful from the start to indicate that therapy has varying durations and intensities depending on a number of factors and that it has an expected ending when goals are achieved or other issues intervene. It can be discussed as similar to what happens in a healthy and functional family. Children are nurtured and protected when young and dependent and then taught skills and encouraged in the processes of separation and differentiation and the ability to function independently and interdependently with others. Even so, it is important for the therapist to recognize the likelihood that a client's dependency needs will be awakened. For some, the therapeutic relationship literally feels like and functions as a lifeline; for others who have been starving emotionally the therapist's undivided attention and empathy feels like "manna from heaven." The client's legitimate neediness and dependency are issues that are acknowledged and provided for over the course of treatment, with the ultimate goals of self-discovery (individuation) and providing a relational foundation and skills (separation) to apply in extratherapeutic and "real-life" relationships. Therapists have a responsibility not to overindulge or overdeny the client, and they walk a "fine line" in being available (but not too available) with reasonable and appropriate limits and boundaries (we discuss this further as a dance of closeness and distancing in the therapeutic dyad in Chapters 9 and 10). Understanding the possibility of a client not progressing due to attachment needs from an empathic and validating perspective and discussing it in ways that do not pathologize or inadvertently communicate blame or fault can provide genuine relief and reduce anxiety about getting better.

A fifth major challenge to the alliance concerns adaptations that clients have made to survive traumatic experiences and to cope with the psychobiological symptoms that come from staying in "survival mode" (Chemtob, Roitblat, Hamada, Carlson, & Twentyman, 1988). Every approach to psychotherapy requires that the therapist construct a formulation of the key clinical issues that treatment aims to address, and regardless of the theory or terminology used, it is nothing less than a statement of what the therapist presumes to know that needs to be changed (e.g., the client's defenses, or "maladaptive" behavior or cognitions) or that serve as a foundation or basis for therapeutic change (e.g., the client's motivations, competences, or resources). In order to develop a truly individualized formulation, the therapist must, over time, increase understanding of the client's unique and defining characteristics that are reflected back to him or her. In turn, the client gains self-knowledge that was either missing or lost. This provides a basis for collaborating with and not simply abdicating all responsibility to the therapist and, over time, for autonomously extending the changes that are rehearsed or mapped out in psychotherapy sessions to everyday life.

Being known by the therapist and acquiring self-knowledge are important in achieving the pragmatic goals of psychotherapy (e.g., changes in problematic behavior, emotion identification and modulation, self-development and relationship skills). If psychotherapy were only an impersonal technical "assembly line" in which every client received the same "one-size-fits-all" procedure, therapists could learn everything they need to know in trade school without the extensive professional training that is now required. Moreover, clients could simply download software applications in which a simulated therapist instructed them to follow a preset sequence of steps without any actual personal interaction. Although impersonal self-directed learning can be an efficient and useful method for acquiring technical information and skills (e.g., see the discussion of the role of psychoeducation and biofeedback in Chapter 6), such a strategy does not provide the client with guided learning experiences in interaction with an attuned and responsive other. Such experiences are particularly crucial for those whose formative early years were marred by traumatic disruptions in their key relationships.

To summarize, in order to form a relationship with a complex trauma client, the therapist must first understand—and be able to communicate credibly—how the client's often extreme symptoms and impairments are the outcome of adaptive attempts to survive severe threats to identity and self-regulation and to attachment bonds. To do this, therapists must move beyond, or see beneath, the often disturbing "clinical presentations" that can shock or discourage them from treating, let alone actually getting to know, such a client. The challenge in Phase 1 is to be able to recognize and help the client become aware of the adaptive as well as the maladaptive characteristics in order to create a solid foundation for change.

SETTING UP THE PRACTICAL ARRANGEMENTS FOR THERAPY IN PHASE 1

Before concluding this discussion of the first phase of psychotherapy, we step back and consider how setting the treatment frame can contribute to—or undermine—the achievement of Phase 1 goals. More detailed guidance regarding these practical arrangements can be found in both general (Cozolino, 2002; Pope & Vasquez, 2005; Willer, 2009) and complex trauma-specific sourcebooks (Chu, 2011; Courtois, 1999, 2010). Next, we discuss elements of the setting or the "treatment surround" that most promote security and safety while providing clarity on other foundational matters.

The Setting

Whatever the setting, it is essential that it be "trauma informed," defined as providing five essential conditions: safety, trustworthiness, choice, collaboration, and empowerment (Fallot & Harris, 2008). Physical security is the bottom line, but unfortunately it often gets taken for granted. It involves, among other things, well-lit and monitored exterior and interior environments, the limitation of access to authorized individuals only, a mechanism for getting help, and a system for providing urgent care or protective services. Privacy and an organized and nonchaotic environment are close seconds. The therapy office and common areas (such as waiting areas, hallways, bathrooms) should be set up to minimize close contact with others or exposure to disturbing sights or sounds. The background sounds or music, lighting, furniture and its arrangement, windows, and objects or artwork should be designed to be calming or neutral rather than evocative. For example, in large institutions in which crowded or noisy elevators, stairways, or walkways cannot always be avoided, exposure should be buffered whenever possible—such as by scheduling appointments at less crowded times (although not at odd times of day or the week, as these may serve as reminders of secretive past abuse encounters).

Within the office setting, even under very difficult circumstances, an ambience of safety and organization should be created. A simple but comfortably furnished office with a white noise machine can be a dramatic contrast to the noise and absence of privacy in a correctional facility, storefront clinic, shelter, or inner-city hospital. Whenever possible and feasible, the door should lock from the inside in order to keep anyone from entering the office during a session, and a "do not disturb" sign should be placed on the outside for privacy and to limit interruptions. The client should have a clear view of the office door and ready and unencumbered access to it. The client and therapist both should have seating that is of equal height so as to not put the client in a lower or physically revealing or disempowered position. Nor should the therapist sit behind a desk. Optimally, comfortable chairs should be positioned in a way that the client has a reasonable degree of personal space and distance from the therapist and can adjust the space to whatever is most comfortable.

The Therapist's Personal and Therapeutic Introduction

The first interaction (by phone and in person) between therapist and client sets the tone for the rest of the psychotherapy. The therapist's personal introduction communicates his or her style and attitude with regard to key issues such as power/status, authority, collaboration, privacy, and respect for gender, ethnocultural, and other individual differences. It is not unusual for interpersonally victimized clients to be particularly perceptive about what the therapist's personal introduction, manner, and choice of words "metacommunicates." Although there is no hard and fast rule about the initial interaction(s), from a complex trauma perspective, the key consideration is the degree to which the therapist is calm, attentive, and emotionally in balance. A personally regulated therapist who is well put together in terms of self-presentation (professional and respectful with an open but somewhat reserved presentation; organized and not disheveled; dressed in modest and appropriate professional apparel; with a neat, clean, and organized office and paperwork; etc.) registers on the client's interpersonal "radar".

In addition to the personal introduction, an introduction to psychotherapy and how it works is especially important to these clients, for whom many previous relationships (including past therapy) have been at best confusing and at worst damaging. The introduction involves explanation of the mutual responsibilities and expectations and discussion of the client's presenting problems. As discussed in prior chapters, right from the first sessions (and sometimes even sooner, in phone or e-mail contacts or through marketing information about the therapist's practice and philosophy), this introduction can involve reframing symptoms and altering self-concept and core beliefs from a trauma-informed perspective. For example, it should convey the message, "You are not crazy, but you do have symptoms. You have communicated that you have strengths and resources. You are much more than your symptoms, and in fact your 'symptoms' can be understood as necessary adaptations to the traumatic circumstance you were in and efforts you made to protect yourself.". Therapy is presented as a collaborative effort, guided by the therapist, who has specific professional responsibilities and specialized knowledge. It is oriented toward enhancing the client's safety, peace of mind, control over key life decisions/choices, ability to use personal strengths to achieve his or her own goals in keeping with personal values, trust in self and selected relationships, and satisfaction with experiences and achievements.

Setting and Disclosing Services, Fees, and Conditions

Ensuring that clients are fully informed and give their consent to the services, fees, and conditions of treatment is essential. With clients with complex trauma, how the therapist sets and discloses these practical parameters can take on special meaning. The extent to which the services, fees, and conditions are reasonable and clearly stated, and the client's perception of this, can have major impact on those who have been previously exploited, betrayed, and deceived. In order for therapy to offer a remoralizing corrective experience, the starting point should be one of informed decision making (as a counterbalance to past misuse), clear and realistic expectations on the part of both therapist and client (to reduce the risk of replicating past betrayals), and full and accurate disclosure (as a counterpoint to past experiences of being manipulated or misled by secrets or outright deception).

The best way to achieve these goals at the outset of therapy is through a concise discussion of what the client can expect from the therapist (and the limits on this) and what the therapist expects or requires in turn. It is particularly important to clarify potential areas that the client may find confusing or in which the client may make unwarranted assumptions, including:

- What the therapy can or cannot reasonably be expected to help the client to achieve
- Frequency and length of sessions
- The therapist's availability for scheduled sessions (i.e., work hours, planned absences)
- How the therapist will handle absences, including informing the client and provisions for clinical coverage in case of urgent needs or crises
- How the therapist expects the client to handle absences or missed sessions, including giving prior notification and rescheduling following missed sessions
- Fees for standard sessions and any additional or modified fees for other services (such as sliding-scale fees or fees for extended-length sessions for consultation with other professionals)
- Payment for missed or canceled sessions
- Charges for additional services (phone calls and e-mails) and unpaid or overdue fees
- Whether third-party payment will be accepted and whether the therapist is a member of insurance panels
- How the client will or will not be responsible for fees or charges (e.g., copayments) not paid for (or for whom the client will be reimbursed) by third-party payers
- Whether sessions can be held other than face-to-face in the clinician's office (e.g., by telephone, Skype, or video conference)
- When and for what reasons the client can contact the therapist in between sessions and by what means (e.g., telephone, pager, voice mail, e-mail)
- Jurisdictional law regarding when and for what reasons the therapist must disclose information to third parties, either at the client's request and with consent or without the client's consent as a mandated reporter
- What information the therapist will or will not disclose to third parties and, when this involves communicating technical information such as diagnoses or functioning or impairment ratings, whether

and how the therapist will share the disclosed information with the client
- Duration of treatment
- If the client is or has been involved in legal proceedings, whether the therapist will provide forensic services, including testimony, reports, or consultation with attorneys in his or her role as treatment provider
- If the client has been or is psychiatrically or medically hospitalized, what role the therapist might take (e.g., admitting/attending, visiting, conducting psychotherapy while an inpatient)
- If the therapist knows of any extended absences or other circumstances (e.g., retirement, end of externship, internship, job change) that would interrupt or necessitate the termination of the therapy
- How and when a treatment is considered completed and how treatment typically ends

As discussed in Chapter 3, it is advisable to provide new clients with a written therapeutic contract that has all of this spelled out, a written informed consent form, and HIPAA disclosure and signature forms. (An example of a group treatment contract is found in Figure 7.1 in Chapter 7. This can be adapted to individual treatment.) Other examples are provided by the major mental health organizations on their websites. These forms are not a replacement for person-to-person discussion, but they formalize the client's informed consent. From a risk management perspective, the dialogue about what can be expected from therapy, the risks and benefits involved, and the alternatives that are available to the client and the formal documentation in signed records are important to be able to refer back to in the event that questions or legal issues emerge.

CONCLUSION

The three-phase treatment model for complex trauma is designed to give the therapist a road map of treatment tasks that are sequenced and approached in a hierarchical way. The foundation of the treatment is the establishment of safety and life stabilization, the initial foci of Phase 1. Establishing a safe setting in which clients can learn and experience emotional regulation and secure attachment is another essential foundation of this phase. The therapeutic interaction addresses the sequelae of interrupted, missing, or abusive experiences with caregivers from early childhood but is done in the framework of an adult-to-adult relationship and with educational and skill-building approaches taking the lead. As stated in the chapter title, this phase of the treatment is measured in the development of safety, skills, and a secure relationship, not time. Most clients are extremely benefited by successful Phase 1 work and its application to their emotional needs and outside lives. Some never move beyond this phase, lacking the emotional or practical resources to do so. Those who remain symptomatic are in need of additional and more trauma-focused attention, leading to discussion of emotion- and trauma-processing approaches that make up Phase 2. These and the tasks of Phase 3 are presented in the next chapter.

CHAPTER 6

Phases 2 and 3

Trauma Memory, Emotion Processing, and Application to the Present and Future

In Phase 2, the therapist guides the client in purposefully developing awareness of and gaining control over trauma memories and the extreme states of physiological arousal and emotional distress they evoke. In Phase 3, the gains made from the trauma processing are applied to present and future life decisions and domains. In this chapter, we describe several approaches that may be used to therapeutically process trauma memories and their related emotions. We emphasize those with the strongest scientific evidence base (i.e., prolonged exposure, cognitive processing therapy, eye movement desensitization and reprocessing, emotionally focused treatment of trauma) and several newer interventions that are clinically promising. The latter are under investigation but are not yet extensively researched. We begin with a discussion of two key features of Phase 2 interventions, and then address the most vexing dilemmas for therapists conducting trauma exposure strategies with complex trauma: what to do when trauma memory- or emotion-processing interventions do not seem to work or appear to have iatrogenic (inadvertent harmful) effects as the result of treatment. We then discuss the application of the gains of Phase 2 to "real life" present and future issues in the third phase of treatment.

PHASE 2: TRAUMA MEMORY AND EMOTION PROCESSING

The interventions in Phase 2 address two cardinal features of traumatic stress disorders: (1) the avoidance of memories of traumatic events, as well as emotions, stimuli, or circumstances that serve as reminders, and associated overgeneralization to trauma-related reminders, and (2) the experiencing of extreme physical, mental, and emotional arousal. Posttraumatic avoidance includes purposeful or more automatic evasion of emotions, thoughts, and physical sensations. These adaptations may or may not explicitly involve memories of the actual trauma, as generalization of what was originally avoided may have taken place. For example, if the perpetrator was a very large bearded man, then men with similar characteristics are suspect, and the survivor will go out of his or her way to avoid large men with beards. This broader form of posttraumatic avoidance has been described as "experiential avoidance" (Hayes, Wilson, Gifford, Follette, & Strosahl, 1996), as well as overgeneralization. Avoidance may begin and continue as a conscious form of coping, but it often becomes habitual, automatic and out of consciousness and control. As such, it can be labeled "behavioral dissociation."

Returning to **Doris**, she specifically refused to associate with anyone who appeared to be angry or to have a drinking problem. In this way, she was able to suppress memories of her father's alcohol-fueled abusive outbursts. She was highly avoidant of feelings similar to those that she felt as a neglected and terrified child, yet paradoxically she sometimes drank to excess (as her father had) in order to blot out these and other bad feelings. Doris seemed completely unaware of how her extreme efforts to be in control of the circumstances and relationships in her life were actually forms of avoidance as well as self-protection. Doris saw herself as "controlling and domineering by nature" and saw these traits as both adaptive ("signs that I'm a strong and effective person") and problematic ("most people can't or won't live up to my high standards, so I don't have many friends"). She neglected to mention that people felt intimidated by or alienated from her when she had been drinking because she was then less inhibited and extremely critical. Thus Doris avoided even recognizing her own extensive repertoire of avoidance tactics!

On the low end (hypoarousal) of the spectrum of physical, mental, and emotional arousal, traumatized individuals experience emotional numbing and dissociative symptoms or states. This characteristic can be deceiving, since hypoarousal can result from such a heightened state of arousal that it exceeds the individual's threshold and is managed by a virtual shutdown of consciousness, as seen in tonic immobility and catatonia. The other extreme of the spectrum involves hyperarousal, also involving dissociation and seen in agitated states of anxiety or in the fear responses that characterize PTSD and other anxiety disorders (notably panic, generalized or social anxiety, and fight–flight responses). Hyperarousal also takes the form of acute emotion dysregulation, including anger (rage or irritability), affective disorder symptoms (reactive depression or mania), rumination (guilt or obsessions), sleep problems, physical tension and pain (manifested in various illnesses and disease states), and impulsivity or disinhibited behavior. The body is highly overstimulated, an uncomfortable state that is difficult to downregulate and is often managed through compulsive and addictive behaviors.

AVOIDANCE + EXTREME AROUSAL STATES = POSTTRAUMATIC EMOTIONAL DYSREGULATION

A distinction between anxiety and fear, demonstrated in clinical research (Luyten & Blatt, 2011), may help explain hypo- and hyperarousal. Anxiety often is associated with hyperarousal, yet hyperarousal is actually characteristic of fear rather than anxiety. Fear and the closely related emotion of anger occur when an individual mobilizes to defend against attack or threat with the classic stress reaction of fight or flight (Marx et al., 2008). On the other hand, anxiety results when fearful circumstances are either anticipated or experienced as unavoidable, inescapable, or unmanageable. Anxiety (as distinct from the underlying fear that leads to anxiety) involves hypoarousal in the form of either anticipatory freezing or involuntary immobility (Marx et al., 2008). For example, rumination and worry contain mixtures of fear (e.g., racing thoughts, obsessive preoccupation, dread) and anxiety (e.g., emotional numbing, psychological resignation, and helplessness). Thus what may appear to be an absence of fear—or even of realistic and adaptive caution and concern—by a survivor of complex trauma who is aggressive or reckless, or emotionally numb or dissociated, actually begins with high levels of fear (physical and mental attempts to mobilize to survive a threat) that over time become infused with protest ("This is wrong!" "This can't be happening!"), resignation ("But there's nothing I can do about it", "I'm helpless"), and ultimately exhaustion ("I don't have the energy to fight back or even to care anymore", "I just need to go away")—defining features of anxiety.

In neurobiological terms, the emotionally unmodulated individual in the throes of these emotional reactions and associated stress reactivity ("survival brain"; Ford, 2009b, 2009c) is at the mercy of the lower reactive regions of the brain (the brain stem and limbic regions) without the "braking functions" associated with the higher cortical regions of the brain that serve as modulators (Panksepp, 1998; Panksepp & Bivens, 2012; Porges, 2011, 2013). Rothschild (2000) described the psychophysiological consequences of traumatic stress, using the metaphor of the braking system in a car. Trauma survivors are like cars without brakes and must learn different mechanisms other than closing down, going numb, or dissociating to "brake" their out-of-control arousal. Ford (2009b) explained the process in the following way:

> As a result, not only emotions but also bodily feelings tend to be experienced as signals of danger or, in and of themselves, as actual threats leading to (1) persistent affective states of anxiety, anger, sadness, and depression; (2) bodily (somatic) discomfort, pain, preoccupation, and loss of physical function (e.g., "hysterical" symptoms, such as paralysis or pseudo-seizures); and (3) associated deficits in basic self-regulation (e.g., feeding, sleep–wake cycles, self-soothing) and behavioral disinhibition (i.e., impulsivity, risk taking, aggression, addiction behavior) that can result in severe and persistent behavioral and physical health problems. (p. 37)

The individual who alternates between hyper- and hypoarousal may seem to be unable to "adapt" but is actually exhibiting complex adaptive capacities driven by a body that has become locked into a state of allostasis (Friedman & McEwen, 2004) and lower brain stem survival mode (Chemtob et al., 1988; Panksepp, 1998; Panksepp & Bivens, 2012; Porges, 2011, 2013). Ford (2009b) describes this entrapment as the individual's being

> literally helpless to understand or change survival-based neural network patterns that result in extreme states of emotional emptiness or distress (*emotion dysregulation*), mental disorientation and confusion (*dissociation*), bodily hyperarousal and exhaustion, and an associated sense of hopelessness and defeat. To the extent that the child was able to develop the neural networks that support a "learning brain" prior to exposure to traumatic stressors, or that the person is able to reengage or augment these neural networks later in childhood, adolescence, or adulthood, we may hypothesize that PTSD and complex traumatic stress disorder impairments are less likely to occur and less severe if they do occur, and that the person is more likely to recover from them. (p. 42; author's italics).
>
> In contrast to *reflective* self-regulation, automatic responses to fear or pain involve *reflexive* or habitual adjustments that maintain a fairly stable (homeostatic) equilibrium. (p. 42; italics added)

Extreme reactivity and lack of modulation put survivors and those around them at risk because they have little ability to control reactions and to modulate emotions long enough to gain perspective and to apply judgment. In fact, it is the inability to modulate strong emotions that is often at the root of violence directed toward oneself and others (this is what survivors experienced with their primary caregivers and significant others who directed their emotional dysregulation at them). In terms of treatment, these *reflexive* or *automatic somatic reactions* become a major focus, especially early on, to shift them into reflective, less automatic and more thought-driven responses, changes associated with the development of the prefrontal parts of the brain in particular. These changes come about over time through ongoing therapist emotional attunement and skills building, In turn, they create the foundation for and result in emotional processing:

> Traumatic stress interventions cannot ameliorate all of the problems associated with the adaptive—but ultimately problematic—shift from a learning brain to a survival brain. However, a focus on enhancing clients' core abilities to engage in reflective self-awareness in the service of consciously regulating emotions and processing information could provide a framework to guide clinical conceptualization, engagement, and education of clients; treatment planning; and monitoring of therapeutic progress and outcomes for clients experiencing complex traumatic stress reactivity. (Ford, 2009b, p. 49)

Many trauma treatment models emphasize the need to lessen or quell the individual's hyperarousal and to develop expanded capacity for emotional tolerance (Ogden et al., 2006; Rothschild, 2003). Briere and Scott (2006) discussed the concept of the "therapeutic window," and Olio and Cornell (1993) described the "therapeutic edge" within which the client has the capacity to tolerate emotional arousal. Too much emotional stimulation exceeds or overshoots the "window" and is demonstrated behaviorally by a return to unhealthy coping methods or shutdown. Too little emotional stimulation undershoots the "window," understimulates it, and leaves the client essentially unchanged. Treatment is geared toward expanding the window (i.e., expanding the client's emotional tolerance) by neither overshooting nor falling short of it. The client is encouraged to incrementally approach and feel rather than avoid or shut down painful or difficult emotions. Over time, the approach–avoid gradient changes from one of avoidance to one of approach as the client builds the capacity to know about and accept the trauma and to face and express associated emotions (such as grief, shame, anger, sadness). What was previously cut off becomes conscious. Whether conducted in prolonged or more graduated forms, numerous exposure-based approaches and strategies are now available to support this process. All are geared toward progressively expanding the individual's "window of tolerance." Quoting Schwartz (2000): "A delicate balance between disruption and stabilization must be continually renegotiated or the traumatized patient and the therapist will be perpetually overwhelmed or stalemated. The therapy relationship must break down old, as well as forge new, linkages between the inner work of the patients and his/her relationships" (p. xix).

Jehu (1988) was one of the first clinical researchers to identify the cognitive errors and predominantly negative cognitions about self and others that victims make on the basis of sexual abuse. He demonstrated how the reversal of these errors can significantly undercut negative affect and mood states. His work was an early forerunner of a variety of cognitive-behavioral, schema, and processing therapies that are now available. Mindfulness interventions are designed to encourage the client to be less self-critical and more accepting and to learn new ways of thinking about him- or herself. Mentalization approaches assist in the development of a more flexible, reflective view of oneself that is based on empathic response and mirroring from others rather than one that is reflexive or reactive (Allen, 2012). Fonagy, Gergely, Jurist, and Target (2002) describe the concept of mentalized affectivity as "a clinical phenomenon that pertains to the mediation of affective experience through self-reflexivity." This is a compelling concept because the aim of changing views of self and the development of a positive sense of self and self-worth and recognition of emotional states is at the heart of psychotherapy. Per these authors, "Mentalized affectivity, which includes the elements of identifying, modulating, and expressing affects, help us to understand how one's relation to one's own affects can be changed" (Fonagy et al., 2002, p. 468).

This formulation may help explain why **Hector** alternates between states of hypoarousal (hopelessness, numbing, withdrawal, exhaustion, dissociation) and hyperarousal (irritability, rage, addictive and reckless behavior, and compulsive self-harm). His past traumatic experiences, along with his formative family, peer, and school experiences (and genetically inherited temperament and personality tendencies), taught him to cope by alternately shifting between states of fear (fight-or-flight reactions) and anxiety (freeze or shutdown reactions). The self-protective or defensive nature of these extreme arousal states differentiates them from similar disorders, notably bipolar disorder, which involves alternating states of hyperarousal (mania) and mixed hyper- and hypoarousal (depression). Bipolar and traumatic stress disorders are similar in that they both involve biological dysregulation of the body's arousal systems, but they differ in that bipolar disorder is genetic, whereas traumatic stress disorders are survival based. It is possible to have both a bipolar and a traumatic stress disorder. Individuals with both disorders need concurrent treatment for each to stabilize and improve. In cases such as Hector's, the primary disorder (and the primary target for treatment) is a traumatic stress disorder with associated major depression and anxiety.

When Hector becomes extremely angry, despondent, or emotionally shut down, he is more likely to benefit from treatment that helps him to recognize or manage fear and anxiety than from treatment that simply stabilizes his moods or attempts to biologically alter what appear to be symptoms of mania and depression. Therapy for mood instability may play an important role in treatment for complex trauma survivors and biological agents such as mood stabilizer medications warrant consideration (see Davidson & Stein, 2008 and Opler et al., 2009, for additional information). However, when these symptoms are largely driven by posttraumatic fear (and associated hyperarousal, irritability, and concentration problems, which can be similar to mania but are instead based on perceived threat reactivity) and anxiety (and associated hypervigilance, sleep disturbance, anhedonia, sense of foreshortened future, and emotional numbing, which are similar to depressive symptoms but are also based on threat reactivity), then therapy is likely to be most efficient and effective when the focus is on the posttraumatic reaction. In Phase 2, the therapist helped Hector to stop avoiding and to begin processing fear and anxiety (and related emotions such as anger, dysphoria, guilt, and shame). This was done by showing him ways to remember traumatic events and manage the emotional distress they caused. Hector learned that he has the capacity to anticipate, be aware of, prevent, or recover from extreme arousal states rather than feeling hopeless and helpless and at their mercy. He was assisted in understanding that his tendency to avoid troubling memories and emotions did not relieve them but actually had the opposite effect of heightening them. In consequence, they persisted and even increased (especially after he was triggered), when they were less subject to containment and regulation. Throughout the course of treatment Hector was taught methods for slowly addressing his traumatic experiences in ways that allowed him to feel his distress in manageable doses, to discuss and accommodate his many related feelings, and ultimately to resolve them.

THERAPEUTIC EXPOSURE AND THE PROCESSING OF TRAUMA MEMORIES AND EMOTIONS

Before presenting various modalities for processing trauma-related memories and resolving their emotional and cognitive aftermath, we discuss the rationale for their use and define and describe what is meant by "processing" and "resolution." Therapeutic exposure and the processing of traumatic memories involve more than simply having a supportive discussion of troubling memories or current emotional difficulties. The process is intended to be therapeutic rather than merely cathartic and to avoid iatrogenically destabilizing the client. It involves a structured process (or protocol) *designed to facilitate not only remembering but also the client's vivid experiencing of trauma-related emotions and physical sensations* (and associated thoughts, beliefs, appraisals, and intentions) *in the immediate moment of the therapy session.* This experiential technique is planned and prepared for, designed to elicit memory and emotions within a high, but safe and tolerable degree of physiological and emotional arousal. This planned procedure is designed to prevent traumatic memories and feelings from emerging unbidden as intrusive recollections and reexperiencing, with their associated states of arousal. Safely experiencing emotions and these states of hypo- or hyperarousal in the company of the supportive therapist as part of a planned protocol helps the client learn how to gain control (Higginson, Mansell, & Wood, 2011). In interventions of this type, the client makes an *informed choice to revisit and reexamine* trauma memories instead of avoiding (or being the passive victim of) their unwanted and uncontrolled reexperiencing. As described later in this chapter, a number of psychotherapies provide different ways for therapeutic exposure to occur, as it is a multifaceted strategy (Abramowitz, Deacon, & Whiteside, 2011) and designed to achieve several types of benefits (Carey, 2011).

Rather than simply a recitation of the trauma story and reactions, therapeutic exposure is hypothesized to reduce fear, anxiety, and dysphoria by demonstrating that the client can engage with the memory and its predominant emotional reactions while in a less aroused state, creating a *condition of emotional disparity.* It is this disparity that leads to the counterconditioning of the original response, allowing for the experiencing of other and often more core emotions, that is, "emotional processing" (Foa & Kozak, 1986). At the present time, there is no universally accepted definition or description of emotional processing of trauma, with its resultant changes in physical reactions, emotions, and thoughts (Carey, 2011). Nevertheless, a number of affect and trauma theorists hypothesize that when core emotions are tapped, acknowledging and feeling them (rather than avoiding or minimizing them) results in changes in emotion awareness, expression, and self-understanding (Fosha, 2000; McCullough-Valliant, 1994). These emotional and cognitive changes further result in alterations in brain activity and related physiological systems (Shapiro, 2012). Paivio and Pascual-Leone (2010) provided the following description:

> Emotional processing of complex trauma involves not only desensitization to painful feelings and memories but also active construction of new idiosyncratic meaning, that is a more adaptive and coherent view of self, others, and traumatic events. Furthermore, processing of trauma memories requires the application of rational/linguistic processes to trauma material that is encoded in the experiential system but has remained unprocessed or has been processed incompletely. An indicator of resolution, therefore, is that trauma narratives become more coherent, personal, affectively focused, and self-reflective. These qualities are reflected in the construct of experiencing. . . . (p. 38)

There is general consensus across various approaches to psychotherapy that emotion processing enables the client to safely experience and appraise in present time the physical sensations, emotions, and thoughts that he or she had interpreted as signals of overwhelming danger and associated powerlessness after the trauma. The therapist helps the client to understand that the direct threat is over (even though it might feel like it is happening in the present, especially when in flashback form) but can be recalled (vs. reexperienced) in the present with a different set of emotions and meanings attached (disparity and separating past from present).

Carey (2011) describes the facilitating of emotional processing (in exposure therapy) as involving "assisting people in psychological distress to consider in detail material they would otherwise avoid . . . whether this occurs *in vivo* or imaginally, or whether a graduated approach is taken in preference to flooding, or whether avoidance occurs due to fear or some other emotion . . . [by] helping people sustain their attention in areas that are difficult" (p. 240). Carey (2011) also notes that it remains unclear what exactly changes biologically or psychologically when distressing emotions are processed but invokes perceptual control theory (Higginson et al., 2011) to propose that sustained attention in the face of distress enables clients to reorganize how they interpret the meaning of extreme states of hypo- or hyperarousal in ways that give them a greater sense of control.

Attachment theorists and those who practice interpersonal neurobiological, somatosensory, and emotion processing approaches (Fosha, 2000; Ogden et al., 2006; Paivio & Pascual-Leone, 2010; Solomon & Siegel, 2003; Siegel, 2012b; Schore, 2003b, 2013; Shapiro, 2012) believe that experiencing the emotion in the company of a therapist who is accepting and soothing provides counterconditioning of the previous indifference or nonresponse. The coregulation of emotion by the therapist, who is physically and emotionally attuned and synchronized with the client, leads to neuronal growth and helps make what was implicit explicit. New neural pathways are stimulated that in turn stimulate brain development, especially the left side (verbal) and the prefrontal cortex (judgment and executive control and functioning).

But *how* do clients actually change the way that they process their trauma memories and associated emotional dysregulation? A limited amount of research has been conducted to clarify what happens when clients emotionally process memories in psychotherapy for any disorder, not only traumatic stress disorders (Carey, 2011). Clinical researchers have hypothesized that processing involves clients becoming able to: (1) habituate to (i.e., tolerate the discomfort associated with) disturbing memories and emotions; (2) learn that they are able to confront traumatic memories safely, thus disconfirming the belief that trauma memories are beyond their capacity to tolerate or control; (3) learn that approaching rather than avoiding fearful trauma-related bodily and emotion states and associated thoughts is possible (i.e., replacing experiential avoidance with acceptance and commitment; Hayes et al., 1996); (4) disconfirm self-defeating beliefs about self and others, while simultaneously strengthening self-confidence in general and as pertains to the possibility of achieving a better life (Linehan, 1993; Linehan, Heard, & Armstrong, 1993); (5) enhance self-regulation skills to reset extreme levels of arousal to a balanced mid-range intensity (from allostasis to homeostasis; Ford & Russo, 2006). As mentioned above, neuronal changes both result from and potentiate these changes.

Ford (2005) offered a deconstruction of emotion processing that begins with the emotion regulation capacities that are often severely compromised when young children are traumatized. Emotion processing is viewed as involving (1) awareness of physical/nonverbal cues associated with emotion states; (2) resetting or shifting these physical states in order to alter emotion states; (3) verbally describing physical/nonverbal states using emotional descriptors; (4) distinguishing between threat-based body–emotion states and learning and exploratory-oriented states; (5) holding "reactive" and "self-enhancing" emotion states in awareness simultaneously and not privileging one over the other; (6) linking emotion states to personally meaningful narratives of memorable life events and using this link to reinterpret their meaning to retrieve what was learned in those past experiences; and (7) actively seeking to recognize, label, and consciously articulate the resultant personal meaning of different emotion states and their combinations. These features of emotion processing are what complex trauma survivors generally describe themselves as *not having been able to do* when they were experiencing traumatic events, precisely because they were too busy surviving to "process" their emotions at the time or later. Therapy involves helping them to *transform emotionally fragmented or empty memories into meaningful life experiences that, although distressing and often tragic, can be "lived with" rather than feared and avoided.* Finding meaning in chaos, horror, and indifference is daunting, but emotion processing provides a set of practical strategies and goals. It is posited that neurobiological changes accompany these changed beliefs and meanings and result in a diminishment of posttraumatic symptoms.

Psychotherapy must address not just isolated negative beliefs but overarching assumptions and schema about self and others (Jehu, 1988; McCann & Pearlman, 1990; Resick & Schnicke, 1993; Young, Klosko, & Weishaar, 2003). These are usually based on cognitions that are overly rigid and that involve cognitive errors. The fact that victimization is not a recent occurrence and is not likely to recur is not a sufficient basis for many survivors to conclude that they are not as bad and the world not as dangerous as their traumatic experiences have led them to believe. To replace posttraumatic beliefs with self-regard, trust, and hope requires major shifts not just in beliefs and cognitions but more fundamentally in the regulation of emotions and physical sensations.

Research findings from a related field, the treatment of phobias, obsessions, and compulsions, point to two key issues regarding the emotion of fear that can inform the understanding of what is involved in trauma processing. First, the most persistent forms of anxiety involve a *fear of fear itself*, or "anxiety sensitivity." What begins as a fear of specific external dangers can become a much broader and more relentless fear of any feelings the individual interprets as signaling vulnerability. The fear of fear itself is really due to either the reality or the resultant self-perception of being helpless or overwhelmed. Second, persistent anxiety tends to involve rumination or thinking about something repeatedly and not being able to redirect attention. Such perseveration is the driving force of obsessions and compulsions which involve repetitive rethinking or reenacting of feared situations. Rumination can become a self-perpetuating or closed loop because the more an individual dwells on feeling helpless or out-of-control, the more his or her anxiety response is reinforced. Therapies for chronic anxiety and obsessive–compulsive disorders, therefore, have focused on helping clients to overcome their fear of fear and to stop ruminating about fear. Their common denominator is guiding the client in purposefully and safely reexperiencing fear while in a state of relaxation and/or while thinking realistic and reassuring thoughts (with specific support and response when in the company of the therapist or of supportive others) instead of while alone in self-defeating fearful avoidance.

What is it that enables clients to relinquish experiential avoidance or rumination? The antithesis of fear or anxiety seems to be confidence (i.e., a sense of being able to understand and have some kind of meaningful control over distressing events and emotions) and contentment or satisfaction (i.e., a sense of pleasure and security) that engenders feelings of well-being and hope. Yet it has been noted that clients with complex trauma do not easily feel confidence and contentment; they usually feel *more* rather than less fearful or anxious if they even imagine—let alone actually begin—to experience such feelings. For these reasons, interventions based on reexperiencing fear have been found to be difficult to tolerate for many such clients (e.g., Cook, Schnurr, & Foa, 2004; McDonagh-Coyle et al., 2005). What must be addressed is *how* they process memories and related emotions, procedural approaches we address subsequently. Before describing the main technical features of these emotion-processing modalities, we provide a therapist's "safety manual" of elements that should be in place before using their evocative and potentially double-edged interventions.

SAFER Strategies

Using the acronym "SAFER" (**S**elf-care and symptom control, **A**cknowledgment, **F**unctioning, **E**xpression, and **R**elationships), Chu (2011) formulated a set of criteria for safely conducting trauma treatment that is particularly applicable to memory and emotion processing.

Self-Care, Symptom Control, and Stabilization

Stabilization is ongoing and should be monitored throughout the entire treatment. If the client is having difficulties in therapy or in daily life that can create an increase in symptoms, memory and emotion processing should be delayed or paused. The therapist needs to engage the client in discussion of what has been triggered (whether by therapy or by extratherapy stressors or life events) and ways to increase coping by applying the skills developed earlier. The client might have dismissed, forgotten, or unintentionally pushed these "to the back of the queue" in an attempt to confront and resolve trauma-related memories and associated issues and emotions. Reinstituting a focus on self-care and symptom management skills can enhance therapeutic processing, because these constitute a key part of therapeutically reworking troubling memories and emotions, that is, being able to apply self-care and symptom management skills *in the moment of processing.*

Acknowledgment versus Avoidance

Memory and emotion processing is fundamentally an act of acknowledging the significance and meaning of troubling occurrences, memories, and emotions. Memories that are recalled without acknowledgment are simply (and perhaps pathologically) being reexperienced with nothing more being done with them (i.e., they are not faced and worked through). To acknowledge an event, a memory, or the emotions attached involves examining it to clarify its full range of impact. Additionally, it establishes a sense of what the memory or emotions now mean about self, relationships with others, and life in general, including the past as well as the present and future. Existential questions about the meaning of life and the reasons for mistreatment and misfortune are common at this point in the process. To the extent that therapists can help clients not just to tolerate troubling memories and emotions but to hold them in awareness, probe them for the specific features that are of lasting significance, and define what they mean in terms of themselves and their lives, these memories and emotions no longer need to be avoided.

Functioning

Therapy must be geared to maintain or enhance the client's functioning, not just to provide symptom relief or a sense of catharsis or personal triumph. Although those are important goals, the "rubber hits the road" with the issue of functioning—the ability to live a life free from or less hindered by the lingering effects of the trauma. Functioning may become impaired during memory and emotion processing due to the distress and confusion that are elicited in facing troubling memories and emotions that previously lacked coherence and evaded understanding. Daily functioning may also be more difficult in Phase 2 because clients are relinquishing a familiar and comforting way of coping—namely, avoidance—and journeying through difficult and unfamiliar territory. The therapist directs and guides the client through this uncharted terrain and monitors and modulates the pace, intensity, and topical focus. Although decreased ability to function is commonly experienced, it is usually temporary. Over time, clients often find that their functioning begins to increase as they are freed from the distractions and the emotional load of unresolved issues and feelings, including the fear and anxiety that long plagued them.

Expression of Emotions and Experiential Awareness

Although catharsis is not the primary goal, memory and emotion processing is essentially all about the identification and related expression of thoughts, feelings, physical sensations, relational patterns, and so on. The therapist helps the client to become experientially aware of the multiple modalities of sensory/perceptual, physiological, cognitive, relational, and affective material that were previously inaccessible because they were encoded in somatosensory modalities and in the right brain (and thus implicitly or procedurally out of conscious awareness) or because of dissociation or other defenses. Verbal encoding and expression (symbolizing) involve the development of the left side of the brain and put into words what has been contained in somatosensory form on the right side. Once verbalized, information can be shared with and responded to by others in ways that are reinforcing to the individual's reality and his or her reactions, thus supporting individual development and differentiation. We return to this concept of multimodal awareness and expression repeatedly throughout this chapter.

Relationships and Response

Ultimately, security and a sense of selfhood, worthiness, and personal accomplishment come from being in relationships with others, rather than being in isolation and without interpersonal contact and response. Psychosocial support by the therapist and others has been found to ameliorate the worst effects of trauma, making it imperative that clients are supported in remembering and developing restorative relationships with others. Memory and emotion processing in the context of response leads to physiological changes beginning at the neuronal level, as described earlier. Clients in a secure and responsive therapeutic relationship (especially when they are distressed and scared) can begin to incorporate the support and its mirroring of them (Siegel, 2012).

With these therapeutic considerations in mind, the therapist can make memory and emotion processing not only safe but also an essential tool for the client's personal integration. Note how each of the SAFER features is addressed in each of the processing modalities described next.

EVIDENCE-BASED TREATMENTS FOR TRAUMA MEMORY AND EMOTION PROCESSING

Based on these approaches to therapy for chronic and persistent anxiety disorders, two extensively researched cognitive-behavioral therapy (CBT) interventions have been developed for the processing of trauma memories (Cahill et al., 2009). These interventions are *prolonged exposure* (PE; Foa & Kozak, 1986; Foa, Hembree, & Rothbaum, 2007) and *cognitive processing therapy* (CPT; Resick & Schnicke, 1993; Resick, Nishith, & Griffin, 2003). Other trauma-memory-processing therapies that have shown effectiveness in scientific studies include *eye movement desensitization and reprocessing* (EMDR; Shapiro, 2001, 2012; Shapiro & Solomon, 2010), *emotion-focused therapy for complex trauma* (EFTT; Paivio et al., 2010), and those that show promise include *narrative exposure therapy* (NET; Hensel-Dittmann et al., 2011), and *imagery rehearsal/imagery rescripting therapy* (IRT; Smucker, Dancu, Foa, & Niederee, 2002).

Prolonged Exposure

PE is thus far the most extensively scientifically validated treatment for the symptoms of PTSD in adults (Mendes, Mello, Ventura, Passarela, & Mari Jde, 2008; Powers, Halpern, Ferenschak, Gillihan, & Foa, 2010). PE involves repeatedly imagining or describing a traumatic event as if it were happening right at the moment, while simultaneously being helped by the therapist to remain fully aware that the event is *not* actually occurring in the present. The usual instructions are for the client to describe in first-person present tense a step-by-step detailed account of what she or he can recall about a specific traumatic event, as well as what she or he thought and felt (physically as well as emotionally). The recounting is repeated several times in several sessions and typically is audiotaped for private reviewing by the client between sessions. This form of *imaginal exposure* (IE) (i.e., imagined and described as if it were actually happening in the present) may be complemented by *in vivo* (i.e., as occurs in day-to-day life) exposure. *In vivo* exposure involves constructing a list of situations, people, places, and activities associated with the traumatic event and purposely "exposing" oneself to those reminders, both in and between sessions. The *in vivo* exposure protocol is similar to systematic desensitization, the behavioral intervention for the treatment of phobias. Both involve creating a "hierarchy" beginning with the least distressing trauma reminders and progressing (over the course of several sessions) to the most distressing reminders and pairing that exposure with a state of relaxation to create a disparity between the original and the current response state.

This procedure combines the recounting of trauma memories with planned exposure to their reminders to provide the client the opportunity to increase emotional tolerance. In this way, the memory is changed from a source of fear and avoidance into one that is still likely to be negative and aversive but is less associated with emotional reactivity and pain, making it more manageable. The metaphor of going through the event as though it were a movie that could be viewed in slow motion "frame by frame" is useful in helping the client to understand that PE is a very careful and unhurried replaying of an event that typically happened quickly and in ways that were overwhelming, making it difficult for the client to respond in the moment and to remember all that occurred. In this procedure, clients are also encouraged to identify "hot spots" (Foa et al., 2007), those moments of peak arousal or distress associated with ongoing negative beliefs that function as triggers for present-day stress reactions. Becoming aware of hot spots gives clients a way to proactively prepare for and manage them to lessen their impact. A by-product is that clients learn new things about what they were like and what actually happened to them, for example, that they were younger and more helpless and/or more competent and resourceful than previously recognized. They might further acknowledge the extent to which they were trapped and helpless and thus unable to change the outcome no matter what, allowing them to shift from a stance of self-blame, shame, guilt, and ineffectiveness to increased self-understanding.

Although PE has the most extensive research evidence base to date and is the one most recommended for treating the symptoms of PTSD, *graduated exposure* modalities have been suggested as a less intense alternative for survivors of complex trauma (Briere & Scott, 2006; Courtois, 1988, 1999, 2010; Fisher & Ogden, 2009; Olio & Cornell, 1993; Steele, Van der Hart, & Nijenhuis, 2005). Graduated exposure is based on the behavior therapy technique of systematic desensitization, originally designed and validated for the treatment of phobias. Instead of beginning with the most (or one of the most) troubling memories, graduated exposure begins with the most mildly distressing memories and progresses to those that are more disturbing. Clients increasingly accommodate emotional distress as they approach rather than avoid what was previously so adverse. Graduated exposure, like the prolonged version, can be conducted *in vivo* (depending on the trauma circumstance) or in imaginal forms. In the imaginal version, clients are assisted to create a hierarchy of traumatic memories, to make the progression from mildly to severely distressing memories efficient and tolerable. *In vivo* exposure homework as prescribed in PE (in which clients gradually seeking out cues or situations that are reminders of past traumatic events beginning with mildly upsetting reminders) can be used in the graduated version. All are paired with relaxation and support to provide experiences of disparity.

Cognitive Processing Therapy

A second scientifically validated approach to helping clients face and come to terms with traumatic memories involves the retelling of the event in a way that is similar to yet different from the method used in PE. CPT (Resick & Schnicke, 1992) involves the client recalling and describing one or more specific trauma memories in writing, a format different from PE and EMDR. The client writes a narrative of traumatic events in as much detail as possible. The narrative becomes owned by the client as her or his "real life story," no longer an incident too terrifying to recall but a terrible or tragic story that is "in black and white" and can be read about and narrated. It can then be closed like a chapter in a book that has been read and finished. The therapist carefully reviews the narrative, looking for themes and descriptive gaps and attending to the client's cognitions and beliefs. These are then reviewed and the client given education about erroneous information, beliefs, or assumptions. Socratic questioning techniques are used to question the logic of various conclusions and to provide alternatives for consideration.

CPT has been scientifically evaluated and found to be effective in treating adults with PTSD (Mendes et al., 2008; Powers et al., 2010; Seidler & Wagner, 2006) and those with complex trauma histories as well (Resick et al., 2003). Because childhood victimization and other trauma can lead to deeply embedded (yet often illogical and false) beliefs about self, relationships, the world, and the trauma itself, CPT provides a strategy to disconfirm posttraumatic schema while strengthening the cognitive network of nontraumatic associations either experientially (i.e., purposefully revisiting traumatic memories and current situations that are strong reminders) or didactically (i.e., analyzing the applicability of posttraumatic cognitions and beliefs to current life circumstances). Clients experience relief as they gain new insights and cognitions about the trauma, themselves, and their actions and reactions, leading to greater understanding and resolution.

Promising Additional Approaches to Trauma Memory and Emotion Processing

Other therapeutic approaches have been developed and applied clinically for trauma memory processing, several created specifically for complex trauma. Although some have long histories of research indicating efficacy, others lack the degree of scientific support that is now available for CBT techniques.

Emotion-Focused Trauma Therapy

EFTT (Paivio & Pascual-Leone, 2010; Paivio et al., 2010) uses a therapeutic examination of emotions associated with past traumatic events to reduce the fear of painful feelings and memories and to construct a new, emotionally coherent understanding. EFTT involves exposure and cognitive therapy techniques similar to those in PE and CPT, but primarily uses experiential/humanistic techniques to help clients experience emotions and reduce experiential avoidance. EFTT's trauma- and emotion-processing methods are illustrated by a core technique, imaginal confrontation (IC), used when clients can tolerate it. In IC, clients imagine perpetrators of maltreatment in an empty chair to which they directly express their thoughts and feelings. EFTT research suggests that IC is most beneficial if clients express specific emotions toward and reparations expected from the perpetrator. It also allows them to develop a more realistic and complex view of perpetrators, including appropriately holding them accountable. These experiential exercises support changes in perspective, enhance self-empowerment and self-esteem, and reduce shame and self-blame.

Eye Movement Desensitization and Reprocessing

EMDR (Shapiro, 2001, 2012) is a second therapeutic approach designed to assist clients in facing, experiencing, and reprocessing memories of traumatic events and experiences. EMDR involves the vivid recall of a specific traumatic incident, similar to the PE protocol; however, in EMDR, it is done imaginally and without the client describing it out loud. A major difference between the techniques is that, as the client focuses on the trauma memory, he or she is simultaneously engaged in saccadic (horizontal, back-and-forth) eye movements or some other bilateral perceptual–motor task or stimulation (such as being tapped by the therapist alternately on the left and right sides of the body, or hearing a tone bilaterally). Clients often report that interposing this competing or distracting repetitive task into the recall of the trauma memory greatly reduces or even eliminates the emotional distress that usually accompanies it. As a result, EMDR may be conducted in less time than typically allotted for prolonged exposure or other CBTs for trauma.

A single EMDR session (or two to three sessions with as few as three to five repetitions of the traumatic memory per session) has been found to have immediate benefits for many clients with time-limited or more "simple" trauma but also for some with complex trauma histories (Powers et al., 2010; Seidler & Wagner, 2006; Shapiro, 2001, 2012), that may be comparable to those reported for PE and cognitive therapies such as CPT (Resick & Schnicke, 1993). Shapiro (2012) reported that, of all processing therapies, EMDR has the most robust evidence base for relieving the classic symptoms of PTSD. The extent to which these benefits extend to the additional symptoms associated with complex trauma disorders is not as well established. The EMDR protocol for the treatment of complex trauma has been extensively modified for use across all three treatment phases and for special problems (Gelinas, 2003; Korn & Leeds, 2002; Omaha, 2004; Schmidt, 2009; Shapiro, 2002, 2012). For example, the application of EMDR to Phase 1 is not to process memories; rather, it is used to help clients build active coping resources. A procedure labeled "resource installation" involves the client actively imagining incorporating strengths and resources from a variety of internal and external sources. Eye movements or other means of bilateral stimulation are used to "set" and establish the resources (Korn & Leeds, 2002). The more traditional EMDR application to trauma processing occurs in Phase 2.

Imagery Rehearsal/Rescripting Therapy

Repetitive intrusive memories and nightmares are haunting to survivors who wish they could forget or at least modify them to be less troubling and tediously unchanging. There is a long clinical tradition of assisting clients to rewrite their memories in psychotherapy, particularly in experiential models such as Gestalt therapy (Perls, 1973) or writing (Pennebaker, 1990, 2004) or narrative models (White, 2011). More recently such an approach has been formalized in two CBT interventions known as imagery rehearsal therapy (Krakow et al., 2001) and imagery rescripting therapy (Long et al., 2011; Smucker et al., 2002). Although these are two different psychotherapy models, they share a core emphasis on having the client reconstruct the narrative (note the similarity to CPT and EFFT) of a traumatic nightmare or waking intrusive memory.

IRT provides an important shift in clients' understanding of traumatic memories and nightmares. Commonly, they have viewed them as permanent, intractable, and "set in stone," because "you can't rewrite history." In fact, all memory (and traumatic memories specifically) have been scientifically shown to be constantly evolving constructions that are more like malleable scripts than fixed and unchangeable "facts" (McNally, 2003). Memory or nightmare rescripting and rehearsal begin by helping the client to achieve a clearer and more detailed and complete narrative of the troubling memory or dream, often revealing new and previously overlooked information. For example, **Hector** had a recurrent nightmare of being helpless while huge monsters tore his body to shreds. When he very reluctantly described the nightmare, he realized that what appeared to be faceless inhuman monsters actually looked more like angry adults, such as his father and the priest who molested him. Although Hector was upset to know that those perpetrators were still, in his words, "haunting me in my dreams," he felt able to think of ways to help himself stand up to and stop the attackers, as if he were a parent helping to protect his own son from adult bullies.

Similarly, IRT applied to waking traumatic memories provides a way for complex trauma survivors to therapeutically reexamine, clarify, and modify their internal narrative of past traumatic experiences. A study by Arntz, Tiesema, and Kindt (2007) showed that adding IRT to PE cut the dropout rate in half and was more effective than PE alone in helping participants to reduce their problems with acting out anger, hostility, and guilt. Gains were reported both at the end of therapy and at a 1-month follow-up. Therapists reported anecdotally that they preferred adding IRT to PE because it gave them a sense of greater efficacy (and less helplessness) when going through the often extremely disturbing details of their clients' trauma memories, thus potentially reducing therapists' vicarious traumatization. Another study by Grunert, Weis, Smucker, and Christianson (2007) found that more than 75% of a group of clients who had not improved in PE were able to fully recover from PTSD with three or fewer sessions of IRT. The authors noted that "non-FEAR emotions (e.g., guilt, shame, anger) were found to be predominant for all 23 PE failures examined in this study, suggesting that a simple habituation model (on which PE is based) is not sufficient to address non-FEAR emotions in PTSD" (Grunert et al., 2007, p. 317; capitals in original). Thus IRT may have particular utility with clients with complex trauma who are not able to engage in or benefit from exposure therapies, especially PE. Or exposure therapies may need to be expanded to focus on other emotions in addition to fear for greater efficacy with complex trauma.

Narrative Exposure Therapy

NET is a brief (typically one to five sessions) psychotherapy that engages clients in imaginal exposure and assists them in reconstructing a personally meaningful narrative of the traumatic events by identifying the specific emotions they experienced at the time (Hensel-Dittmann et al., 2011; Neuner, Schauer, Klaschik, Karunakara, & Elbert, 2004). NET has been tested with a unique range of severely traumatized and underserved populations in impoverished and war-torn countries (Schauer, Neuner, Catani, Schauer, & Elbert, 2010). Although there have been no large-scale studies of NET, several scientific (randomized controlled trial) studies have shown NET to be superior to (1) interpersonal therapy with young adult Rwandan genocide orphans (Schaal, Elbert, & Neuner, 2009), (2) brief psychoeducation with 60- to 70-year-old survivors of political imprisonment and torture (Bichescu, Neuner, Schauer, & Elbert, 2007), and (3) supportive therapy or brief psychoeducation with political refugees (Neuner et al., 2004).

In the largest study to date, Hensel-Dittmann and colleagues found that a 10-session version of NET was superior to stress inoculation training in reducing PTSD symptoms with adult civilian survivors of torture and war, although neither therapy was successful in reducing depression or other psychiatric symptoms. A children's version, KIDNET, was found to be more effective than wait list in reducing the PTSD symptoms and improving the functioning of 7- to 16-year-old refugee children (Ruf et al., 2007). Thus NET, which combines elements of PE and CPT in a brief and efficient memory-processing intervention, may provide an important approach to psychotherapy for adults and children who have experienced complex identity and cultural trauma.

Additional treatments that are "hybrid" adaptations of some of these have been developed and have preliminary and accumulating empirical support. These are discussed next.

Trauma Affect Regulation: Guide for Education and Therapy

As a foundation of the treatment, Trauma Affect Regulation: Guide for Education and Therapy (TARGET) provides education linking affect dysregulation with PTSD symptoms (Ford & Russo, 2006; Ford et al., 2011, 2012). Clients learn that their susceptibility to rapid intense emotional reactivity and difficulty in regaining equilibrium are the result of biological adaptations and alternations related to PTSD. Restoring affect regulation is described as requiring seven practical steps or skills summarized by the acronym "FREEDOM": Focusing the mind on one thought at a time; Recognizing current triggers for emotional reactions; distinguishing dysregulated ("reactive") versus adaptive ("main") Emotions; Evaluations (thoughts), goal Definitions, and behavioral Options; and self-statements affirming that taking responsibility for Managing intense emotions is crucial not only to personal well-being but also to Making a positive contribution to primary relationships (e.g., as a parent) and the community. The FREEDOM steps are learned and practiced incrementally with modeling and coaching by the therapist, via imaginal rehearsal in session and *in vivo* individualized homework assignments, using a template (the "Personal Practice Exercise for FREEDOM") that walks the client through each FREEDOM step as it applies to preparing for or analyzing posttraumatic emotional dysregulation.

TARGET also provides a creative arts activity designed to enhance positive and negative emotion recognition in the context of autobiographical narrative construction (the "lifeline"). The procedure includes the use of collage, drawing, poetry, writing, and music to depict life experiences that the client views as emotionally significant (including but not limited to traumatic events). The FREEDOM steps are applied as the organizing framework for each lifeline event, with the client assisted in identifying trauma-related triggers, feelings, thoughts, goals, and behaviors and counterbalancing them with resilient feelings, thoughts, goals, and behaviors.

Seeking Safety

Seeking Safety (SS) is an individual or group therapy designed for adults or adolescents with comorbid (or co-occurring) PTSD and substance abuse (Najavits, 2002a, 2002b). It uses principles and educational materials adapted from dialectical behavior therapy (DBT) and CBT interventions such as SIT, cognitive therapy, and motivational enhancement therapy that were designed and validated for the treatment of either PTSD or substance use disorders. To cover this wide range of skills and to link them to psychoeducation about the interplay between PTSD and substance abuse, Seeking Safety usually involves more sessions (e.g., 25–30) over a longer time period (e.g., 6–12 months) than most trauma-memory or emotion-processing interventions (but it is comparable to the length of DBT). SS does not usually have a formal memory-processing component, although participants have many opportunities to relate trauma memories to the education and skills taught in each session. This model has shown evidence of efficacy in several studies with highly traumatized underserved populations such as delinquent girls (Najavits, Gallop, Weiss, 2006), homeless female military veterans with psychiatric disorders (Desai, Harpaz-Rotem, Najavits, & Rosenheck, 2008), adults with chronic substance use disorders (Hien, Cohen, Litt, Miele, & Capstick, 2004; Hien et al., 2010), and incarcerated women (Zlotnick, Johnson, & Najavits, 2009). This method may have particular application to complex trauma survivors, having been shown to reduce PTSD symptoms in the most distressed of participants (Hien et al., 2010). As traditional addiction programs have been deficient in including an emphasis on trauma as part of the recovery process, Seeking Safety makes an important contribution in this regard.

Skill Training in Affect and Interpersonal Regulation

Skill Training for Affect and Interpersonal Regulation (STAIR; Cloitre, Cohen, & Koenen, 2006) is sixteen to twenty-session individual psychotherapy designed specifically to help women with complex trauma histories and severe chronic PTSD. The intervention has two goals: (1) teaching skills to help clients regulate their often extreme and unstable emotion states and (2) providing psychoeducation and skills in assertive and effective communication to manage conflict and develop intimacy in personal relationships. STAIR has shown promise in two large randomized clinical trials of women with child-abuse-related PTSD (Cloitre, Koenen, Cohen, & Han, 2002; Cloitre et al., 2010). STAIR was found to be most efficacious in reducing PTSD severity and enhancing affect regulation when followed by a modified brief version of PE, but it has not been evaluated as a stand-alone therapy except for short-term outcomes (Cloitre et al., 2002, 2010). Additional research is underway.

Summary: Memory- and Emotion-Processing Therapies

Trauma-memory and emotion processing can be accomplished in a number of ways with several well-validated interventions described in training manuals designed to enable clinicians to deliver the intervention accurately and effectively. In addition to these evidence-based memory- and emotion-processing therapies, other creative variations have been developed to help clients process the emotional, biological, and cognitive impact of complex trauma (Ford, 2009b, 2009c). These include experiential psychotherapies such as Adaptive Information Processing/EMDR (F. Shapiro, 2012; R. Shapiro, 2010); Accelerated Experiential-Dynamic Psychotherapy (AEDP; Fosha, 2000; Fosha et al., 2009; McCullough et al., 2003), sensoriomotor psychotherapy (SP; Fisher & Ogden, 2009; Ogden & Fisher, 2013; Ogden et al., 2006), somatic treatment (Levine, 1997, 2008; Rothschild, 2000), contextual therapy (Gold, 2000, 2009), contextual behavior therapy (Follette et al., 2009), affect or emotion-based therapies (Fosha, 2000; Fosha et al., 2009; Paivio & Pascual-Leone, 2010), psychoanalytic treatments (Bateman & Fonagy, 2004a, 2004b; Kohlenberg & Tsai, 1991; Spermon, Darlington, & Gibney, 2010), and attachment-based (Basham & Miehls, 2004), attachment and neurophysiologically based (Schore, 1993b, 2013; Siegel, 2012a, 2012b; Solomon & Tatkin, 2010), and emotion-focused therapies for couples in which one or both have been traumatized (Johnson, 2002; Johnson & Courtois, 2009), to name only a few of the most widely disseminated models (see Courtois & Ford, 2009, and Courtois, 2010, for a more complete overview of complex-trauma-processing therapies). These interventions utilize theory-driven techniques to encourage therapeutic discussion of past or recent distressing events that may be actual traumas or experiences that are thematically similar to past traumatic events to help clients become more fully aware of their emotions, bodily states, thoughts, and avoidant behavior patterns in a very specific and structured manner.

The goal in all processing models is to help clients reinstate a full and accurate awareness of trauma-related emotions, bodily reactions, thoughts, behaviors, and consequences, but, what is more, to help them to recognize that what they felt, thought, and did in reaction to past traumatic circumstances does not have to be ongoing in the present or repeated in the future.

This involves both *realization* and *presentification*, per Van der Hart, Nijenhuis, and Steele (2006). Such traumatic stress reactions, defenses, and adaptations were necessary then. They became automatic despite the fact that they were no longer needed. Clients are encouraged to purposefully reenact (e.g., in a role-play fashion derived originally from Gestalt therapy and psychodrama) or carefully observe (e.g., by keeping a detailed self- monitoring diary of what led up to and followed in the aftermath of symptomatic reactions) their current emotionally charged or dissociative experiences in order to change them. Armed with new awareness, clients can then create and experiment with alternative ways of feeling, thinking, and behaving when they are experiencing traumatic stress reactions in the present. Although exposure to or creating a narrative of specific past traumatic events is not required in any of these therapies, these methods help clients achieve a better understanding of the origin of otherwise puzzling symptoms or intrusive memories.

PREPARING THE CLIENT FOR TRAUMA AND EMOTION PROCESSING

It is now a given that traumatic memories must be faced directly and then processed for them not to be replayed as reexperiencing and avoidance symptoms. Facing memories challenges clients' known and comfortable ways of coping and years or decades of habitual avoidance. Because avoidance/dissociation may have been the only viable way for survivors to avoid troubling memories, raising the necessity to face them may seem irrational and unnecessary and may even feel coercive. "I don't really have a choice; my therapist and other important people in my life just want me to 'get over the trauma' and 'get better.' " Thus even considering trauma memory processing may lead to a reaction of anger and confrontation (e.g., "What right do you [therapist] have to make me go through those awful memories all over again?") or attempts to put the therapist on the defensive (e.g., "Why do you think that you can help me when you don't know what I've been through and you don't seem qualified to do this [risky] type of therapy?").

Many trauma survivors were essentially brainwashed by perpetrators who told them what they thought or felt or that certain thoughts or actions were indications of their culpability or defectiveness. Subsequent messages that are well intentioned but that essentially second-guess the client are likely to be interpreted as similarly controlling, condemning, or threatening. For this reason it is important for the therapist to learn from the client what she or he was taught or has come to believe about remembering or disclosing past trauma. With that knowledge, the therapist can provide reassurance that therapy can help the client to gain mastery over those memories but that the choice to approach them belongs to the client. It is just as important to help the client understand and work through these past demands for secrecy and fears of disclosure as it is to process the traumatic events themselves, as the two are often intertwined.

Technical Considerations in Conducting Phase 2 Trauma and Emotion Processing

In addition to the technical guidelines provided for the various trauma- and emotion-processing models, several transtheoretical clinical considerations are essential for safe and effective work: (1) determinations for moving into Phase 2, (2) tactics for encouraging engagement, and (3) tactics for optimizing affective intensity and physical arousal. Due to the multitude of symptoms and the lack of skills experienced by the average client, most complex trauma requires more rather than less time in Phase 1; however, no specific amount of time or number of sessions must be completed before moving into Phase 2. As noted earlier, some clients never go beyond the first phase and are satisfied with the progress made and the support gained.

Once the tasks of Phase 1 have been accomplished, clients who remain symptomatic then face the question of whether to engage in emotional processing. To do so, they should have sufficient resources (personal and interpersonal) and life safety and stability to be able to provide voluntary informed consent. Some clients feel pressured internally or by external sources (e.g., family members who want them to be less symptomatic or to be done with treatment, financial pressure, etc.) to face and divulge traumatic memories, regardless of the emotional cost to them. The therapist must help them discern whether such pressures are in play. They should also seek to uncover and understand the client's beliefs and fears about facing the trauma. Clients tend to benefit from validation of their intense desire to "get it out" or "get it over with," with sensitive redirection to focus first on the method under discussion (described to them in detail) to make an informed decision about proceeding or not. Clients need to be redirected from premature and impulsive "purging" or "dumping" because the gains achieved by such catharsis (if any) tend to be short-lived and often lead to upsurges in symptoms and regressions in functioning rather than resolution.

Other clients are terrified or at best anxious or suspicious about revisiting the past. They tend to benefit from permission not to disclose anything until they decide they are ready and are convinced that processing can be done safely. In general, the therapist can best encourage these clients to do processing work by carefully explaining that the goal of reviewing troubling memories in writing or imaginally is to develop increased understanding and for the memory to lose its potency to trigger the reexperiencing and numbing symptoms of PTSD. It is useful to add a caveat that the processing of traumatic events and aftereffects does not erase the memories, nor does it cause them to become emotionally neutral. It does result in their becoming more like memories of normal (nontraumatic) events, no longer triggering unanticipated and upsetting reactions. What processing can accomplish is to provide the client with experiential evidence that it is possible to reflectively review troubling memories, to feel the impact but in manageable amounts, while being able to think clearly about what is happening and how the event(s) ended and life continued on—rather than being trapped in the vicious cycle of PTSD symptoms.

Informed consent for trauma and emotion processing is an extension of the informed consent obtained at the beginning of treatment (involving either an amendment to the original document or a separate one). Once some emotional processing has begun and the client has achieved sufficient emotional stabilization and skills to be able to anticipate, recognize, and cope with distress, therapist and client can discuss more formal processing procedures. The client needs specific information about several key points:

1. What he or she will be asked to do to maintain a sufficient intensity of physical arousal and emotional engagement for processing to occur without becoming overwhelmed (including ways to reduce arousal or emotional intensity without disengaging from processing).
2. What he or she is likely to experience emotionally. The client should be informed that he or she might feel worse in the short term but that the increased emotional load is of limited duration and is the mechanism that allows resolution.
3. What the therapist will do in order to ensure emotional safety and support.
4. What the known potential risks and benefits of the procedure are.
5. What control he or she will have over ending the protocol if it is overly aversive or overwhelming, or if he or she simply chooses to do so.

Although it is not therapeutically optimal to discontinue the review and processing of troubling memories because the client feels unable to tolerate the distress or dissociation elicited, it is essential that the client always have the choice to stop, pause, and regroup if she or he does not feel safe, appears unsafe, or begins to decompensate. In order to prevent this from happening, the therapist can utilize a number of tactics for optimizing arousal and engagement while conducting this aspect of treatment.

Informed consent is an affirmation by the client of these points, as well as an explicit agreement that she or he agrees to proceed with the trauma and emotion processing work. On the other hand, informed refusal is just that.

Tactics for Optimizing Affective Intensity and Physical Arousal

Therapeutic exposure can be conducted in a variety of ways in order to best match each client's tolerable and therapeutic window of emotion intensity and arousal (Carey, 2011).

• *Flooding* involves having the client reexperience full memory with as complete and intense an awareness of her or his physical sensations and emotional reactions as possible. This is the approach typically used in PE (especially implosive flooding).

• *Systematic desensitization* involves a more gradual increase in arousal and emotional intensity, using a "graduated hierarchy" of memories and arousal and emotion states—starting with the least distressing aspects of a troubling memory and progressing to points in the event in which the client was most hypo- or hyperaroused or distressed—that the client and therapist construct prior to beginning their actual review of memories. This method is used routinely in CPT and the emotion-focused and experiential psychotherapies.

• *Narrative reconstruction* is involved in all of these procedures. It calls for the development of a first-person story-like description of how the event(s) began, unfolded, and ended, with as much detail as possible. The ultimate goal is for the client to put the pieces together in a temporal sequence (instead of the typically fragmented and disjointed memories) and to reassociate emotions, sensations, and thoughts that have previously been dissociated or split off.

Across all approaches, memory and emotion processing is safest and most effective if the client is encouraged to and is able to stay within a personally manageable "window" of affective intensity and bodily arousal. When he or she moves out of this space and exhibits hyper- or hypoarousal, the therapist must help with a return to homeostasis and encouragement to expand emotional tolerance. Briere and Scott (2006, 2012) recommend several ways to remediate "window errors" (p. 137) in line with recommendations made by others such as Fisher and Ogden (2009), Ogden and Fisher (2013), and Van der Hart et al. (2006):

- Help the client immediately use self-calming or emotion regulation skills developed in Phase 1.
- Use intonation and carefully chosen words to convey calm confidence that the client has the skills to be able to move through the memory to achieve a sense of closure.
- Calmly remind the client that she or he is not alone and not actually in the traumatic circumstances but is being safely guided through revisiting them with the therapist present and in support.
- Redirect the client to a less distressing or dysregulating aspect of the event in order to titrate the arousal intensity without interrupting the processing and narrative building.

To these we add gentle encouragement on the part of the therapist, "nudging" the client to face or to describe "a bit more, and then just a bit more." For example, the therapist might repeat the suggestion to "put what you're seeing, hearing, feeling, and thinking into words, as long as you feel able to continue to experience the memory." This statement helps the client to focus on actively making sense of her or his personal experience rather than simply reexperiencing it as intrusive and intolerable. The therapist thus serves as a guide in supporting the client in acquiring a sense of personal authority over the memory (Harvey, 1996), while reinforcing the progress in reprocessing traumatic material.

Tactics for Enhancing Engagement

Trauma and emotion processing is most effective and efficient if the client is actively engaged as a participant as well as an observer. This enhances a sense of control that stands in sharp contrast to the typical feeling of helplessness during the actual trauma. In contrast to the actual time of the trauma, when it is difficult if not impossible for the victim to step back and self-observe, therapeutic processing offers a very different vantage point from which to understand the circumstance and its accompanying physical, emotional, and cognitive responses. The intent of active engagement is not to heighten the client's arousal or emotional intensity for its own sake but to put the client in the position of being both an active participant and a mindful observer. Active engagement is different from being emotionally overwhelmed and in a state of shock or detachment. The latter interferes with the ability to make sense of the flood of impressions, sensations, and emotions.

Tactics for enhancing engagement in trauma and emotion processing include behavioral or experiential techniques in which the client is encouraged not just to imagine but actually to enact the troubling memory or event. *In vivo* exposure is an example: the therapist directs the client in purposefully encounter reminders of traumatic events, that is, situations, people, places, or activities that trigger emotional distress or shutdown. This usually is done using a systematic desensitization format in which the client progresses through a hierarchy of current-day activities to those that are triggering and previously had elicited overwhelming distress or numbing. In another technique, engagement can be enhanced behaviorally through experiential exercises in which the client confronts people in a role-play format—for example, the empty-chair technique in which the client role-plays a conversation with a perpetrator in which thoughts and feelings that were unspoken or unacknowledged are disclosed and limits and boundaries set for any current or future interactions.

Somatic tactics for engagement help the client become aware of and reflect on the possible meaning(s) of physical reactions and sensations and body states that occur during emotional processing. For example, in sensorimotor psychotherapy (Ogden et al., 2006; Ogden & Fisher, 2013), the therapist carefully monitors subtle nonverbal signs of somatic changes reflecting hypo- or hyperarousal when the client is asked to access the memory "frame by frame." The therapist selectively comments on these physical signs and state shifts as a way of bringing them to conscious awareness thus allowing them to be assessed as to their meaning (i.e., unspoken thoughts, emotions, and intentions).

Affective tactics for engagement involve helping clients to develop or expand their emotion vocabulary, their confidence in and willingness to express rather than hide, discount, or avoid their emotions, and their ability to use emotions as information rather than regarding them as useless distractions or harmful burdens (Ford, 2005). Techniques from emotion-focused and experiential psychotherapies focus attention on conflicted, disavowed, dissociated, and disinhibited emotions (i.e., rage, resentment, shame, grief, terror) and on positive emotions (i.e., confidence, contentment, pride, interest, determination, love) to normalize the full range of emotions and to identify them as means of self-definition rather than as useless or threatening. For example, the TARGET intervention guides clients in distinguishing between emotions that reflect either a state of stress reactivity ("alarm") or a state of self-awareness and confidence ("focus") so they learn that both types of emotion have purpose and function and that the ability to have both and to have ambivalent and mixed emotions is normal. Similarly, the emotion regulation modules in DBT (Linehan, 1993), SS (Najavits, 2002a, 2002b), and STAIR (Cloitre et al., 2010) assist in the recognition and modulation of emotion states.

Motivational tactics for engagement involve identifying and building on the client's goals and values to underscore that the processing work is worth the effort and discomfort involved. The motivation may be self-focused (e.g., to be able to feel free from onerous reactions or strong and courageous enough to overcome and transcend traumatic memories; to increase self-confidence and self-esteem) or other-focused and altruistic (e.g., to be able to be a better partner or parent; to be able to protect others from experiencing trauma; to be a role model for others who have experienced trauma and are struggling to recover).

Strategies for Enhancing and Maintaining Reflective Self-Awareness

Although processing requires mid-range arousal and consistent engagement, the ultimate goal is for clients to develop the ability to be *reflectively self-aware* when experiencing traumatic stress reactions (Ford, 2009b). The psychoanalyst Harry Stack Sullivan coined the term "participant observer" to describe how therapists can provide a role model by being actively involved in the therapeutic interaction even as they are able to step back (figuratively) and observe the dynamics of the client's inner life and the therapist–client interaction. Subsequent advances in the evolution of psychodynamic psychotherapy, such as Kohut's self psychology (Kohut &

Wolf, 1978), the British school of object relations (e.g., Winnicott, 1971), Bowlby's (1969) seminal work on attachment and loss, and Fonagy's mentalizing model (Allen et al., 2008; Allen, 2012), have converged on the importance in both child development and psychotherapy of developing the client's capacity to be mindful and to be able to engage in self-reflection. For an individual to be self-reflectively aware requires the development of increased attentiveness to and understanding of his or her physical sensations, emotions, thoughts, and choices, beginning with the incorporation of the mirroring of attuned others.

During trauma and emotion processing, the therapist models reflective self-awareness. This involves inquiry about the nature and source of emotions and thoughts that the client identifies and describes while processing a troubling memory (e.g., possible reasons why certain feelings or thoughts might occur and how they make sense under the circumstances). It also includes modeling how to develop and test theories regarding the motivations and intent of people to help make sense of their actions. The therapist also helps the client to extend her or his "working models" or "theory of mind" of self and other to hypothesize how the client's feelings and thoughts affect those of others and vice versa. Inquiries of this sort help clients to understand the influence they have on others—especially important for those who have believed themselves to be worthless or powerless in relation to others and those who are largely oblivious to their ability to influence others.

Determining When to Stop

Trauma and emotion processing may be done in as little as a single session (as reported in some cases of EMDR), especially for one-time or limited duration trauma, but most often requires repetition in many sessions (some of extended duration) over several weeks or months. Two criteria are particularly important in judging when "enough" processing has taken place. The first is whether the client feels no longer as troubled by the memory. Although the client's desire to continue or stop should always be taken into consideration, it is important to discuss and assess the reasons behind any request. Then it remains important to assess whether this sense of resolution has generalized beyond the therapy context to the client's daily encounters and moods. If the primary reasons are fatigue or difficulty tolerating the distress elicited, it is better to pause and discuss what can make the procedure more tolerable. If the client continues to avoid triggers or experiences symptom flare-ups or downturns in mood that seem to involve unfinished emotional business of a focal trauma memory, additional discussion and processing of aspects of the troubling memories are important to consider.

The second criterion is whether the client is able to develop a personal lifeline, including an understanding of his or her life that is coherent and has a narrative structure (notwithstanding that there may still be gaps).

Clients from insecure and disorganized backgrounds usually lack coherence in understanding their experiences and putting them into words. As discussed in the prior section, processing requires the development of a theory of mind, both in relationship to oneself and to others. The first involves developing explicit beliefs about how mentally processing of past experiences can result in a sense of calm and resolution; the second involves an increased understanding of the motives and actions of others.

To the extent that the client has formulated a complementary theory of what others involved in the event (including victimizers, other victims, caregivers who did or did not provide help and protection, and any bystanders) were thinking and feeling and how their actions (or inaction) followed from these possible states of mind and emotions, the client's sense that the event is understandable is likely to be greatest. Traumatic events often include unexplainable aspects, but they also involve logical sequences of feelings, thoughts, and actions that are the survivors' (and also the victimizers') attempts to adapt to and have some control in largely uncontrollable situations. When a client is able to understand the logical connections within a traumatic event, especially the psychological components and how they fit together, the memory begins to resemble other nontraumatic memories even though it can still retain a distinct emotional impact. To make sense of previously inchoate memory, the higher-order areas of the brain (prefrontal region) regain some inhibitory control over the emotional (limbic) areas of the brain (Ford, 2009a, 2009b). This does not neutralize the emotional impact; rather, as it is more understood it is no longer the threat it was.

Tactics for Preventing and Managing Crises

Crises and decompensation can occur in Phase 2 (as throughout the treatment) in a variety of ways, including hypervigilance or emotional numbing, dissociative self-fragmentation, suicidality, self-mutilation, risky or self-defeating behavior, violence or relational aggression, and deterioration of comorbid psychiatric symptoms and disorders. Such crises occur for many reasons, some of them external and situational, making them beyond control and ability to anticipate, and some due to the client's behavior, making them preventable or manageable if reported or noticed early enough. A common reason for crises to develop during this treatment phase is impatience in the therapist or client that can result in overwhelming the client's. The therapist can help impatient or fearfully impulsive or compulsive clients from lapsing into (or remaining in) a state of partially self-induced intrusive reexperiencing by modeling patience and validating the importance of every apparently "small" step the client takes toward being more self-regulated ("make haste slowly" or "take just a slice of the experience until you feel something"). Typically, clients don't want to be overwhelmed or to go into crisis—although there may be some secondary gain for some—yet at times they may overestimate or "overshoot" their actual capacity in a rush to get the process over with. The best approach is a return to the skills of emotional modulation before beginning or resuming exposure and processing activities.

Where the therapist is the one who is impatient with the pace of treatment, self-assessment is in order. Therapist intolerance might be due to personal or professional issues, some of which are unrelated to the specific client and some of which might not be in the therapist's control. To whatever degree possible, the therapist experiencing personal or professional stress must determine whether he or she is able to be emotionally available and supportive to the client once processing is underway. If not, then processing should not be undertaken, or the selected techniques should be those that evoke the least amount of intensity. Although the therapist should be careful about overdisclosure of personal information, explaining to the client that he or she is overburdened or stressed is appropriate. Another reason for therapist impatience may be countertransference to the client's impatience. It can be resolved, in part, by jointly pacing the work. It can be important for the therapist to get consultation or supervision to clarify whether the problem is technical or whether he or she is holding overly high expectations on one hand or is in a position of dread and avoidance on the other, or whether other factors are at play. Relational issues and countertransference are discussed in Chapters 8–10, and the vicarious trauma or compassion fatigue that can contribute to or result from trauma-related countertransference is discussed in detail in Chapter 10.

Unfortunately, the treatment itself sometimes results in the development of a crisis—for example, when it does not simply expose the client to troubling memories but inadvertently activates or intensifies intrusive reexperiencing. In such a situation, it is vital to pause, step back and refocus on self-regulation skills to strengthen the client's capacities for secure attachment (in the therapy and in daily life) and to collaboratively develop a working theory with the client about why the procedure is triggering intrusive memories (Briere & Scott, 2006, 2012). Repacing the exposure or replacing prolonged exposure with more graduated and attenuated approaches is usually in order. Optimally, the client comes away from the setback with a better understanding of personal triggers and how to maintain rather than lose control when triggers occur.

The cases of Hector and Doris provide vivid illustrations of how crises can develop in Phase 2 work, as well as how they can be effectively handled.

Hector: Dealing with Suicidality in Prolonged Exposure Therapy

After a considerable period devoted to stabilization and sobriety, Hector and his therapist successfully initiated PE to help him work though a military combat trauma memory that he found particularly shaming. This procedure was implemented only after extensive preparation, with special attention to periodic spikes in suicidality when he found himself ruminating about this memory. They developed a shared plan for him to "check in" about any increases in feelings of guilt and shame and in his urge to escape during the course of the exposure work in order to catch and defuse (using his emotion regulation skills) any early warning signs of suicidality. Hector was reassured to know that he could signal if he felt even the smallest precursor symptoms, either by asking the therapist to pause while he identified emotions and thoughts that he could draw on to prevent dissociative detachment or by nonverbally indicating he needed help from the therapist in regaining a sense of being in a safe place with a trustworthy person.

When Hector attempted to listen to an audiotape of his traumatic memory at home as part of the agreed-on exposure protocol, he began to dissociate and feel suicidal. Nevertheless, he persisted in listening and had a full flashback of being in the traumatic event. His roommate found him staring at a loaded gun (which he had locked up separately from the bullets and had no recollection of unlocking or loading), muttering, "it's time, it's time. . . . " His roommate called the police, who took Hector to the emergency room, where he was hospitalized for 5 days. He was able to be discharged safely at that point—about one-third the length of stay that usually was required when he had previously been suicidal.

At their session the day after his discharge, his therapist asked Hector what he thought had happened and after Hector just shook his head and did not speak, offered the possible explanation that "you may have felt extremely alone, even abandoned, when you listened to the tape of that traumatic event. This likely reminded you of your experience early in life of being left alone while scary things were happening. I was mistaken in not realizing how traumatizing it was for you and how trying to process alone would restimulate those feelings. We can modify our plan so that you are not alone when you're doing exposure work."

This illustrates a "repair" of the therapeutic alliance as described by Briere and Scott (2006, 2012) and attachment theorists, in which the therapist takes responsibility for not providing sufficient guidance and support but simultaneously formulates a plan for addressing the client's distress so the exposure can continue. Hector and his therapist did not rush back into processing but spent most of the next two sessions shoring up their preparation plan, including adding several ways in which Hector could imaginally reestablish secure contact with the therapist when they were apart any time that he felt that would help him to feel confident and supported and not just when recalling a traumatic event. When they resumed, Hector was able to relive the event more vividly and fully than previously, and he realized that his fear of facing the event alone was a critical trigger. Hector also noted that he seemed to feel more generally trusting of his therapist and of other key people in his life. He stated with some poignancy, "I know none of you will ever leave me, because I'll always keep you inside me."

Doris: Dealing with Dissociative Dysregulation in EMDR

After Doris learned about EMDR from a friend, she insisted that it was the solution to all of her problems and pressured her therapist to "Get on with it, don't make me waste any more of my life waiting to finally feel normal!" Her therapist helped Doris work on a number of somatic, affective, and cognitive strategies for recognizing the precursors of dissociation, explaining that EMDR required the client to be present in the moment in order to have the most rapid and full benefit. Doris reluctantly experimented with these skills in therapy sessions and in daily life, frequently characterizing them as "fluff, just the opening act before the real event, when you finally *let me do* EMDR." The therapist realized that Doris's perspective was colored by magical thinking and idealization—of the technique in this case, with the therapist and their interaction correspondingly devalued.

However, when Doris had had several weeks of consistent attendance and engagement in therapy and was able to manage problems in her day-to-day life and her emotions with self-regulation skills, the therapist agreed to proceed. Per the EMDR protocol, the therapist cautioned Doris that, although the technique can provide a great deal of relief from distressing memories, this outcome could not be guaranteed. Even if it did, the continuing challenge would be for her to be aware of and regulate her bodily, emotional, and mental reactions when circumstances triggered traumatic memories. The therapist provided further perspective on the benefits by suggesting that whether or not Doris felt relief, she could gain understanding and self-knowledge from the memory work, which could help her further build her confidence and hopefulness.

Doris described her experience in doing EMDR initially to be "powerful; it's almost like the pain I've been carrying just melted away. I felt cleaner and freer than I ever have." Her therapist recognized this as likely a continuation of her idealization and likely to be short-lived. She helped Doris to pay close attention to physical sensations and to articulate her specific emotions and thoughts as she experienced different parts of the traumatic event. Doris experienced vivid "in the moment" awareness of her internal experience, along with the seemingly overblown sense of relief and bliss. This lasted until she encountered a point in the memory in which she perceived her mother as "turning on me like she wanted to kill me, turning into the hideous monster that's been in my nightmares all my life!" At that point, Doris became very still, her eyes glazed over, and she very slowly hunched over and put her hands over her head and in front of her face as if to protect herself from blows from above. When she did not respond to requests to describe what is happening "outside you and inside you" and was clearly not consciously aware of or following the saccadic movement protocol, the therapist spoke to Doris in a calm but somewhat firmer and louder voice to begin to reestablish their connection and to ground her in the present time and place.

> "Doris, I see that you are remembering being very frightened of your mother, and we can help you be safe if you can focus on not being alone

right now. You are facing a terrifying experience that has stayed with you for many years but you are not alone as you were then. You and I together have found the little girl that you were back then and we will help her. You and I are making sure that the little girl inside you—a younger and more scared version of the same person that you are now—get the help she needs to understand why your mother was so upset and angry back then and we will protect you today."

The therapist noted that as she spoke, Doris was able to briefly glance in her direction, as if beginning to realize that she was not alone and checking to see if the therapist was calm or angry. The therapist therefore continued:

"I'm just going to move my chair a little closer to you so I can be close enough to help, but not so close that I scare you. As I move over, you can know that you are not alone and you can begin to let the little girl inside you know. You are still very scared and feeling helpless with your angry mother, but I see that you can tell that this is not happening all over again—you can hear me and you know me and my voice as someone who helps you and is not angry with you. You can begin to see that my face and my body are not tense and angry. I'm moving very slowly to be near you but will not make you do anything you don't want to. [The therapist notes a somewhat longer glance, with a very intense and questioning gaze from Doris.] That's it, come back to the present and know that you are here with me in a therapy session and that it's 2011. As you let yourself see me more clearly and as you hear my voice, you can decide if you feel safe letting me help you."

The therapist continued to help Doris gradually reinstate awareness of familiarity and trust in their relationship and in the safety of the office atmosphere. At one point, Doris sharply shifted her demeanor, becoming enraged, as if she were enacting her mother's rage toward the therapist. The therapist firmly but calmly helped her to know that the anger she had experienced from her mother was not going to hurt her (the therapist), nor was it going to cause the therapist to abandon helping "adult Doris" get "child Doris" safely through the terrifying event. Doris challenged the therapist's capacity to stand up to this anger, even screaming expletives at her, but the therapist responded only by speaking more firmly to let Doris know that that anger did not belong in their relationship. She could choose to let go of the rage without either hurting her mother (by transferring the introjected angry self back into her mother, which she protectively did not want to do because she did not want to lose her mother's caring) or being a monster in retaliation toward her mother.

Doris rapidly went back to the "little girl numbed" state and gradually showed signs of calming, letting down her guard, and feeling comforted. As she did, the therapist continued to help her back to the present. She continued to describe how they were working together to provide the safety, security, strength, and protection that Doris had lacked as a child. After about 20 minutes of intensive grounding and refocusing, Doris "came back" as if waking from a dream. At first, she denied any memory of the interaction. The therapist reconstructed what had happened, focusing on the meaning of each part of the experience. In this way, the therapy was able to transform a potentially countertherapeutic resurgence of dissociated memories and self-states into a reparative experience. Doris could understand her needs more fully, including for her own safety, connection, and competence in the face of her mother's unpredictable rage and also for her mother not to be harmed or lost to her due to her reciprocal anger. Doris also was able to experience herself as having those feelings and achieving previously unarticulated (but evident to the therapist) hopes and goals. From Doris's perspective, the experience helped her to understand why, as the therapist had suggested, there was more to EMDR than simply feeling pain from disturbing memories, and how EMDR needed active participation in order to meet past traumatic challenges. As she said in winding down the session, "Now I see why I can't do this all by myself or just my way. When I let you help me, I'm not giving up my independence."

As we wrap up this section, we note that new methods for Phase 2 processing within the context of group treatment have been developed (Mendelsohn et al., 2011). Approaches to group therapy for adults with histories of interpersonal victimization (Taylor & Harvey, 2010) or PTSD (Lubin & Johnson, 2008; Shea, McDevitt-Murphy, Ready, & Schnurr, 2009; Wampold et al., 2010; Zlotnick, Capezza, & Parker, 2011) have shown mixed evidence of effectiveness, at best. The approach that has most consistently demonstrated clinically significant benefits is CBT with trauma-memory processing. Although a large randomized clinical trial study with male military veterans with PTSD failed to support the CBT/trauma-memory-processing model (Schnurr et al., 2003), adaptations to the memory-processing protocol have made it more suitable to group therapy (e.g., primarily conducting imaginal recall of trauma memories in carefully structured homework exercises), with promising results in a small randomized clinical trial with motor vehicle accident victims with PTSD (Beck et al., 2009) and in an open trial with more than 100 male military veterans with chronic PTSD (Ready et al., 2008). Relationally focused approaches to helping survivors to move from Phase 1, stabilization, into Phase 2, integration of trauma memories into their overall life narratives, are currently being field tested (Campanini et al., 2010; Fallot & Harris, 2002; Lubin & Johnson, 2008; Mendelsohn, Zachary, & Harney, 2007). These models are consistent with the evidence supporting narrative approaches to individual therapy for trauma survivors (e.g., CPT, NET, STAIR) and offer a complementary alternative approach to CBT.

LOSS AND MOURNING AS SPECIAL ISSUES IN PHASE 2 PROCESSING

Interpersonal victimization and other types of complex trauma involve not only an assault on the self and involves major loss—of the self as it might have been or as it was before; of control, trust, innocence, and naiveté regarding self and others; of life assumptions and of a sense of safety in the world (Janoff-Bulman, 1992), along with other more tangible losses. Victimized individuals frequently view themselves as pre- and postevent selves, profoundly altered by what happened to them. The recognition of loss might be evident earlier in treatment but is especially likely to occur in Phase 2. Whatever the procedure used to address the trauma and however it is applied, emotion processing of trauma evokes the recognition of what has been lost and with it feelings of sadness, rage, grief, mourning, anguish, and despair. As significant as these losses are to the individual who experienced them, they may not have been identified or recognized because they are private and personal rather than public and are therefore less visible to others and not easily quantified. For example, the loss of identity and self-esteem, sense of personal worth, faith and trust in self and others, spirituality, sense of body ownership, and body integrity are less outwardly dramatic and noticeable than the loss of home and property. And yet they are so much more significant and profound.

Boss (2006) pioneered the study of *ambiguous loss*, defined as an indistinct loss lacking a clear ending. The very uncertainty that surrounds ambiguous losses makes them highly stressful. They are not visible or concrete, not publicly recognized for the most part, are ongoing, and have no formalized certification process or mourning ritual that demarcate their ending and that allow a good-bye. Although the losses accrued through child abuse and other forms of interpersonal victimization that make up complex trauma were not specifically discussed by Boss, they fit her formulation and provide a means of understanding the many subjective losses that can occur, including the loss of self and such issues as the interruption of the individual's "normal," preordained, or God-given soul or life trajectory, major losses indeed.

Related concepts of *complicated grief, bereavement* (Neimeyer, 2001), or *complicated mourning* (Rando, 1993), *traumatic bereavement*, (Kaltman & Bonanno, 2003) and *disenfranchised grief* (Doka, 1989) are useful in understanding clients' losses. Ambivalence in primary attachment relationships that have been abusive, exploitive, or neglectful contributes to difficulties with bereavement, especially after the death or loss of perpetrators or other family members or after less concrete and public types of losses. Of particular poignancy, despite a lack of conscious awareness, the client might nevertheless be engaged in a compulsive pattern of seeking out lost objects and lost opportunities in a futile search for what was denied or previously lost. Repetition compulsions or traumatic enactments and reenactments are ways to unconsciously attempt to gain what was lost, was previously unavailable and to be acceptable to others, thereby changing the past. Unfortunately, these strategies put clients at risk for continued harmful and hurtful relationships when they result in reenactment-based revictimization and additional abandonment or disregard; furthermore, unless the losses are accepted and resolved, clients may spend their lives in a futile search for what was and continues to be unavailable.

To process and heal trauma memories and emotions, the client must grieve past losses as part of the emotion processing and stop the self-sacrifice involved in trying to heal the family or take care of anyone else. *Accepting the loss means, in part, admitting to its reality and to the inability to control the circumstances.* Paradoxically, attempts to control and make up for loss can result in more loss. Yet, as losses are accepted the genuine but formerly disowned pain comes forward, along with grief and mourning. The client grieves for losses that are about him or her as a person (i.e., "original," undeveloped, or unrecognized, pretrauma self, or lost innocence) and for other losses of significance (i.e., the absence of healthy and attentive parents, lost childhood, lost security, lost career opportunities, lost relationships, compromised health and mental health, and so forth). In another paradoxical twist, some clients must accept trauma-based successes, because some have been able to use survivor skills to their advantage and have enjoyed personal recovery, been successful parents and spouse/partners, and achieved career and community success as a result. Such "posttraumatic growth" may be hard to accept and disavowed, as it may be accompanied by feelings of unworthiness or of being an imposter.

Grief and mourning are natural and painful processes that, when they result in emotional resolution, free up stores of emotional and physical energy that can be applied to present-day and future life. During the later part of the therapy process and after processing, the client is encouraged to look forward rather than back and to use this newfound clarity and energy to build a self-defined future, one not based on the needs or expectations of others or of caretaking. Emotional energy is thus withdrawn from past trauma and reinvested in the self and in new ways of being, increasing the likelihood of healthier and more reciprocal relationships.

Additionally, during this phase of treatment, the client might begin to consider specific actions with regard to abusers or others such as disclosures and discussions, the development of better personal boundaries in relationships, or separation from or reconnection with others. At this stage, these are all based on enhanced awareness and understanding derived from trauma processing and resolution that supports new skills for self-definition and assertiveness with others. Whatever the actions, clients are on a more solid footing when they are considered after emotion processing when they are more stable and less in the throes of posttraumatic reactivity.

PHASE 3: CONSOLIDATING THERAPEUTIC GAINS

The client's challenge in Phase 3 is to apply the knowledge and skills gained throughout the treatment to daily life and the future. The goal of this phase is to consolidate therapeutic gains and move toward ending the treatment. This does not imply complete recovery or freedom from all posttraumatic symptoms or impairment. Instead, this phase should be understood by therapists (and communicated clearly to clients) as applying treatment gains to the goals that motivated the client in the first place (or additional goals determined during the course of treatment). In this phase, survivors are challenged to apply their new learning—from the all-or-nothing ways of evaluating themselves and the world that are based on trauma and interrupted development (Foa, Ehlers, Clark, Tolin, & Orsillo, 1999) to a nuanced and realistic understanding of their life options based on *who they are and what they want.*

This phase involves checking out practical options for change and for life ownership that may not have been possible previously due to the impact of symptoms, injunctions from the past, and the client's lack of awareness that change was even possible. This is also when clients assess what resolution and the termination of treatment mean to them. Some wrap up therapy rather quickly, whereas others have a number of additional issues that need further work before ending. Unlike Phase 2, for which there are several well-validated or clinically promising therapy interventions, specialized interventions for Phase 3 have thus far received less clinical attention (except for some specific topics such as sexuality and sexual functioning, career development, etc.) and very little by way of scientific study, a situation that is now changing.

This section provides an overview of the tasks of Phase 3 and some of the most common issues that arise. This phase can be understood as the next logical step beyond healing the psychic wounds of trauma to reversing posttraumatic decline and creating a more enriched and satisfactory life. The client with complex trauma is no longer "just" a distressed survivor but can lay claim to increased self-esteem and ability to differentiate self from others and have relationships that are reciprocal and trustworthy. In Phase 3, the challenge is to extrapolate and deploy in daily living the knowledge and skills gained or strengthened earlier in therapy and to deepen and broaden their application. This is done with even more intention after the client has achieved emotional resolution of the trauma and a lessening of symptoms. This intentional application means *responding to life events and making choices from a position of increased self-knowledge, along with healthy self-regard and positive and appropriate selfishness, thoughtfulness, and mindfulness.* These are then assessed and applied to the development of healthy and more intimate relationships with others.

Phase 3 continues the integration of distressing and previously disowned memories and feelings into a coherent rather than disjunctive personal narrative, allowing increased understanding of responses and reactions to and from others and applying this new information to present-day life circumstances. Old maladaptive mechanisms, patterns, and symptoms that continue to have impact can be analyzed and replaced with ones that are more appropriate to the present day. Not infrequently, radical redefinition of the self and relationships results as the client increasingly understands the family and the social group and community patterns and dynamics associated with past traumatization. At root, *this phase of the treatment encourages self-knowledge and understanding in context* (L. S. Brown, 2008, 2009; McMachin, Newman, Fogler, & Keane, 2012) that, in turn, leads to the capacity for self-compassion, empathy, and forgiveness that, of necessity, results in the development of a more positive self-concept to replace the shame and self-hatred of old. Furthermore, it also provides a potential path to choosing and sustaining relationships based on improved self-esteem, assertiveness and mutuality, and the development of trust and security. These replace relational patterns that required deference, superficial compliance, and dependence/codependence in return, opening different life choices that were previously unavailable, untenable, or unattainable.

For clients with a history of secure attachment experiences and whose lives were not totally overtaken by posttraumatic reactions, being emotionally regulated and engaging in relationships with a secure sense of attachment is essentially "a return to normal" rather than a radical shift, and so may be a fairly easy next step. However, for those whose lives and relationships were anything but normal, this third phase is likely to be lengthier and beset with additional problems, including exposure to other stressors and more losses. Unfortunately, when abuse has occurred within a closed system (whether the family, a political or ethnocultural context, a religious tradition or institution, a chain of command or another work setting), recovery may involve separating from the system and the people within it. This is analogous to what happens with substance abuse creation when the newly sober need to replace addicted and addiction-supportive (or codependent) people and contexts with new companions who support them and their sobriety.

Clients with complex trauma are frequently required to make difficult decisions involving separating from and limiting or cutting off contact (on a temporary or more permanent basis) with those in their family and social system who do not support their recovery and who instead persist in unhealthy and dysfunctional behaviors and interactions, including additional abuse. Change can be very threatening to relationships that are based on old patterns. It may be the case that the client's increase in health is met with a controlling or abusive response and a dictate to "change back" to the way things were. Depending on the degree of danger that is either ongoing or that emerges in the form of current abuse, violence, and coercion, the client may need to fully separate in order to be safe. When individual or groups of family members or a family atmosphere pose serious threats to safety, therapists have an equally serious obligation to understand the protective reporting laws pertaining to child, adult, and elder abuse and domestic violence in his or her practice jurisdiction. In some cases, the therapist will have little or no option than to make a report. In others, the law is less clear-cut, and reporting is left to the therapist's discretion, creating professional and ethical dilemmas. In such fraught and anxiety-provoking circumstances, the therapist may benefit from consultation and support from other professionals.

Adapting Phase 1 Interventions to Phase 3

Following the increased resolution and control over trauma memories and their reminders or triggers, the safety, stabilization, and self-regulation interventions used in Phase 1 (Chapter 5) are revisited in the third phase in order to solidify and reinforce them and broaden their application. Safety planning, self-care, and emotion regulation become a way of life rather than preventive or ameliorative tactics used primarily for coping. The therapist helps the client to examine areas of her or his life and to plan ways to apply self-regulation and interpersonal skills proactively, with increased confidence in the ability to discern the trustworthiness of others (based on observation and interactions and direct teaching about assertiveness and communication and the difference between acquaintances, work colleagues, friends, and intimates). Phase 3 constitutes an updating of the gains of the initial phase, but with a new self-knowledge and self-determination, and a sense of pride (vs. shame and helplessness), and hope and optimism (vs. hopelessness) for the future. In his contextual model of treatment developed predominantly to meet the needs of college students with complex trauma histories, Gold (2009) described Phases 1 and 3 as the "book-ends of treatment." His model emphasizes these phases over Phase 2 emotion processing, as he found that his treatment population predominantly benefit from skill building and information to make up for what was never taught due to pervasive neglect in the family of origin. His model is therefore largely cognitive; however, he has found that this cognitive understanding and the application of skills help many clients to redirect their lives in healthier ways. His modification is an example of how the treatment can be tailored or customized to more specifically target the needs of the client population.

Adapting Phase 2 Interventions to Phase 3

The memory- and emotion-processing skills of Phase 2 are directly applicable to daily living and to therapy as well, as the client becomes a more active partner in the treatment while continuing to address and make determinations about current issues that are stressful, unsatisfactory, and disappointing or that continue to elicit traumatic stress reactions. The careful, detailed review of physical states, beliefs, and affective and cognitive responses to stressful events that is the hallmark of trauma processing provides an excellent template for clients to use in addressing present-day events and choices. Rather than simply talking about events that occur between sessions, a processing approach enables clients to break those events down into their component parts to achieve a fuller understanding of their reactions and how to regulate associated emotions and maintain (or develop) a working model of secure attachment. In addition, processing interventions provide a template for the continued organizing of fragmented and confusing life events into a coherent narrative that has personal meaning and utility. The methods used to process traumatic or emotionally significant memories provide a foundation from which the client can approach life more systematically, intentionally, and mindfully. Accordingly, the interventions of the previous phase can be viewed as tools for clients to use in Phase 3 to help them not just to go through life on automatic pilot but instead to translate their experiences into personal meaning through the process of mentalization (Allen et al., 2008; Allen, 2012) that is then applied to decision making and life orientation.

Deciding If, When, and How to Return to Phase 1 or 2 after Moving On to Phase 3

Having progressed through the first two phases of therapy, clients often believe they will not, or should not, ever have to "go back" and work further on the symptoms that were addressed earlier or the trauma memories or posttraumatic emotions dealt with in trauma processing. As discussed earlier, it is important for them to understand that reworking skills, issues, or challenges that had seemed to be resolved earlier does not represent a "regression" or a "failure." Nor is it uncommon for the resolution of some issues to result in the emergence of others or for external events over which the client has no control to retrigger symptoms or otherwise cause a relapse. In the case of clients with DID, part-selves who had achieved some degree of co-conscious awareness and integration might redissociate under the stress.

Obviously, whatever the source, events such as these can be quite disruptive to progress and can be frustrating and disillusioning for both members of the therapeutic dyad. As discussed previously, this phase-oriented treatment model is best introduced as one that is fluid and flexible rather than static, as one that recursively returns to previously learned tasks and skills as needed in order to relearn or reinforce them (Courtois, 2010; Ford, 2012). It is modified according to the needs of the client, including the starts and stops and relapses that are created by all sorts of circumstances, some beyond the control of the client. In these cases, self-management and emotion regulation skills are revised and reapplied as necessary, hopefully with increased effectiveness as the client becomes more adept with repeated practice in different contexts. The client is also encouraged to gain increased understanding that random, unexpected, and stressful events occur in the lives of all human beings (and not to the survivor alone or only to trauma survivors) and that these cause coping challenges for anyone when they occur.

Although Phase 3 primarily focuses on moving forward in life and in relationships outside of therapy, this process invariably involves reworking some of the previously addressed issues. So the issue of whether and when to return to the previous issues is rather straightforward: whenever the skills and knowledge acquired in those earlier phases is relevant to dealing with current-day life. The more challenging question is *how* to return to Phase 1 or 2 in order to most effectively help maintain and consolidate the gains that have been achieved. The best approach seems to be to blend Phase 1 and 2 interventions into the ongoing work of Phase 3.

For example, after doing EMDR in Phase 2, **Doris** came to believe that she would never again be overwhelmed by the feelings of intense anger that had caused her to feel powerless and ashamed and that had wreaked havoc in her relationships. However, after her therapist was gone for 2 weeks, Doris was shocked to feel infuriated when the therapist was 15 minutes late in starting their first appointment after her return. Doris found herself screaming, "You think you can treat me like dirt, make me wait until you're good and ready and then act like everything is fine when you know perfectly well that you've cut me to the core. I was so happy to get to see you again after all this time and then you made me wait!" The therapist focused on staying calm while helping Doris to feel validated for her feelings of hurt, abandonment, and disappointment. She was able to explain what had happened to cause her to be delayed and to apologize. Doris was able to recall what she had learned earlier in treatment, specifically that she often slipped into perceiving other people from the perspective of a little child who felt (as she actually had in her own childhood) powerless, abandoned, and unable to defend herself except by venting feelings of rage.

In Phase 1, Doris had learned that her rage was an exaggeration of her healthy assertive desire to express her outrage and to protect herself and that impulsive and unmodulated expression could be problematic, if not harmful. Furthermore, in Phase 2 EMDR work on her trauma memories, Doris had been able to experience the feelings of terror, loneliness, and shame that she had experienced as a child and to gain empathy for herself by understanding that those feelings were an expectable reaction to the rage she had experienced when her parents took it out on her and on one another. As her therapist stayed calm she regained her emotional balance as she remembered the ongoing security in the therapeutic relationship. Doris felt her rage subside and was able to use the insight she had gained in Phase 2 to verbally discuss rather than vent the hurt and fear underlying her anger. The next several sessions were productive in reviewing this incident and helping Doris apply what she learned from this (as she described it) "meltdown" to similar situations in her life and in outside relationships. The therapist helped Doris to draw on emotion regulation skills and acknowledged her right to her feelings; these things and the increased security of the working model of relationships she had acquired in Phase 1 (in this case, with the empathic repair associated with her therapist's explanation and apology and her calmness and emotion regulation in response to Doris's rage) allowed Doris to process the contemporary dysregulation incident using the same careful and detailed narrative reconstruction approach she had learned earlier.

It also would have been possible for the therapist to formally use EMDR with Doris to process either the in-therapy incident or a past experience that paralleled current events (e.g., a traumatic abandonment by her mother and her resultant rage and hurt). The formal reinstatement of Phase 2 trauma-and emotion-processing techniques is particularly helpful with clients in Phase 3 who become so emotionally dysregulated or disorganized in their attachment working models (with the therapist or in other key relationships) that their safety and stability or their ability to remain engaged in therapy is threatened. In such cases, Phase 1 interventions become the first priority, and Phase 2 formal trauma and emotion processing provides a bridge back to Phase 3, attention to current adjustment and functioning.

Other Significant Issues in Phase 3

A broad range of life issues, many of which are related to the client's age, life stage, and related developmental tasks can emerge at this point in treatment. (Specialized resources on all of these topics and issues—italicized subsequently—are included in Self-Help Resources and Workbooks [in the online supplement to this book].) For example, young adults (and even some adults in midlife and later) might focus on *career and occupational/vocational development* (or a change of training and focus) and have a broader range of choices once they have solidified their self-esteem and their right to self-determination and personal preferences. Previously, they might have been deterred or restricted by a number of posttraumatic symptoms and adaptations and by injunctions and prescriptions in their families or cultures or by personal characteristics and other life choices.

The *development of trustworthy relationships*, interdependence, and a viable support system apart from abusive others may accelerate during this treatment phase, in turn hastening the client's independence. For those for whom *intimate relationships* were overly threatening, they might now seem much more likely. *Intimacy* based on trust, respect, and mutuality is ever more possible with the ongoing application of previously learned self-regulation and communication skills. *Healthy sexuality* can be a hard-earned achievement for incest and sexual abuse survivor clients in particular. A number of specialized resources are now available. Clients may need specific support and education in *child-rearing and parenting issues* as they may have had no viable models to learn from. At this stage of treatment, clients might ponder actions such as *disclosures to others, confrontations of abusers and/or nonprotective others, ethics and other complaints to licensing boards and professional organizations and other actions, such as lawsuits*, against individuals or organizations in jurisdictions where statutes of limitations have been extended to allow such courses of action, especially for abuse/trauma that occurred in the distant past. Extensive discussion should occur prior to taking any of these actions because they can lead to significant counterreactions that can interrupt the client's life and therapeutic progress. Such courses of action, therefore, require discussion as to their pros and cons and cost–benefits before they are pursued. They are best undertaken at this stage when the client is most stable and is beyond major posttraumatic symptoms and repercussions. See Courtois (2010) for extensive discussion of issues such as these in cases of incest that is applicable to other forms of complex trauma within closed settings.

As discussed earlier, *interactions with past abusers and with involved others, including family members or membership groups*, also come under increased scrutiny during this phase of treatment, with courses of action determined. Increasingly, previously abused adult children are being expected to provide medical, practical, and financial care for aging parents or others who may have been their primary abusers or abetters. Responsibilities such as these also are best undertaken after discussion and preparation (L. S. Brown, 2012). It is important that clients not be exposed in the same way they were when they were younger and that they have safety plans and exit strategies in place if relationships within the family or other settings continue to be abusive in any way. In some cases, abusers take the opportunity to express their regrets for past behavior and offer apologies, permitting reconciliation. In others, no acknowledgement of wrongdoing is forthcoming, much less apology, and abusive interactions may continue unabated.

Addressing these challenges often leads to discussion of *existential issues, spirituality, religious beliefs, and personal meaning making* (Harvey, 1996; Herman, 1992b). Clients question core beliefs about themselves, other people, the world, the meaning and purpose of life (Foa et al., 1999; Frank, 1973; Janoff-Bulman, 1992), and the existence of God. These are existential/spiritual questions for which there are no simple universal answers, and therapists should not attempt to provide (or press clients to accept) any particular "answer." Although it is possible, and generally desirable, for clients to achieve a sense of resolution and closure with regard to the existential/spiritual conflicts that trauma engenders, this outcome is a spontaneous form of posttraumatic growth that should not—and, indeed, cannot—either be forced or prescribed. Each client must come to his or her own conclusion about the deeper meaning—if any—of the events they have experienced and of their own spiritual and existential beliefs. Therapists can best help in this endeavor by diplomatically and empathically "staying out of the way" in terms of their own beliefs, instead providing the client with the opportunity to think through these questions and by accepting the client's right to disillusionment and despair. This can be done by respectfully drawing the client's attention to the spiritual or religious beliefs that have been important at different times over the course of the client's life in different relationships with family and community. The ensuing discussion often includes not only affirmation or dismissal by the client of religious/spiritual beliefs and commitments but also a frank appraisal of feelings of spiritual disillusionment, detachment, and despair. It is also the case that many clients find comfort and solace in spirituality and religious beliefs and practices. Ultimately, the client's conclusions about spirituality and life are best viewed as a work in progress rather than a chapter in a book that must be finished and closed in therapy.

As they tackle and discuss these issues, some clients might revisit thoughts of suicide. At this point in treatment, this is likely due to the client's questioning whether he or she wants to live with new knowledge rather than being an expression of the wishes of others or of the client's own desire for self-destruction or self-punishment. Despite this difference in motivation for living or dying, careful attention must be given to client safety.

Clients might also consider other courses of action labeled "survivor missions" in the trauma literature. These courses of action are pursued when individuals decide to do something to fight oppression and victimization. Many trauma-related programs and services are based on the determination and contributions of survivors who make meaning of their experience by fighting back, providing services, and promoting change.

The *end of treatment* is a time of great poignancy for therapist and client. Because it inevitably revisits other losses, it, too, needs careful discussion and preparation. Therapists must allow enough time for leave taking with careful attention given to the form that any posttherapeutic contacts will take. It is advisable for therapists to maintain the same boundaries that were in place during treatment so that clients can return for a "check-in or tune-up" or for the resumption of treatment without concern for having developed any form of dual relationship.

Application to Cases

Phase 3 provides clients with complex trauma with guidance and support as they translate the gains in emotion regulation, self-confidence, and relational security acquired in the stabilization and processing phases of therapy into their ongoing lives and relationships. For **Hector**, Phase 3 involved only individual psychotherapy because he had previously had negative experiences in group therapy—in his words, "with a bunch of other vets who got totally crazy venting about their horrible war experiences and made me more upset and suicidal." Hector focused on understanding and coming to terms with an issue that he had not recognized until he explored trauma memories with PE in Phase 2:

> "I never understood why I couldn't get over feeling guilty until I realized that I was like a judge, jury, and executioner who condemned myself to hell for messing up and not saving my buddies who were killed or hurt. When I went back and walked through the worst times, I could see that I did everything I possibly could and more! And I saw that I was putting myself down just the way I felt put down when I was a kid growing up, so the one person I never really 'saved' was me! I realized that I was condemning myself just the way Father ______ blamed me for the abuse and condemned me. Then I started to feel some compassion and respect for myself, starting for when I was a little kid, rather than being fixated on hating myself. You helped me to see that the 'guilt' was really feeling ashamed and embarrassed, like there was something that had always been wrong with me which turned up again when I was under fire and didn't feel scared but felt incredible pressure to make everything all right for everyone else—to prove I wasn't totally worthless. I saw that I handled those situations pretty well even though I was an emotional mess, and I stayed an emotional mess because I couldn't face my own self-hatred and not because I didn't do right as a man and a soldier. Now I can see the real enemy isn't someone else who's gonna hurt me or anyone I care about—I can handle that—but it's the critical voice inside me telling me I'm no good and damned to hell. And I don't believe that anymore, because I know it's not true, it's just what I heard and learned to think about myself when I was a kid. It's not my voice, and I don't have to let it—the self-hatred—ruin me and my life anymore."

Not every client is as insightful and articulate as Hector, but many are. For Hector, Phase 3 involves consolidating what he learned in Phase 2, and applying this knowledge to reconsidering how he defines himself, his relationships, and his prospects for a meaningful and satisfying future life.

CONCLUSION

Phase 2 involves therapeutically revisiting troubling memories of past or more recent traumatic events in order to replace experiential avoidance with direct exposure to encourage emotion processing. In all of the procedures presented in this chapter with the exception of EMDR, the detailed description of the objective characteristics of the traumatic events is important in therapeutic memory work. Such description serves as the means for accessing subjective reactions and adaptations. When troubling memories are reflectively examined and placed in context, the client can develop increased understanding of their personal meaning and develop a more coherent and logical narrative. Emotion processing to the point of some acceptance and resolution and the related diminution of the most onerous symptoms set the stage for the final phase of treatment directed towards a number of life domains and posttraumatic redirection. We now turn to Chapter 7, in which we review systemic therapies (group, couple, and family) as they apply to complex trauma. Although these can be used in all phases of treatment, they are most often applied in Phases 2 and 3.

CHAPTER 7

Systemic Therapy across Phases

Group, Couple, and Family Modalities

Therapists have other treatment options to consider in addressing complex trauma, namely, systemic interventions provided in group, couple, or family therapy modalities. Systemic interventions are usually incorporated late in Phase 1 and early in or throughout Phases 2 and 3, most often as an adjunct to individual treatment. As discussed in this chapter, the individual therapist may serve in the dual role of both individual therapist and group cotherapist (potential dual roles that should be assessed carefully before assuming them and discussed ahead of time with the client), or the systemic therapy may be provided by a different therapist or cotherapy team (preferable in terms of couple or family therapy because the "client" changes with the addition of spouse/partner or other family members in ways that are different from group treatment in which the client is treated as another member of the larger group). There are no hard and fast rules for adding a new treatment modality; however, specific attention must be given to how the client would react to having the same therapist in a different setting or whether it would be better to involve another therapist in the additional treatment. Consideration should be given to not undermining the bond with the primary therapist, since, in most cases, individual therapy will be supplemented rather than replaced by the additional treatment. However these modalities are organized in terms of the therapist, the goal is to sustain and enhance the gains in trust and relational security, as well as the symptom relief and improved functioning achieved in individual therapy, without inadvertently undermining these accomplishments by creating dual roles or divided loyalties.

As emphasized throughout this text, the relational impact of complex interpersonal trauma is profound and is itself complex. Mistrust and isolation from, conflict with, and/or caretaking for spouse/partner, family, friends, coworkers, across the full spectrum of relationships are persistent relational styles. Therefore, although individual psychotherapy is the most commonly used approach, therapy that brings these clients together with one another (i.e., group therapy) or with their primary partners (i.e., partner/couple therapy) and family members (i.e., individual or multifamily therapy) is an important concurrent or adjunctive modality to consider in a complete treatment plan (Courtois, 2010; Johnson, 1989, 2002). Each of these psychotherapies requires specialized training and expertise and poses a different set of challenges to the therapist (or cotherapists), even as they provide potentially unique advantages to clients with complex trauma.

GROUP THERAPY

On a practical level, group therapy has a large number of benefits for trauma survivors in general (Foy, 2008; Klein & Schermer, 2000; Young & Blake, 1999). This is also the case for those with complex trauma histories, as described by Alexander, Neimeyer, Follette, Moore, and Harter (1989), Courtois (1988, 2010), Ford, Fallot, and Harris (2009), Harney and Harvey (1999), Harris (1988), Mendelsohn et al. (2011), Parker, Fourt, Langmuir, Dalton, and Classen (2007), and Scott (1999) including those who routinely dissociate and or who are diagnosed with dissociative identity disorder (DID; Fine & Madden, 2000; International Society for the Study of Trauma & Dissociation [ISST-D], 2011). Group therapy directly and experientially addresses interpersonal and relationship difficulties and gives a unique opportunity for "give and take" and for *in vivo* interaction and feedback. Being a member of a group in which safety, respect, honesty, privacy, and dedication to recovery are operating norms provides unique opportunities for traumatized and shamed clients to see and hear and to be seen and be heard by their peers who also struggle (albeit each in his or her unique way) with the anxiety, sense of rejection, betrayal, exploitation, and abandonment that are so common (Leehan & Webb, 1996). Group therapy provides the opportunity to join others with similar histories to gain perspective on the past and its impact on the present, as well as becoming more authentic and reclaiming personal memories and sense of self with the explicit support of others who have had similar experiences. The discovery that a group of peers can be genuinely supportive of personal growth while being trustworthy and nonexploitive is major. Crucial features of psychological and interpersonal growth include individuation and differentiation not supported in the family of origin or in other victimizing contexts and relationships. These can be difficult or even impossible to evoke or rework in the same way in individual treatment. Individual therapy often lays the groundwork for involvement in group, though, for some survivors, group participation is a necessary precursor to individual work, as they trust others like themselves more than they trust authority figures. Some cannot imagine being in a closed and private setting with a therapist/authority figure, as their fear and mistrust are too substantial and create major impediments.

Group therapy has many benefits and provides a specialized context for learning social and interactive skills that were not part of clients' upbringing (Courtois, 1988, 2010; Klein & Schermer; 2000; Young & Blake, 1999); yet, group also has some drawbacks and is contraindicated for some. The screening based upon established selection criteria should be applied to any group that has an open-process format rather than one that is strictly didactic, educational, and is more structured (Tables 7.1 and 7.2 describe benefits of and contraindications for group therapy for trauma, especially for the complex variant). Due to the complicated individual and interactive dynamics that occur in group therapy, the use of a cotherapy team is strongly endorsed across various group models. Screening interviews conducted by both therapists (optimally together) are recommended offering the opportunity to meet and assess potential members and to answer questions. Cotherapists must seek to screen out members who are either not ready for such an experience and/or who would be disruptive to the group process by virtue of impulsiveness and lack of control over emotions or behavior or of learned patterns of compliance and aggression in their interactions with other members. The use of screening interviews followed by pretreatment preparatory sessions assist potential members with information and informed consent.

Types of Groups

Harvey (1996) developed a *task-by-stage (or phase) model* that she labeled the *ecological model of trauma treatment* that follows the sequenced model for individual treatment of complex trauma. Harney and Harvey (1999) then applied this model to group treatment, and Mendelsohn et al. (2011) have recently published a book devoted to Phase 2 treatment conducted in a group setting. The Trauma Recovery Group, an ecological model developed by the staff of the Victims of Violence Program at Cambridge Hospital in Massachusetts, and other similar group models begin with a pretreatment group oriented toward building motivation, developing treatment goals, and identifying and modifying therapy-interfering behaviors (the latter adapted from Linehan's [1993] DBT model).

Harris (1998) developed Trauma Recovery and Empowerment (TREM) for treating chronically mentally ill women in group settings. The duration of most groups is relatively short term in the range of 6 months to 1 year, but some open-process groups in a psychodynamic format may go on for a number of years. Longer term groups obviously give more opportunity for in-depth exploration of relationship styles and beliefs; however, groups of midrange duration have been identified as those having the most benefit. Some groups are organized to treat a homogeneous population (e.g., incest

TABLE 7.1. Benefits of Group Therapy for Trauma Survivors

- Education, peer role modeling, and practice, with coaching from the group leader, in skills for understanding and communicating assertively and effectively with peers.
- Learning through the sharing of personal experiences that victimization is widespread and that the individual is not alone in having experienced it, thus breaking down the sense of stigma and isolation.
- Learning through the sharing of personal experiences that survivors and their experiences are all unique but that survivors share many common experiences and dilemmas with others.
- Learning that PTSD and complex traumatic stress symptoms are adaptations that once worked and that now can be changed.
- Learning that being a survivor is a fact but not a source of shame.
- Learning that PTSD or related traumatic stress disorders are a condition that a person "has," but not an incurable illness and not a definition of who the person "is." Abuse does not equal the person.
- Experiencing and learning to express and regulate a range of emotions in a range of relational scenarios.
- Receiving therapeutic guidance and peer role modeling in identifying, differentiating, labeling, and modulating these emotions from group leaders and other group members.
- Learning and practicing skills for modulating bodily arousal through experiential exercises in which members share experiences and practice bodily awareness skills.
- Developing a sense of empathy for oneself and others through active listening and being listened to empathically by peers and the group leader.
- Learning and practicing relational and social problem-solving skills to apply to the management and resolution of problems in relationships (both within and outside of group).
- Learning ways to give voice to personal suffering and pain and achieving validation for the struggle without criticism, encouragement of dependency, or maintenance of the role of the "sick one."
- Feeling inspired by the resilience of other survivors and learning that personal efforts to achieve a worthwhile and satisfying life can likewise inspire others.
- Learning that the complex interpersonal dynamics in groups can be discussed and resolved rather than just suffered or survived. Adults have resources, rights, and capabilities that were not available in childhood that can be applied to problem solving in social situations.

TABLE 7.2. Contraindications to Membership in Open-Process Group

- Inability to discuss abuse or trauma experience without having an intense (and initially uncontrollable) anxious, dissociative, or depressive reaction or strong posttraumatic symptoms of emotional flooding, numbing, and/or hyperarousal (as opposed to the more occasional or moderate reaction).
- Inability to regulate emotions and self-soothe.
- Inability to control strong impulsive tendencies.
- Inability to control interpersonal aggression.
- Inability to tolerate the interpersonal demands and sharing required of group participation or a highly negative orientation to the possibility of success in group treatment.

(*continued*)

TABLE 7.2. *(continued)*

- Active psychosis.
- Active and uncontrolled dissociation and uncontrolled switching of self-states associated with dissociative identity disorder.
- Active risk taking and severe self-injury.
- Active homicidality or suicidality.
- Active and severe substance abuse or other addictive process that is not acknowledged and/or under treatment and that creates serious personal risk.
- Lack of motivation to change.
- High dread of self-disclosure.
- High dread of hearing the stories of others.
- High degree of denial.
- Paranoid, sociopathic/antisocial and highly narcissistic/borderline personalities and behavioral patterns.
- Other, individual cautions or circumstances.

victims, male or female survivors, rape victims, clergy abuse victims, adolescent victims, a specific refugee population or cultural group), whereas others are more heterogeneous (e.g., mixed gender adult survivors of childhood trauma, adult children of alcoholics).

Many group treatment models for traumatized individuals and for those with complex trauma histories in particular are now available for use in different treatment settings (i.e., inpatient, residential, day treatment, mental health agency, private practice). Because groups can potentiate clients' feelings in ways that easily result in overstimulation, it is imperative for therapists to involve their clients only in groups that are in their range of tolerance in terms of relationship dynamics between members and the group's content and emphasis.

In the Harney and Harvey (1999) phase-oriented model, as in many others (Courtois, 2010), groups organized to meet Phase 1 goals are quite structured and presented in educational/didactic form. They are not in open-process format. The structure limits and contains (but does not suppress) whatever emotions are generated. In these structured groups, clients learn about trauma and traumatic stress reactions and learn skills. They may be asked to complete worksheets and to engage in therapeutic tasks between group sessions, which they report on in the next session and then discuss with other members, or to practice skills or engage in role plays in the group setting. Group discussion might also be organized around topical themes and issues (sometimes in response to a lecture, a reading on a relevant topic, or a topic suggested by group members).

Once clients have more emotion modulation capacity and their lives are increasingly safe and stable, their participation in a group that is more open ended and process oriented is often warranted. The open-process group, by virtue of its minimal structure and its open-discussion format, is typically overstimulating to and beyond a dysregulated client's ability to tolerate. As with individual treatment, some clients have sufficient skills and resources to quickly complete or entirely skip skill building and move directly into a process group. Some of the more organized treatment programs (such as the Women Recovering from Abuse Program (WRAP) program at the Women's Hospital in Toronto, discussed later) are so structured that the client must complete and graduate from the introductory skill-building groups before moving on to the next treatment level. Whether clients remain with the original group or enter a completely new open-process or structured group with different members, all have more opportunity to interact with one another in a format that moves beyond a didactic focus but does not abandon it entirely (as some process groups are organized around themes and how they apply to the group members, their relationships, and their lives and some continue the focus on skill building and role playing). Open process allows more opportunity for interaction and gives increased attention to relational dynamics and patterns between members and between members and the cotherapists. Over time, as in individual work, groups in the second phase are directed toward trauma recounting, processing, and resolution, but with the specific help and support of the cotherapist team and other group members. All members are encouraged to "give as well as take" as part of their group interaction, even when doing so is uncomfortable. Members are usually more used to being in the giving/supportive role vis-à-vis others than in receiving mode. In a related vein, it is usually much easier to extend kindness and understanding to others than to receive it in return, a disparity that can be observed, questioned, and discussed.

Phase 3 groups, in parallel to individual treatment, are focused on posttrauma life organization and relationships and may simply be an extension of the Phase 2 group or may be organized as an entirely new group with different emphases and tasks. As with Phase 2 groups, those addressing Phase 3 issues generally involve a more open format, although some are structured around themes or issues or around particular therapeutic tasks or skills. In some programs, participation in more heterogeneous therapy groups is recommended at this point in treatment.

Expectations and Ground Rules

From the outset (and in every session that includes new members), the therapists must be explicit in the expectation that the group is a place in which members must feel secure that their privacy and unique experiences and views will be protected and respected by others. Privacy and confidentiality are essential, but freedom from criticism is equally important and unfortunately is not the norm in some groups. Individual members may have very different opinions and beliefs in conflict with those of others, but the conflict should always be one of valid (and often informative) individual differences and not one in which any individual or her or his experience or views are treated as inferior or faulty, or attacked in an *ad hominem* manner. Members should be taught to distinguish between feedback, criticism, and advice giving and taught skills in feedback and assertion. Also, a norm of group members being responsible for their own recovery is advisable and group members deterred from providing advice and engaging in problem solving with one another rather than focusing on feelings and group process (see Table 7.3).

Consistent with this point, trust is a critical and ubiquitous issue that can be experientially addressed in group therapy. It is important for the leaders to consistently highlight trust as a highly legitimate issue for discussion but not a foregone conclusion either in the negative (e.g., "no one ever can be trusted") or positive (e.g., "everyone should be unconditionally trusting of others") direction. Indeed, discussion of how members may have come to either or both of these conclusions and how both points of view can be true under certain circumstances but not under others can be a central and very productive focus that the group may revisit frequently over its course.

As discussed, complex interpersonal trauma results in deep mistrust of authority figures, a stance that might occur in conjunction with a simultaneous longing to be rescued by them and relieved of the burdens of having been parentified. In group therapy, the cotherapists can become the foils for the full range of feelings about and transference reactions to parents (see Chapter 9), as members become stand-ins for siblings. For some clients, it is less frightening to work through issues related to parents and other family members in the supportive presence of their peers. For others, it will be preferable to work on these issues in the privacy of individual therapy.

Cotherapists are responsible for analyzing the dynamics between members in the group and for helping members to understand them. For example, a parentified client may intentionally or inadvertently avoid working on personal issues by assuming a familiar role of caregiver, protector, or rescuer of others. At times, this behavior can put him or her at odds with the group leader, becoming a "third leader" (i.e., developing a position of rivalry with the leaders and symbolically moving from the sibling "generation" to the adult "generation," in keeping with a highly honed parentified role) or challenging the leader's competence or authority and fomenting dissent among others. Such a dynamic, when identified and discussed, can be an opportunity for that client and other group members to become aware of how their attachment styles and habitual roles (and their mistrust of authority figures) continue in their present-day relationships. Discussions of this sort depend, in part, on the cotherapists' ability to nonjudgmentally validate the distrustful member's attempts to ensure

TABLE 7.3. Sample Group Ground Rules

We welcome you to membership in this group and we look forward to working with you. Groups function best when "rules of engagement" or ground rules are specified. The following are requirements for this group that will be in effect until the group decides to change them, and we ask that you agree to abide by them during the time of your membership. After a time, you and other group members may want to revisit and change these according to the specific needs of the group and as you and the others take more ownership of how you want the group to function. Be aware, however, that some of these guidelines are nonnegotiable due to state law or other professional standards; as co-leaders of this group, we will inform you of these requirements when these issues come up for discussion.

Confidentiality. Privacy and confidentiality are very important issues in a group such as this one. Outside of group, you may discuss anything about *your own experiences* with anyone you choose, *but any discussions must completely protect the privacy and identity of other group members.* State of __________ law is explicit about this. If you happen to run into another member outside of the group setting, you must also respect confidentiality; for example, if you are with someone else, you do not make an introduction nor mention your mutual group membership, although he or she may make a self-introduction (but *not* as a fellow group member), as that would compromise confidentiality.

Attendance. Consistent attendance develops stability and security and enhances trust among members. Irregular attendance and nonattendance are often interpreted as abandonment or as a sign of disregard and works against stability and consistency, important elements in recovery work. *As a condition of your acceptance into this group, you have agreed to make a commitment to ongoing attendance.* Please make every effort to attend all sessions, even if it is difficult (emotionally or otherwise) to do so. The structure of this group model is designed to allow you to first gain an intellectual understanding of material *before* discussing personal meaning to help make it easier to engage in discussion. Material in one session builds upon material from the week before and, in missing sessions, you will start to lose the sequence of the material and the structure on which the group format is built. You also start to "lose the thread" with other group members. We will follow up with you to discuss any nonexcused or excessive nonattendance. If any outside circumstances make it difficult or impossible for you to keep this commitment, please be sure to discuss them with us and bring it up for group discussion. Be aware that absent reasonable and unavoidable reasons for nonattendance or for group discontinuation, you will be charged for and responsible for payment for all sessions.

MORE ON THIS GROUP'S STRUCTURE

Participation and Communication. Please participate to the best of your ability and strive to communicate in the group even when doing so is uncomfortable. If you feel you cannot readily verbalize, communicate that fact to the group. Co-leaders and other group members will encourage you to state your opinions and feelings routinely as a part of the group process. This may be quite contradictory to how communication was handled in your family or in other settings and may feel foreign or contradictory at first. You are free to decline opportunities to talk until you are comfortable, but you will be encouraged over time to verbally participate.

Group is designed as a place to give and receive feedback; problem solving and advice giving are often ways to avoid issues and discussion. *Feedback involves giving information for personal reflection and exploration in a thoughtful, assertive, and nonaggressive way. Advice giving often involves telling people how to solve their problems and usually has the effect of cutting off exploration.* You will be encouraged in giving feedback and response and redirected from advice giving.

(*continued*)

TABLE 7.3. *(continued)*

The emotion of anger sometimes presents a special communication problem. It is possible to express anger without being aggressive. Participation is enhanced if members know that what they have to say will be accepted without an angry, condemnatory response and without judgment. Group leaders will intervene if communication becomes hostile and aggressive and will ask other members to give feedback. If it becomes apparent that you cannot interact without hostility or without being passive–aggressive or retaliatory, you may be asked to leave the group or to engage in outside adjunctive (anger management or assertiveness) training.

If you find yourself overwhelmed, we ask that you first try to communicate that in group to receive support and/or to lighten the intensity or change the focus. If you feel you are unable to stay in the room, first tell the group that you need to leave and go the waiting room or restroom, but otherwise remain in the suite vicinity. Once you have become resettled, return to the group before the group's end. *Do not just leave.* Leaving abruptly and without communication creates anxiety and feelings of abandonment on the part of other members.

Humor is encouraged as a way to lighten the heaviness of the topics that are covered; however, at times, humor can be used in a cutting or sarcastic way. We encourage gentle and supportive humor.

Graphic Discussions of Abuse Experiences and Emotional Discharge. You are invited to discuss your abuse experiences in detail as a part of the group; *however, please refrain from graphic recounting until you receive permission from other members as to their ability, readiness, or willingness to hear about abuse and victimization in that degree of detail.* Graphic depiction can, at times, be overwhelming, and other group members should be asked for their agreement to hear graphic depictions before anyone goes into detail and discharges intense emotion in recounting experiences of abuse. We do encourage description of abuse experience and emotional discharge as a part of the group process, but we encourage modulation and planning. Co-leaders will teach emotional expression and affect management skills.

Boundaries. Trauma, particularly when it involves abuse, is a violation of personal and emotional boundaries; therefore, the identification and maintenance of boundaries becomes an important control issue. The following are ground rules regarding boundaries:

Physical Touch. Physical touch or contact can be a difficult issue for trauma/abuse survivors. Although touch is not absolutely prohibited, you should offer a general reassuring touch only after receiving permission and it should be limited and of short duration. Understandably, some members will be uncomfortable with any physical touch and will decline contact. This is their prerogative (and yours as well). Please also maintain an awareness of the physical boundaries of others in group and make efforts not to infringe on others' "personal envelopes."

Contact Outside of Group. Within the group model used here, the development of outside friendships and relationships apart from the group [is not allowed] or is allowed, but with several caveats:

1. Contacts are initially made to provide mutual support outside of the group setting and direct discussion about life and treatment issues by the individuals having outside contact is encouraged or discouraged.
2. Those having outside contact do so in a limited way (i.e., do not become overly involved outside of the group or develop a special or exclusive friendship). The development of intimate and particularly sexual contact between members is explicitly prohibited.

TABLE 7.3. *(continued)*

3. Outside contacts are disclosed in group so that they are not secret from other members.
4. Discussion about other group members' issues outside of the group is prohibited.
5. Every group member has the right to decline contact with others outside of group.
6. Co-leaders reserve the right to change this ground rule if, in their opinion, it is interfering with the group process and group members agree to abide by the change. Members are expected to notify the co-leaders if the safety of another group member is at issue, such as suicidal feelings or thoughts or self-harming behavior. These communications to the therapist are not acts of betrayal but rather involve the maintenance of safety and appropriate concern for one another. All members must agree to this.

Communication between Members between Meetings. Another issue involves members having phone and e-mail contact or texting between sessions. This [is not allowed] or is allowed as long as it is a voluntary exchange of this information among members and is in keeping with the restrictions noted above. Members have the right to decline to participate in outside contacts of all sorts. Please be aware that the confidentiality of e-mail or texting is not guaranteed, so discretion in communication is called for. Cotherapists should be included in all group e-mail correspondence.

Conflict between Members and/or Members and Co-Leader(s). All relationships have the potential for disagreement, strong feelings, and conflict. *The salient issue is not to avoid conflict but rather to communicate respectfully (although in possibly heated ways) until some common group resolution can be reached.* The structure of this group model is designed to provide containment of discussion topics and emotions. As a part of their responsibilities, co-leaders will seek to facilitate communication and respectful conflict resolution when issues arise.

Appreciation of Survival Skills as a Group Norm. Each of you has survived very difficult and abusive circumstances using a variety of coping and surviving skills. We encourage recognizing and supporting these, as well as the strength of each member, even as we may suggest changes in coping strategies. We will also support positive experiences, relationships, and emotions as a matter of course.

Problem Coping. If you or someone close to you perceives you as reverting to old negative ways of coping, for example, cutting, drugging and drinking, eating, aggressing, zoning or spacing out, or sexualizing, you or they should try to let your therapist, the group co-leaders, and the group know as soon as possible so you can receive assistance. Co-leaders will ask you to determine precipitants to the behavior and to replace maladaptive coping with substitute behaviors. They will also offer the opportunity for check-ins and support.

Group Cotherapist Roles and Responsibilities. Our responsibilities include the provision of information, facilitation of communication and group process, and the provision of feedback to members. We also monitor emotional and physical safety (the responsibility of all and not only the cotherapists) and, at times, will stop the group process and discussion if it becomes aggressive and/or otherwise does not seem to be safe. We explicitly encourage open communication between us and between members and make attempts to model clear, open, and respectful communication.

(continued)

TABLE 7.3. *(continued)*

Cotherapist Absences. At times, one or the other co-leader may have a scheduled absence. We will notify you ahead of time, and members can decide whether to have a session when only one group leader will be in attendance. We anticipate that group sessions will be held when only one therapist is present for group continuity; however, there may be times when it is important for both co-leaders to be present.

Release of Information to Your Primary Therapist, Psychiatrist, or Other Allied Professional. *An open release-of-information form to your primary therapist, psychiatrist, or other involved allied professional is a condition of participation in this group.* We will contact outside therapists only in the event of an emergency or as we deem necessary to coordinate treatment. Whenever possible, we will notify you in advance of our intention to contact your therapist. It is your right to retract your permission; if you choose to do so, we retain the option to terminate your participation in group treatment.

the safety of all members, a stance that results in ongoing testing of the therapists. Using a reframe such as this, group process can focus on the distrustful member's adaptive goals and help all members recognize and reevaluate posttraumatic roles and reenactments with the specific intent of letting them experience other roles (e.g., being the recipient of the caring and caretaking of others, rather than always being the responsible one) and being in interaction with authority figures who are, in fact, responsive and deserving of their trust.

Group therapy for complex trauma involves many reenactments of traumatic experiences, adaptations, and relationships in the group interaction, often in indirect or symbolic form. Even when the discussion does not involve the processing of a specific memory, cotherapists must be aware of and ready to help group members titrate the intensity of disclosures they make in the course of group discussion and their reactions to hearing the stories of others and identify the possible historic antecedents to their present-day emergence. Although there is no clear and firm determination of whether to explicitly encourage the retelling of specific trauma memories in group therapy, it is crucial for the group leaders to help all members (whether the discloser or the listener/witness) to avoid becoming emotionally flooded. Disclosure and discussion in group are not the equivalent of the therapeutic procedure of flooding described in Chapter 6.

Group therapy is not generally designed for intensive cathartic disclosures of traumatic events—although, as noted before, this can happen spontaneously, and the support of group members may be critical in allowing the disclosing client to ventilate and receive affirmation—newer group models have developed that involve trauma-processing activities (including PE) in a group context (the specific focus is discussed in recently published treatment books by Lubin and Johnson, 2008, and Mendelsohn et al., 2011). In group, however, unless the activity is undertaken with careful planning and informed consent of all members, the cotherapists may be hard-pressed to provide either the disclosing member or the other members with the careful one-to-one guidance and support that is an essential component of the PE or flooding protocol as conducted in individual therapy. Group members can end up feeling overwhelmed, burdened, abandoned, or violated by an intensive trauma memory disclosure, whether they are the disclosers or the witnesses; therefore, group ground rules should specify that graphic descriptions need to be agreed to ahead of time and disclosure and resultant emotional reactivity need to be modulated to the degree possible.

Graphic material should be presented only with the permission of other group members and with appropriate stops in place if any member becomes emotionally overwhelmed. In our experience, asking permission before the recitation of details is usually enough for members to be able to tolerate it. Group models that incorporate PE, including memory disclosure and emotional reactions, as a mandatory part of the process (Mendelsohn et al., 2007, 2011) and preliminary clinical findings from studies investigating one such approach are promising (Ready et al., 2008). This finding is in contrast to the results of a previous large study that showed that PE was no more effective than a problem-solving approach in the process (Schnurr et al., 2003). Ready and colleagues (2008) designed therapy so that trauma memory exposure work was done primarily on an individual basis by group members, rather than as a part of the group discussion. Group members took turns sharing a detailed description of a past traumatic event that they taped and repeatedly listened to between sessions (each to his or her personal recording only). Group sessions were focused on education, helping group members learn skills for safe emotional processing of their traumatic experiences and those of others, thus enabling them to support one another in doing the home-based exposure therapy exercises. The Mendelsohn et al. model (2011) utilized a different approach. It involved highly individualized goal setting and the processing of the trauma narrative in the relational context of the entire group.

Research information from the Women Recovering from Abuse Program (WRAP) of the Women's Hospital in Toronto offers preliminary research support for another and related model, one of a highly organized outpatient group therapy program of 6 weeks' duration (requiring daily attendance) that includes a variety of types of task-oriented groups applied sequentially and hierarchically. The researchers were able to document changes in posttrauma symptoms and, very significantly, in the group members' attachment styles (from insecure to "earned secure"). A description of this specialized treatment program is found in Parker et al. (2007), and additional studies of this model are currently ongoing.

However the group is conducted, the norm for its ending is to spend time discussing the loss it entails and the gains made. In open-ended groups, session time is reserved so that a departing group member can express sentiments about the group and his or her participation and can receive feedback and good wishes in return. Saying good-bye or farewell is important and should be encouraged, as some members tend to want to avoid such leave-taking sessions and the feelings of loss and abandonment that come to the fore. As is the case with individual therapy, the group treatment contract (see Figure 7.1 as an example) should include the client's agreement not to leave abruptly without giving notice and attending one last session to provide a conclusion and wrapping-up opportunity. Some members never learned to have endings in their families of origin, where cutoffs and nonrecognition or nondiscussion of significant losses such as deaths, divorces, stillbirths, and so forth, were the norm. Working against this avoidance and instead experiencing feelings of loss or abandonment in a context of support conform to the overall treatment goals and contract.

Members of these groups consistently affirm the importance of being able to "find their voice" and "tell their story" in the context of a respectful and validating gathering of peers to their developing greater internal clarity, hope, empowerment, self-esteem, and a sense of belonging associated with being accepted by others with experiences similar to theirs (Courtois, 2010; Fallot & Harris, 2002; Mendelsohn et al., 2007, 2011). The opportunity to disclose and reflect carefully on key memories (including but not limited to traumatic experiences), along with discussions of the impact of the past on current behavior and relationships in the context of mutual support and understanding, is of great benefit when done within the "window of tolerance." The cotherapists are responsible for keeping the group focus on emotional processing (see Chapter 6) by encouraging reflective processing as much as the "telling of the story." As in individual therapy, it is common for the listeners (in this case the cotherapists and other members) to feel the emotions that the disclosing member split off in the interest of self-protection. In group, these feelings can be reflected back for the discloser to consider and can open up new channels of feeling at more intensified levels.

As illustrated in the interactions in the simulated group session presented in this chapter, there are several potential approaches to helping members titrate the emotional intensity of group participation. One method explicitly models and teaches emotion regulation skills (e.g., Bradley & Follingstad, 2003; Ford & Russo, 2006; Wolsdorf & Zlotnick, 2001; Zlotnick et al., 2009) beginning in the stabilization phase of therapy and continuing through the second phase of memory work (Ford et al., 2005). Another embeds memory work in a context of building a complete personal life story or narrative, including but not limited to traumatic experiences (Fallot & Harris, 2002; Ford & Russo, 2006; Lubin, Loris, Burt, & Johnson, 1998; Mendelsohn et al., 2007). A third approach provides a detailed structure for memory work that includes sufficient practice in and outside

GENERAL INFORMATION AND FEE POLICY FOR PROSPECTIVE AND ONGOING PATIENTS IN GROUP THERAPY

The following information is provided to establish a clear mutual understanding of the professional and business aspects of our treatment relationship. Please read this information carefully and feel free to ask about anything that is unclear to you, to ask for additional information, and/or to share any concerns about these issues. Bring this policy statement with you to your next session for discussion. When you sign the document, it will represent a binding agreement between us.

GENERAL INFORMATION

A. Psychological and Mental Health Services. Individual and group psychotherapy varies depending on the personalities of therapist and client(s), the particular problems and issues being addressed, the length of the treatment, and the strategies and methods selected. Group therapy, like other forms of psychotherapy, has both benefits and risks. Risks sometimes include experiencing uncomfortable feelings, giving or receiving uncomfortable feedback, and/or working with unpleasant life events. Psychotherapy often leads to a significant reduction of distress, better relationships, and the resolution of specific problems. In order to be most successful, hard work is required, both during our sessions and between them, on the part of all group members, including the cotherapists.

B. Intake and Assessment. In addition to the screening interview that you participated in pregroup, the first few group sessions provide a time to evaluate whether this group can meet your needs and your treatment goals. During these early sessions, we will ask you to generally discuss with other members: (1) your reasons for wanting to be in the group and what you hope to achieve; (2) your current problem(s) and symptom(s), current and past personality and interpersonal functioning, past/current individual and group treatment (and whether you currently or in the past are in individual treatment with either of the group's coleaders—these ongoing relationships need to be discussed as they constitute preexisting relationships and might have some impact on group dynamics), family background and history, and personal strengths and assets; (3) any special circumstances that might affect your ongoing participation in the group, for example, time limits, work and travel schedules, and so forth. These first few meetings will allow you the opportunity to assess whether the group members and treatment issues seem to be a compatible fit for you. If so, we ask that you make a commitment to regularly attend group (unless the group decides to disband or otherwise alter its schedule).

In addition to the verbal exchange of information, we request that you complete a one-page intake form and a personal history questionnaire of about 12 pages, along with open releases of information for us to talk with your current individual therapist and/or to request summary records of previous treatment.

C. Confidentiality. In general, the confidentiality of all communications between a patient and a psychotherapist is protected by law, and we can only release information about our work to others with your written permission. Under DC law, we are limited in what information can be released, even to insurance companies. Be aware that once information is released, we cannot guarantee that it will remain confidential. Additionally, DC law is quite explicit about the confidentiality of members participating in group psychotherapy. A copy of the DC law regarding group participation is attached for your information. Any communication made to one co-leader of the group will be shared with the other in order that we both operate as co-leaders with the same basis of information.

(*continued*)

FIGURE 7.1. (*continued*)

In most judicial proceedings, you have the right to prevent us from providing any information about your treatment. However, in some circumstances, such as child custody proceedings and proceedings in which your emotional condition is an important element, a judge may require our testimony if he or she determines that there is no privilege or it has been waived.

There are some situations in which, as a licensed Psychologist and Social Worker, we are legally required to take action to protect others from harm, even though that requires revealing information about a patient's treatment:

- If we learn during treatment that a child, an elderly person, or a disabled person (by name) is being abused, we must file a report with the appropriate protective services agency.
- If we learn that a client is threatening serious bodily harm to another we are required to take protective actions, which may include notifying the potential victim, notifying the police, or seeking hospitalization.
- If a client threatens or engages in self-harm or is suicidal, we may be required to seek hospitalization or to contact family members or significant others who can help provide protection.

D. Professional Records. We maintain records regarding treatment strategies and progress as a professional obligation. We will release records or information about your treatment to other professionals with a release of information form signed by you. We will also review your records with you at your request.

E. Patient Rights. You have the following rights in therapy: (1) to ask questions about our philosophy of therapy, our experience with the problem at hand, your treatment plan, and the procedures used; (2) to seek a consultation regarding your treatment from another credentialed professional (we ask that you discuss this with us prior to seeking such a consultation; at times, a meeting involving the consultant and both of us is advisable and helpful); (3) to end therapy at any time without moral, legal, or financial obligation beyond payment due for completed sessions (although we are asking for a commitment of ______ months to this group). Should you decide between sessions to withdraw from therapy, you agree to attend at least one additional session to discuss your reasons with us and other group members. Therapy termination can sometimes be the result of misinterpretation, miscommunication, and the painfulness of the material under discussion and an abrupt termination can feel like abandonment to other members, each of whom has invested in the group membership and functioning. We encourage open communication before a final decision is made.

F. Other. If a problem of any type (e.g., financial, scheduling, therapy approach, communication) arises during the course of our work, please bring it up for discussion.

As a condition of being in treatment with us, do not undertake any other form of simultaneous therapy *without first bringing it up for discussion and mutual decision making*. Additional therapy of any sort should be coordinated with your main therapy. *Signed releases of information to facilitate communication between treatment providers is a condition of participation in this group.*

Another condition of treatment with us involves no *unplanned major disclosures, confrontations, and/or cutoffs of family members or other significant individuals*. Such action should be discussed, decided upon, and prepared for to minimize adverse outcomes (both to you and possibly to us) and therefore should not be undertaken impulsively.

FIGURE 7.1. *(continued)*

This psychotherapy practice has a specialization in the treatment of adults abused as children and the treatment of posttraumatic conditions. If your therapy involves issues of delayed or recovered memories, we will provide you with additional written and verbal information on these topics, with cautions and strategies regarding memory for traumatic circumstances. Considerable controversy surrounds these topics, making it very important that we have a mutual understanding about how these issues will be addressed in treatment.

FEE INFORMATION AND SCHEDULING

Group will meet on Tuesday evenings from 5:00 to 6:30 P.M.

A. Initial Session. ___________ per 50 minutes.

B. Group Therapy. ___________ per 90-minute session, payable by session for 5 or more members; ___________ per session for less than 5 members.

C. Reduced-fee hours. We are able to negotiate some reduced fees as needed.

D. Other. Other professional services you may require, such as report writing, telephone conversations that last longer than 10 minutes, attendance at meetings or consultations with other professionals that you have authorized, preparation of records or treatment summaries, or the time required to perform any other service, will be billed on a prorated basis of our individual therapy fees.

In unusual circumstances, you may become involved with litigation that may require our participation; however, we are unable to serve as both an expert witness and a treating therapist in any litigation. In the event that we must participate on your behalf, you will be billed for our professional time, even if we are compelled to testify by another party. Fees for these services will be negotiated separately; our fees for testimony are higher than for psychotherapy due to the additional demands imposed by this type of work.

E. Fee for Service. Our practices are fee-for-service, meaning that we do not accept insurance or belong to any managed care panels. You may submit our bill to your insurance company for out-of-network payment.

F. Payment. All fees are payable at the time of service. You will receive a personal statement at the end of every month. We are *unable, for professional and personal reasons, to allow back balances to build.* Please discuss it with us if financial circumstances make it difficult to pay your bill on a weekly basis.

If your account is more than 60 days in arrears and suitable arrangements for payment have not been made, we have the option of suspending or discontinuing treatment. Interest will accrue on balances unpaid after 60 days at a rate of 18% per year, 11/2% per month.

In the event of an unpaid bill, legal means can be used to secure payment, including collection agencies or small claims court. (If such legal action is necessary, the costs of bringing that proceeding, including attorney fees, will be included in the claim.) In most cases, the only information that is released is the patient's name, the nature of the services provided, and the amount due.

(continued)

FIGURE 7.1. *(continued)*

G. Scheduling. Fees will be charged for all missed sessions, regardless of the reason for the absence, except: (1) if you give sufficient forewarning, *at least* 24 hours in nonemergency situations. (2) three sessions per calendar year, which you might use in the case of vacation, business trips, illness, and so forth. This three-session limit will be waived in the event of prolonged illness or work-related absence and by discussion. (3) "Snow days" or other circumstances beyond our mutual control.

Occasionally, telephone contact is needed when issues come up or a crisis develops between regularly scheduled sessions. We are often not immediately available but do monitor voice mail frequently. We will make every effort to return your call on the same day you make it with the exception of late nights, weekends, and holidays. If you are difficult to reach, please leave some times when you will be available. If you cannot reach us, and you feel that you cannot wait for a return call, you should call a local hotline or the emergency room at the nearest hospital and ask for the psychologist or psychiatrist on call.

Phone calls over 10 minutes in duration are billed, pro rata, at our normal individual-therapy hourly rate. Fees are added to your bill when 50 minutes of telephone time accrues. Phone contact is usually kept brief unless you are in a crisis or unless a session by phone has been scheduled in advance. If the reason for your call involves a group issue or dynamic, we will offer you support but refer you back to the group to discuss it.

H. Vacation. Our schedules include professional and vacation time each year during which we are out of the office. We will discuss upcoming absences with group members and decide whether group will be scheduled with one cotherapist. Occasionally, we need to reschedule or cancel appointments on short notice for professional commitments or personal reasons. We will attempt to give notice for changes wherever possible.

When one of us is away, you may feel free to contact the other as a backup therapist. Each of us maintains additional backup coverage during vacations and other absences.

CONSENT TO TREATMENT

I acknowledge that I have received, have read, and understand the "General Information and Fee Policy for Prospective and Ongoing Patients." I have had my questions answered adequately at this time. I understand that I have the right to ask questions throughout the course of my treatment in this group and may request an outside consultation. (I also understand that the therapist may provide me with additional information about specific treatment issues and treatment methods on an as-needed basis during the course of my treatment and that I have the right to consent to or refuse such treatment.) The cotherapists might also seek or suggest outside consultation.

I understand that I can expect regular review of treatment to determine whether treatment goals are being met. I agree to be actively involved in the treatment and in the review process. No promises have been made as to the results of this treatment or of any procedures utilized within it.

I further understand that I may stop my treatment at any time but agree to discuss this decision first with the cotherapists and other group members. My only obligation, should I decide to stop treatment, is to pay for the services I have already received and to attend one final group meeting to discuss my reasons and to terminate with other members.

I have been informed that I must give 24 hours notice to cancel an appointment and that I will be charged if I do not cancel or show up for a scheduled group.

I am aware that I must authorize the cotherapists in writing to release information

FIGURE 7.1. *(continued)*

about my treatment but that confidentiality can be broken under certain circumstances of danger to myself or others. I understand that once information is released to insurance companies or any other third party, my cotherapists cannot guarantee that it will remain confidential.

My signature signifies my understanding and agreement with these issues and with the additional information conveyed in this statement.

Patient Signature ______________________________ **Date** __________
Printed Name: ______________________________
Address: ______________________________
Cotherapist Signature: ______________________________ **Date** __________
Cotherapist Signature: ______________________________ **Date** __________

FIGURE 7.1. Sample group treatment contract for men's adult survivor weekly therapy group.

of sessions to permit members to experience a sense of mastery of previously avoided anxiety or fear (Ready et al., 2008), as well as of grief and shame (Ford & Russo, 2006; Mendelsohn et al., 2007, 2011).

As noted earlier, group treatment is not for everyone and careful screening is required. The severely dysregulated trauma survivor is a bad fit in group therapy. In supportive or interpretive groups for adults with traumatic grief (Piper, Ogrodniczuk, Joyce, Weideman, & Rosie, 2007) and interpersonal therapy groups for women with chronic PTSD secondary to childhood abuse (Cloitre & Koenen, 2001; Courtois, 2010), the presence of one group member with poor object relations or borderline personality characteristics (especially uncontrolled reactivity and aggression toward others or the inability to tolerate sharing the leaders' attention with other members) has been associated with diminished outcomes for all group members. In addition, Cloitre and Koenen (2001) have described an "anger contagion" phenomenon whereby all members of groups with a member designated as borderline personality reported increased anger following the group. These findings are consistent with those of Follette, Alexander, and Follette (1991), who reported that women with sexual abuse histories who had experienced more severe molestation or had higher initial levels of psychological distress or depression had poorer outcomes than other members in both supportive open-format and structured dyadic discussion groups.

Linehan (1993) describes behavior such as this as "therapy interfering," and her DBT explicitly teaches group members new skills and ways of interacting that are valuable for complex trauma survivors in groups (as they have been shown to be in individual therapy for women in therapy for PTSD related to childhood sexual abuse; Cloitre et al., 2010). It is important for group leaders to screen potential members in advance in order to determine their readiness to handle the stresses and triggers that occur in this setting (see Table 7.4 for a listing of potential screening questions). It is not a favor to the prospective member—any more than to other group members—when an individual without baseline self-regulation and interpersonal skills is included. For that individual, a course of preparation in individual therapy or participation in groups that have an educational or skill-building focus may be necessary precursors. It is advisable for cotherapists to consider that group participation is not possible for all who seek to join, as some may not be able to share time with others or hearing their stories, in addition to difficulty with self-modulation. They may be able to tolerate only individual treatment, at least initially and possibly permanently, and might find even an affectively contained form of individual therapy overwhelming unless intensity is carefully monitored by the therapist (e.g., focusing on empathic validation; using a relatively neutral affective approach of a primarily educational and/or supportive intervention). On the other hand, they may benefit from structured psychoeducation in a group format such as a DBT skills group that does not focus on or even permit descriptions of past traumatic experiences (Wagner et al., 2007).

TABLE 7.4. Sample Screening Questions for Potential Process Group Membership

The co-leaders can make some or all of the following comments by way of introduction to the screening session: There are no right answers and the potential member should try to answer as honestly and completely as possible. The potential member can choose not to answer, although the preference is for him or her to do so because the cotherapists are trying to assess readiness for group inclusion and participation. The potential member is invited to ask for clarification if questions are unclear or not understood. The interview can be stopped at any point, whether to regroup and then resume or to not be completed if the potential member determines it is too stressful or it is not the right option at this time. Cotherapists encourage potential members to ask questions in order to help determine whether the group experience and the co-therapists and their approach would be a fit.

- "What are your reasons for wanting to join this group? What do you want to get out of it?"
- "How did you hear about the group? Have you ever had a group experience of this sort or do you know of anyone who has? How was it?"
- "How do you feel being here today?"
- "Tell us about yourself, your current life—family, school, work, friends. How are things going in your life at the present time? How are you functioning? Any areas that are going particularly well? Problem areas or crises?"
- "What was it like to grow up in your family? Are you in contact with your family at present? How do you feel about your family?"
- "Have you ever discussed the abuse or other trauma with anyone before? What happened? What were the reactions? How did you react?"

(*continued*)

TABLE 7.4. *(continued)*

- "How do you think it will be for you to disclose your trauma experience in a group and to hear others discuss theirs?"
- "Tell us, to the degree that you can and to the degree that is relatively comfortable for you, in general about your abuse or trauma experience. Who abused you? How did the abuse begin and end? How old were you? For how long, and how often? What kinds of activities were involved? Were you told anything by the perpetrator? Were you threatened? Bribed? Tricked? Was force used? How did you cope? While it was ongoing, did you ever tell anyone, or did anyone find out about the abuse or trauma? Their reactions? Yours? Did you have more than one experience of abuse and other forms of trauma?"
- "How has it been to have us ask about these things and to be talking with us about them today?"
- "How do you think the abuse or trauma affected you at the time it occurred and since then? How do you think it affects you today?"
- "What are your feelings about being in a group with other abuse and trauma survivors? Do you have specific fears or concerns about dealing with your history with others? Specific things you are seeking or are excited about?"
- "Have you been in or are you currently in individual or group therapy? Tell us about that therapy—what you are (or were) working on, the therapy relationship, how you feel (or felt) about the therapy and the relationship, and so on. [If in past and/or current individual therapy (the latter is often a requirement for group inclusion):] May we contact your therapist? Are you willing to maintain an open release-of-information form between us and your therapist for the duration of the group?"
- "Tell us about your medical history and also about any substance abuse problems. Are you currently in treatment for any medical or addiction problems, and are you currently on any medications? What and in what dose? Are you currently under the care of a psychiatrist or a primary care physician? Are you willing to maintain an open release-of-information form between us and your psychiatrist or physician for the duration of the group?"
- "Tell us about your degree of safety. Any current threats to your safety from yourself or others? Domestic violence? Suicidal feelings or ideation or plan? Past attempt(s)? When, where, how serious? Safety plan in place? How would you deal with suicidal feelings if they emerged during or after a group session?"
- "Tell us how you typically deal with strong feelings, especially anger and shame. Do you have ways to self-soothe and to stay safe?"
- "Tell us about your support system. Who do you turn to when you need support or comfort?"

Note. Adapted from Courtois (2010). Copyright 2010 by Christine A. Courtois. Adapted with permission from W. W. Norton Company, Inc.

Severe problems with dissociation can make group participation difficult; however, group therapy is an indicated intervention for many persons with dissociative disorders (including DID; ISSTD, 2011; Fine & Madden, 2000) if the affective intensity is carefully modulated by the co-leaders. Classen, Koopman, Nevill-Manning, and Spiegel (2001) found that both memory processing and a present-centered approach to group therapy with women survivors of childhood sexual abuse were associated with improvements in dissociation, as did Wolsdorf and Zlotnick (2001) in their affect management group therapy and as discussed by Boon, Steele, and Van der Hart (2011). Co-leaders should help all members to understand dissociative responses and to identify some of the observable changes that can occur when a member dissociates—ranging from mild dissociation, indicated by "spacing out," a blank stare, or physical stilling to dissociative switching of self-state, indicated by more overt changes in style, behavior, eye contact, voice tone, memory, and so forth. Dissociation can also be explained as a condition of complex trauma responses that all members experience to a greater or lesser degree. Co-leaders must be prepared to help ground and reorient members who dissociate and to teach these forms of interruption and intervention to all members. This can be a positive learning experience, demonstrating experientially that dissociation can be recognized and managed without becoming a serious crisis or causing anyone more than temporary discomfort.

These ideas are in keeping with recommendations for effective engagement and alliance formation and maintenance in group interventions with members who are severely dissociative, including: (1) knowing how to identify subtle, as well as obvious, instances of dissociative alterations in awareness and personality (Steele & Van der Hart, 2009), (2) skills in grounding members when they or other group members are significantly dissociating—for example, sensorimotor strategies for assisting the client to regain a sense of immediate safety and awareness of self, circumstances, and others (Fisher & Ogden 2009); and (3) the ability to "gently confront" dissociative defenses (Scott, 1999, p. 35) and empathically relate to the member while acknowledging rather than challenging dissociated parts of the personality if these structural splits emerge, for example, in the form of dissociative flashbacks or intrusive memories, as well as in more obvious (e.g., DID) shifts in self-state (Schwartz, Schwartz, & Galperin, 2009; Van der Hart & Steele, 2009).

Group members with co-occurring substance use disorder or severe mental illness may experience periods of behavioral, emotional, or interpersonal dysregulation and crises (e.g., relapse, suicide attempt, self-injury) that pose threats to their safety and are stressful for other group members. An integrated rather than fragmented approach to their overall care, as well as their group participation, is essential in these cases, as illustrated by the findings of the Women, Co-Occurring Disorders and Violence multisite study (Veysey & Clark, 2004), in which members reported greater benefits following comprehensive, integrated, trauma-informed service interventions (such as Trauma Recovery and Empowerment (TREM), Seeking Safety, Addictions and Trauma Recovery (ATRIUM), and similar models; Veysey & Clark, 2004) than with core services that were delivered in separate interventions or by several providers (Morrissey et al., 2005). Group therapy that teaches self-regulation skills has been found to be effective with adults and adolescents with PTSD and problems with addiction, many of whom contend with complex-trauma-related distress (Ford & Smith, 2008; Najavits et al., 2006).

Group Therapy Vignette

This vignette involves members who were prescreened and are working on present-day relational issues and linking difficulties with their previous trauma (late Stage 1 and Stage 3 issues).

LEADER 1: Last week we worked on the issue of trust, and I appreciated the very open and direct feedback that members gave to me. You were also open to how I responded and to considering how trust was betrayed in past experiences. Does anyone have thoughts or reactions after having had a chance to think about last session in the past week?

MEMBER 1 (**Doris**): I hope I wasn't too rude last week. I think I really put you through the wringer and it really was all just my old stuff with my father coming out.

LEADER 1: Thank you for letting me know this, Doris, I think that shows once again your compassion and integrity, just as we discussed last week. But I also think that you're being quite hard on yourself and too easy on me—you raised some important concerns about whether I was being too hard on other group members, which I really needed to look at in order to make sure this group is a safe place for everyone. So you may have been working through some issues with your father, but you also were modeling how to assertively stand up for yourself and the whole group, which is really valuable to all of us.

MEMBER 2 (Carol): I think Doris really was too hard on you, Doc, and you're being too easy on her. I don't feel safe if anyone attacks anyone in group and she really attacked you last week.

MEMBER 3 (Jen): Now you're the one who is attacking Doris, Carol. And kissing up to Doc, like you'll earn brownie points, something you seem to like to do.

MEMBER 4 (Sandra): (*Bursts out crying.*) This is just like being in my dysfunctional family again!

LEADER 2: We're all seeing how important safety and trust are, and how they bring up really deep emotional issues for each of us. (*Turns to Member 4.*) Sandra, I want you to know that we want to make this group different in healthy ways from what you went through growing up, but there are times when those old patterns can happen even when we're trying hard to understand them and not repeat them. But that's what we're working on, and you're being really courageous in helping us get it right.

MEMBER 4: Thank you for that, I don't want to be a baby, but I just can't take any more of what I went through in my family growing up. And I didn't mean to criticize you, Jen.

LEADER 1: What do you think about that, Jen? I think Sandra is saying something very similar to what you're saying, but what do you think?

MEMBER 3: Well, I guess I was being kinda harsh, but it really upset me that Carol was making Doris out to be the bad guy—that's just what my mother did to me, and my husband too and now my daughter. I don't want to go through any more of that.

LEADER 2: So, like Doc said, it does sound like you really agree with Sandra, Jen.

MEMBER 2: I was just trying to be honest so we don't whitewash things that happen in the group. I didn't mean to attack Doris, Sandra, but listening to you and Jen I see why you took Doris's side and called me out on this. Doris, I'm sorry I criticized you, you didn't deserve that.

LEADER 1: Doris, how do you feel about what Carol is saying? Then maybe we can go back and talk about why you're hard on yourself because I wonder if that might have started with other people criticizing you in ways that were much harsher than the direct and, as Jen said, somewhat harsh, feedback Carol was giving you. Is there anything you'd like to say to Carol?

MEMBER 1: I think Carol just got caught up in being competitive with me, but she was right that I was treating you like you were my father abusing me and my sisters judging me all over again.

LEADER 2: Let's all step back for a moment and look at the important step you are taking as a group—discussing issues and supporting one another even when you feel triggered and you slip back into old patterns. But what makes this different is how honest you are being with one another while taking responsibility both for making this group not like the bad parts of your family experiences and for slips when you fall back into those dynamics.

LEADER 1: I agree completely and I'd add that I think this group is becoming safe because you are willing to stand up for your point of view even if it means dealing with a leader or another member in a way that creates conflict. But equally importantly, this means all of us, including me and Leader 2, take responsibility for the slips when they happen. We are also openly dealing with conflict with one another and learning to do so in ways that are direct but not aggressive.

MEMBER 4: I really like that way of looking at things. It's not all a bed of roses because we're all just human and we've had some bad influences in our lives, but we don't have to look the other way or keep secrets if someone is out of line.

MEMBER 1: Yeah, and people like me who can be potty mouths can learn to be kinder without having to just shut up and let bad things happen.

MEMBER 2: Well, I guess that goes for me, too, so you're not alone, Doris. I'm with you about not just standing aside when shit happens but I don't want to be creating more crap.

MEMBER 3: That makes three of us, Carol, I've had to eat too much shit and I know sometimes I just can't seem to stop dumping it out on other people, but I can work on that here.

MEMBER 4: Well, just so you know, I'm not always nicey-nice either. I can be way meaner than anyone in this group has been when I feel trapped and cornered. I was starting to feel that way today, but then I thought that I don't have to blurt things out because of the calm way that Doc and Leader 2 handle our outbursts. So I just felt sad and cried instead of getting angry.

LEADER 2: But I noticed that you didn't hide that sad feeling, Jen, which is a big step that everyone is working on—being able to show feelings is an important part of making this group very different from your families. And when we sometimes slip up, we can discuss it.

LEADER 1: And on that note, I want to check in with two of you who have been quiet so far today. I know you each have been observing very carefully and it would be helpful if you could share any observations or reactions that you have.

Commentary

The leaders helped members regain affect regulation by modeling characteristics of secure (trustworthy and responsive) attachment relationships, beginning with their own ability to self-regulate. Both remained calm and collaborative as a cotherapy team and helped members regain a sense of trust by validating their core goals and values and refocusing them on their legitimate concerns from earlier in life. They started with a discussion of the reenactment that had taken place in the prior session and that reemerged in a new form at the outset of this one (including the one member's attempt to disavow her previously conflicted stance by idealizing a group leader). The leaders did not allow themselves to join with the splitting (idealization and devaluation), but instead helped the members reaffirm their own and other members' strengths in the context of a shared goal. The leaders also paid attention to members' affective states and distress, moving sequentially to first help the member (Member 4) who was the most distressed and unable to maintain a tolerable degree of arousal and then, successively, to help the others regain emotional balance. They also paid attention to members who were not actively participating, communicating that they were not forgotten or ignored and reframing their participation as keen observers.

One or both of the leaders also would have intervened to help any members who were observed to be overly quiet and possibly dissociating and/or moving into a state of emotional numbing and detachment (hypoarousal). Although this vignette is only a brief snapshot, it demonstrates how much can be accomplished in group therapy with complex trauma and that this often occurs in what appear initially to be extremely dysfunctional interactions with members exhibiting "therapy interfering behaviors" (Linehan, 1993). Those behaviors are carefully monitored and directly addressed by the therapists to make the interaction a corrective emotional experience rather than simply professional control and limit setting. This is the case when therapists intervened with a focus on affect regulation and attachment security, consistent with the core issues and needs of clients with complex trauma.

COUPLE THERAPY

Many survivors, either unintentionally or more purposefully, choose as their romantic/sexual partners or spouses individuals who match (by either similarity or dissimilarity) their attachment style. At one end of the spectrum are partners who are emotionally detached (and therefore safe, but emotionally sequestered in a way that makes them unavailable emotionally to their partner) but who are otherwise solid, loyal, and reliable. At the other end are those who are needy, immature, unreliable, unresponsive, and/or overtly abusive, often mirroring people with whom the survivor has had past relationships. If, however, a survivor finds a partner who is dependable, loving and responsible (with a secure attachment style), the relationship might provide a needed "safe haven" that gives the survivor a base for improved self-concept, self-worth, and relationship skills and the subsequent development of an "earned secure" attachment style. Sadly, in some cases, survivors may be unable to believe that they deserve or can trust such a healthy relationship and either fail to commit to it or sabotage it in some way. Pushing away from or ending a healthy relationship can seem like the safest and most self-protective course, as getting close involves getting vulnerable.

Related to this, survivors often fail to disclose their past trauma, its extent, and its consequences to their intimates, fearing that they will be stigmatized or rejected if their experiences are known in any detail. The client's expectation and fears may be of exploitation, infidelity, or rejection or abandonment (especially after the partner or spouse finds out about what happened in the past and discovers his or her core "badness"). It may make it easier to be the one who leaves than to be the one who is left. Of course, this strategy of avoidance, nondisclosure, and the expectation of inevitable abandonment leaves the partner in the dark, leading to further problems when and if the history emerges. Some partners are resentful that their partners have been less than honest with them; some may regard their partners as damaged goods and distance from them rather than support them; and still others might be relieved to know about what happened and be empathically supportive in response.

Given these difficult, debilitating, and somewhat unique dyadic relational problems, couple therapy should be considered for clients with complex trauma whose primary relationships are troubled, but seems sustainable and has the potential to offer much-needed emotional support. In the past, therapists have quite consistently failed to consider these clients within the context of their primary relationships and, as a result, tended to work with the client independently without regard to the repercussions on loved ones, a position criticized early on by Johnson (1989), who called for more integrated care. Therapists also may have failed to tap an important source of support where one was available, and, in some cases, alienation between partners resulted as the left-out member of the dyad came to feel resentful even while being relied on. Couple therapy is contraindicated however, when there is active ongoing domestic violence. A number of couple-treatment models that are applicable to this population have become available in recent years, all based on an understanding of attachment dynamics (Basham & Miehls, 2004; Catherall, 2004; Johnson, 2002, 2004; Monson & Fredman, 2012; Solomon, 2003; Solomon & Tatkin, 2010). These treatment models have been recently supplemented by texts devoted to military couples in which one or more partners have been traumatized as a result of their combat experience and multiple deployments (Everson & Figley, 2011; Herzog & Everson, 2007; Sneath & Rheam, 2011; Snyder & Monson, 2012).

Most often, couple therapy does not replace individual treatment, and the individual modality may provide important preparation or support for couple work; however, it is equally possible that couple therapy can facilitate stronger engagement in individual treatment. Providing guidance and an active role in resolving communication and intimacy problems can help the partner and survivor (it is often the case that both have histories of complex trauma) better understand how their traumatic pasts have affected them both as individuals and as a couple and how they can work together on the development of secure attachment for them as a couple and as a foundation for the entire family. Couple therapy provides an ideal *in vivo* opportunity for both partners to clarify and revise negative models of self and others and self-defeating patterns of engagement with key people in their lives.

When working with this population, the therapist may have to help the couple with affect regulation and to contain chaotic, dysregulated, and overwhelming emotional responses such as intense anger or hopelessness—expressed not just by one but also by both (but not to the point of active violence)—and identify the typical relational dynamic of the couple (Johnson, 2002; Johnson & Courtois, 2009). Traumatic reactions such as flashbacks and emotional numbing must also be considered. The therapist should determine whether the couple, as individuals and together, understands the definition of trauma and posttraumatic reactions. If not, education should be the first order of business. Then the couple can be taught strategies and skills for response, soothing, and containment. Education and skills training counteract the conclusion on the part of one or both partners that traumatic stress reactions are too dangerous and uncontrollable to be safely experienced or to be anticipated, interrupted, and controlled. The therapist must help partners to understand why the survivor might have difficulty trusting or accepting assistance and to jointly develop methods that are acceptable and tolerable to both. Compassionate response and soothing can serve as crucial antidotes to repetitive posttraumatic emotions and reactions.

As in the individual modality, it is helpful for couple therapy to proceed in phases involving a hierarchical progression of treatment tasks. It should be noted that, at times, ongoing domestic violence and other forms of aggression between partners or toward children might be occurring. In Phase 1 couple work, akin to the focus on safety and stabilization in individual therapy, the therapist conducts a formal violence and risk assessment. The goal of the initial work, as in individual treatment, is to end all aggression and violence and ensure basic safety of all members of the family. Specialized resources are now available for working with domestic violence and child abuse (see Self-Help Resources and Workbooks in the online supplement to this book). It should also be acknowledged that some relationships are so dysfunctional or distressed as to be unsalvageable. In cases in which violence or emotional abuse is ongoing and unremitting, couple therapy is not the option of choice. In less charged situations, the task of treatment might be to help the couple separate in the healthiest and least harmful ways for all involved.

Once safety is determined, the therapist seeks to identify and deescalate negative cycles of interaction and to access underlying feelings and hopes. The partners learn to recognize how their interactions originate in and perpetuate negative cycles such as "demand-and-withdraw" (Johnson, 2002; Johnson & Williams-Keeler, 1998), which are likely to represent the expression of symptoms of traumatic stress and resultant coping mechanisms in one or both partners. This identification strategy further helps partners recognize core emotions that are embedded in (but often obscured by) the obvious emotional distress that they voice or act out with one another. For example, when hurt, fear, shame, or guilt are the elemental emotions with which they are grappling, couples often fight with great intensity and anger or withdraw in stony silence. The therapist encourages the couple to experiment with identifying and sharing these core emotions in guided interactions with each other that usually involve feelings of hurt and grief and fear of being further rejected or abandoned. As each partner becomes more willing and able to interact with the other on the basis of their deeper emotions and understanding (along with associated hopes, values, goals, and commitments), relational safety and stability tends to increase enough for them to communicate in more detail about the trauma and then to engage in trauma-related emotion processing. As in individual treatment, Phase 1 might be the longest phase devoted to basic skill development (communication skills and the ability to increase levels of recognition of the needs of each partner and of increased trust and intimacy—including sexual interactions and sexual functioning).

Phase 2 has parallel tasks in both couple and individual therapy. The focus shifts to helping the couple to talk more directly about how one (or both) partner's experiences and posttraumatic adaptations have influenced their relationship. Because it is not unusual for both to have trauma histories that have not been disclosed in any detail due primarily to shame and fear (or for other reasons, such as dissociative forgetting), the therapist must assist partners in talking to each other and gradually disclosing what they have kept secret. Often, once a partner has more information, he or she is more understanding and accepting of the other partner's symptoms. Couples may discuss specific traumatic events that one or both have experienced as a means of developing a shared narrative that helps them gain a mutual understanding of the event(s) and the influence these exerted on their relationship. Couples are also assisted in processing the trauma in less direct ways by helping each other recognize, interrupt, and alter posttraumatic coping patterns that undergird reenactments of traumatic events in the relationship. In this way, a partner who formerly felt helpless can now feel useful in comforting and providing needed support and specific agreed-upon interventions.

Aggression, in its verbal, emotional, and physical manifestations, constitutes another major area of intervention. The therapist helps the couple recognize that aggression is usually a learned behavior, a reenactment of abuse and other previous experiences of victimization, and that at times it is the consequence of identification with the aggressor, who was a role model for the negative behavior. The therapist helps the enraged, critical, or otherwise intimidating partner in identifying aggressive behavior, shifting from a stance of externalizing blame to one of accepting responsibility and replacing it with assertiveness. As this partner takes on more responsibility and changes attitudes and behaviors, the therapist then reengages the withdrawn partner. That partner often benefits from the development of skills in assertiveness to enable her or him to move out of the position of victimized, withdrawn member of the couple.

In Phase 3, the couple is encouraged to take the new knowledge and to jointly discuss ways to prevent traumatic stress reactions from undermining the security of their attachment and to extend this to their parenting and their relationships with other (including abusive) family members. Using their shared understanding of posttraumatic reactions and their associated impacts on relationships, they can rework interactions that have previously led to the escalation of conflict or withdrawal and replace them with ones that are responsive and that foster movement toward rather than away from one another. Couples can also be assisted in learning how and when to talk to their children about their experiences and how to manage relationships with family members who were or who remain abusive. Both can be daunting tasks and may require extensive discussion and planning.

Where it has been absent, couples are also encouraged to reestablish physical and sexual intimacy, starting with soothing touch and increasing physical contact at a pace that is comfortable and that helps each partner have control. They are encouraged to recognize the roles that posttraumatic reactions and coping mechanisms have played in creating difficulties in their sexual interactions. At times, a referral to a sex therapist is in order, and specific resources are available that might be incorporated as part of the couple treatment, such as Maltz's *Sexual Healing Journey* (2012), which includes a variety of exercises that partners undertake alone and apart. This book also offers a great deal of information to partners about their loved ones' responses, sexual or otherwise, as does the book *Allies in Healing* (Davis, 1991) and other resources (Courtois, 2005). Specialized resources on specific topics as related to a history of trauma, such as drug and alcohol addiction (Najavits, 2002), codependency (Black, 1981), sexual addiction (Canning, 2008; Carnes, 1991; Carnes & Delmonico, 1996), or addiction to pornography (Maltz & Maltz, 2008) are also now available and can help each partner normalize to some degree the various difficulties each one faces.

As part of this phase, as well as in the two preceding phases, attention is also paid to parenting and other family issues as they emerge. Parenting skills training might be in order, and books are now available that offer specific suggestions and strategies for parents to employ (e.g., *Parenting from the Inside Out* [Siegel & Hartzell, 2003], and *Attachment-focused family therapy* [Hughes, 2007]). The bottom line is the development of a healthy and respectful family environment that is safe for all members.

Whether one or both partners have ongoing relationships with their families of origin is another area of concern if one or both sets of parents were (or still are) troubled, or inadequate as parents, addicted, and/or were the original abusers and enablers. The degree of dysfunction or health in these individuals and other family members and any potential for dangerous interactions in the present must be assessed. In most cases, it is not the therapist's place to determine whether the couple maintains contact with members of the family of origin or not—that is for the couple to decide and to plan contact that is safe for all. Of course, the exception is ongoing present-day violence, especially toward children, which requires a report to child protective services by the therapist. In such a case, the couple might also be encouraged to make their own report as a means of empowering them to break the cycle of secrecy and family violence.

Additional information about disclosures and discussions, confrontations, reports to authorities, and possible actions (such as permanent separations from family members, criminal reports, lawsuits, etc., with parents or other family members and responsible others) can be found in Barrett, 2003; Courtois, 2010; Davis, 1991, 2002). Whatever the circumstance and selected courses of action, the couple must be advised of and prepared for possible consequences so that they can anticipate and plan for them together. Their joint efforts at creating safety and supporting one another create a new relational template for them.

Couple Therapy Vignette

Joyce is a 37-year-old woman who sought therapy a year ago because she began to have panic attacks after the birth of her third child (a daughter). She had been molested by a paternal uncle starting at age 7 when her mother was pregnant with her younger sister. It stopped when she disclosed the sexual abuse to a teacher, who reported it to social services. Her father defended his brother and blamed Joyce for being "a liar who made the story up." When her mother defended Joyce, the parents became so estranged that Joyce's father left and subsequently remarried and started another family. Although Joyce's mother steadfastly supported her in an ensuing trial in which the uncle was found also to have molested two of Joyce's older cousins, her mother also "never forgave me for breaking up the family—she blamed me for 'ruining your sister's life and my marriage.' She was a lonely woman who devoted her life to putting my sister on a pedestal and never was involved in a relationship with a man again."

Joyce asked her therapist for help when she found that she couldn't stand to be intimate, not just sexually but also emotionally, with her husband Simon after their daughter's birth. This distancing continued even when she was no longer having panic attacks after receiving medication and having some EMDR sessions. Her individual therapist referred them to a therapist he knew to be experienced in working with couples in which one or both were trauma survivors. The following vignette is from a session that took place after 3 months of couple therapy in which Joyce has recognized that her daughter's birth triggered intrusive reexperiencing reactions that were fragmentary flashbacks of both the molestation and her mother's rage at her disclosure.

THERAPIST: Simon, your wife told you that she loves you deeply and that she needs you. You looked away and told her that she doesn't ever show it anymore and seems to only want you to be a "lodger" in the house who helps take care of the children and who pays the bills. You've been very supportive of Joyce as she's gone through this painful reliving of the hurtful experiences with her uncle and parents, and you've been very clear in letting her know how much you miss being close to her. It seemed to be a different message when you turned away. It's like you're giving up. (*Joyce nods tearfully.*) Can you talk with Joyce about how you're feeling and what's changed for you?

SIMON: I have needs, too, and it seems like all we talk about in here is Joyce's abuse and what she needs from me. You both only seem interested in her needs, like I don't matter.

JOYCE: I know I've let you down, and I feel like a horrible selfish person for asking so much from you and not giving you what you need, Simon. I just don't know how to get through this emotional wall that I feel between us. I know it's my fault and I'm hurting you. (*Sobs.*)

THERAPIST: Joyce, I see how much you want to feel close to Simon again and how hard it is for you not to blame yourself when you feel blocked emotionally. But what Simon is saying, which takes courage on his part, is that he is caught between wanting to support and love you but that he needs attention too. He needs not to feel so separated from you and to know that his needs matter to you.

JOYCE: I know I've let him down terribly, and I feel like such a failure as a wife. Now I'm ruining my own marriage, after I ruined my parents' marriage!

THERAPIST: Joyce, this self-blame and fear that you ruin relationships is the issue we've been working on, and you've addressed in your own therapy. But I think Simon is offering another way to work on this issue, where it doesn't just belong to you alone and you're not to blame, but you actually have the power to help him in a way that no other person can. Simon, what you're communicating to Joyce is that it is painful for you when you feel her pulling away from you, because she's that important to you. I don't think that's the message that's coming across to Joyce, and she may be thinking that you just want her to put her needs aside and to meet your needs. As a result, Joyce has been having a hard time feeling how much you love her—not because either you or she have been doing anything wrong, but because you're not sending her the message you intend and she's so afraid of losing you that she's losing track of what she used to know about your love for her.

SIMON: So you're saying I have to just keep putting aside *my* needs until Joyce gets over her feelings about her past abuse? I can't keep doing that. It's just too much to ask anyone to do! And I'm tired of being seen as an abuser because I'm a man.

THERAPIST: That's exactly the problem: Joyce has found that she can't put aside her need to heal the wounds she sustained as a child, and you've been extremely supportive, but you're feeling the loss of the emotional foundation that Joyce's caring has provided for you. It does sound to me like you deeply miss Joyce's emotional presence, not that you want her to put her needs aside and just take care of your needs. Do you see the difference? Could you tell Joyce why you miss her, so she'll know that what's important to you is her love for you?

SIMON: After all this, I can't believe she doesn't know I love her! (*Turns to Joyce.*) What do I have to do to prove I love you, put all my needs aside forever and only take care of yours?

JOYCE: No, that's not what I want! I just don't know how to get through this and I can't do it without you, but I don't want to ruin your life because I'm so selfish and needy!

THERAPIST: Joyce, I think Simon is saying that he wants exactly the same thing for you that you want—and he wants it for both of you, so you both can be free of these old binds. If you just stop for a moment, and look at Simon, really look at him and see this man as he is right now, not anyone else, as the man you married and who you never want to lose. (*Pauses briefly.*) Do you feel blamed or exploited or abandoned by him?

JOYCE: (*Looks at Simon, then back to the therapist, and starts to talk to the therapist.*) I . . .

THERAPIST: (*in a very soft but firm voice*) Wait just a moment, can you turn back to Simon and really look at him? Do you see blame or demands, or loss and love? (*Pauses and looks toward Simon.*) Simon, as Joyce is looking at you, and focusing on really seeing you, I think this is exactly what you've been saying you've been missing—Joyce really seeing you. As she does, know how much you love her and how much she loves you. In spite of how much it's hurt you to feel her withdraw from you emotionally while she's been healing from her childhood, can you see her love for you in her eyes?

SIMON: (*Looks toward Joyce, who has stopped crying and is looking intently at Simon; then his face shifts from angry to sad, and turns back to the therapist.*)

THERAPIST: I want to ask you to let yourself stop trying to be strong and solve all the problems, but just for a moment look at Joyce and take in what you see her showing you about her feelings for you. Joyce doesn't have to do anything except let you see what she feels for you, and you don't have to do anything to rescue her. Just take in her feelings for you. (*Pauses.*) I think maybe you've both been missing this for a long time, while you've each been working so hard with much courage and dedication to each other and to healing old wounds. It's easy to lose track of what you do for each other without having to try to meet anyone's needs because you deeply care about her and the love between you is precious to each of you.

JOYCE: I've felt like I had nothing to give to Simon. (*Therapist nods in Simon's direction.*) Okay. (*Turns toward Simon.*) I've felt like I've had nothing to give to you, Simon, I've been so selfishly obsessed with my own past that I've abandoned you and treated you like an abuser instead of like the man I love and always want to be with.

SIMON: I used to know that, but (*tears in his eyes*) you went so far away inside yourself that I haven't been able to find you, like you left me and I don't know why you had to go!

THERAPIST: (*softly*) Does your wife seem here now, I mean emotionally, for you, Simon?

SIMON: (*Looks back at Joyce inquiringly, then softening.*) Yes, maybe, I think so. . . .

THERAPIST: What does that feel like for you, Simon? What does that mean to you?

SIMON: This is what I need, I can be as strong as Joyce . . . (*Therapist looks from Simon to Joyce, signaling him to focus on her; Simon turns to Joyce.*) . . . As you need, I just need to feel you with me, that you can show me you love me so I don't feel alone while we go through this.

JOYCE: I can do that. That's what I want to do for you because I love you and I know you love me. We've had so much to deal with since our daughter was born. Our children need both of us, too.

Commentary

Simon and Joyce repeatedly revisited moments in which her sense of exploitation and blame activated old feelings of being helplessly victimized and at fault for ruining relationships she counted on, undermining her self-confidence. Simon's fear of losing her made it hard for him to ask her for reassurance without feeling weak or demanding. He realized that he had old fears, not based on trauma per se but on the difficult family situation he experienced when his parents were preoccupied with caring for a younger brother born with muscular dystrophy. As Joyce could see that Simon also had old emotional wounds that needed attention, she was able to feel less like the defective, deficient partner and more like an equal whose love and compassion meant as much to Simon as his did to her. The therapist intervened to interrupt a potential crisis in the relationship by helping both partners reinstate their sense of security based on their mutual love, using their experience in the immediate interaction as a way to refocus them together on acknowledging their devotion to one another, rather than their trying so hard to meet each other's needs. This session was a turning point in working through a number of misconceptions that each partner had transferred to the relationship.

Subsequent sessions were devoted to the processing of both of their troubling memories—many of which they recognized as important only when the therapist helped them to see how they were reenacting them. That connection between the past and present provided a basis for the couple to refocus on their actual feelings and relationship in the present and to interrupt intrusions from their pasts instead of playing them out with one another.

FAMILY THERAPY

A family member who is a survivor of trauma (of any type, but especially complex or cumulative trauma) alters the family system in profound ways, some of which are not readily identifiable without the direct report of family members. Family therapy as applied to this population is a relatively recent innovation and is consistent with developments in similar populations, namely, military families in which a member has been traumatized in combat or families with a member who was traumatized in an accident, a natural disaster, or by a death or major illness (Catherall, 1992, 2004, 2005; Everson & Figley, 2011; Figley, 1989; Matsakis, 1998; Zayfert & DeViva, 2011). Family therapy helps to restore relationships between all members, including but not limited to relationships with the traumatized member. It can offer information and support to a family that allows its members to more effectively contribute to (and not inadvertently undermine) the survivor member's recovery and the functioning of the entire family. Although complex traumatic stress disorders are not "contagious" per se, family members are profoundly affected when even one member is struggling with severe emotion dysregulation, traumatic stress reactions, and attachment disorganization. Family process and dynamics (as described in Chapters 1 and 2) can be transmitted from generation to generation, behaviorally and through messages and injunctions to all family members. By definition, when the traumatic events occur within the family as the result of the actions of its members (e.g., incest, domestic violence), every family member is potentially traumatized, whether directly or vicariously.

The adverse effects on family members can be particularly profound when complex trauma began in early life. Additionally, individual family members may themselves have received different levels of actual exposure to potentially traumatic events and may have experienced different types and degrees of posttraumatic reactions (Ford & Saltzman, 2009). An individual's reactions to his or her own trauma certainly influence response to the trauma experienced by other members and the provision of sustenance and support.

Trauma responses also affect the ability to successfully parent children. If insecure attachment styles and processes are not interrupted, then they are likely to be utilized in child rearing and transmitted to offspring. As a result, the family members to whom a traumatized person looks for help and protection may themselves have different needs related to their own direct or vicarious stress reactions, including those associated with living with a traumatized family member. These stress reactions can lead to major breakdowns in communication, conflicting needs, discord, and reenactments of traumatic events in subsequent family interactions. Such reactions can also unfortunately be compounded when the traumatized individual or others in the family are addicted and turn to substances to cope or are violent or emotionally or sexually abusive. When parental abuse is already occurring within the family, family dynamics are skewed and roles and relationships between members get distorted (Courtois, 2010). Nonoffending caregiver(s) and other family members (i.e., siblings) are exposed to trauma when they witness abusive events or their aftermath. They might also feel they failed to prevent the abuse in the first place or did not adequately protect other family members from its influence. It is an ironic truth that, due to family loyalty, when abuse is perpetrated within the family, it brings less response and protection from family members than when it is perpetrated by someone on the outside (Courtois, 2010).

When one or both parents are in the throes of traumatic stress reactions, their ability to adequately parent their children and to maintain family routines and roles is reduced (Jordan et al., 1992; Ruscio, Weathers, King, & King, 2002). This is the case for children directly victimized by a traumatic event (Nader, Pynoos, Fairbanks, & Frederick, 1990), for those who indirectly learn about a family member's violent or traumatic experience (Pine, Costello, & Masten, 2005), and for nontraumatized children whose parents are troubled by their own past traumas (Brand, Engel, Canfield, & Yehuda, 2006). Parental withdrawal, overprotectiveness, excessive preoccupation with the trauma, or ongoing anxiety and depression, as well as frank posttraumatic symptoms can directly or indirectly exacerbate a child's traumatic stress symptoms (Meiser-Stedman, Yule, Dalgleish,

Smith, & Glucksman, 2006; Scheeringa & Zeanah, 2001). Conversely, a child's traumatic stress reactions can elicit posttraumatic stress symptoms in parents who were not previously trauma-exposed (Cohen, 2008; Pat-Horenczyk, Rabinowitz, Rice, & Tucker-Levin, 2008).

On the positive side, family relationships also are indispensable to the traumatized person's recovery, as they simultaneously provide essential support for the restoration of emotional security, physical safety, and hope. Not surprisingly, children, adolescents, and even adults often look to their parents, siblings, and other adult relatives as sources of support during a variety of potentially or actually traumatic situations. In these circumstances, children in families that are cohesive, caring, and emotionally involved are more likely to recover (Fairbank, Putnam, & Harris, 2007). The support and protection provided by parents and other attachment figures are essential to the security and safety needed to recover.

Family systems approaches to psychotherapy aim not to just change individual family members but to restructure, rebuild, and restore healthy family relationships. Family therapy for PTSD has been described as aiming to repair the family "system" in order to enhance the social support available to and utilized by the family (Catherall, 1992, 1998, 2004, 2005; Figley, 1989; Riggs, 2000). Family systems models attempt to facilitate the development of several features of family relationships that support an ongoing emotional connection. These include: the safety of all members in the family (as the responsibility primarily of the parents but also of all members); healthier roles for family members; explicit and reasonable expectations of one another; open and sensitive discussion of troubling past experiences in place of "secrets" or other forms of avoidance in dealing with the past; a balance of individuality and togetherness ("relational boundaries" among individual members and between the generations that includes strong but inclusive leadership by parents and a clear distinction between the roles and responsibilities of adults and children in the family); open, respectful approaches to affection and communication; and effective family problem solving.

Family therapy is designed to help members develop ways of interacting with and understanding each other that convey respect, affection, inclusion, and support for each member, including his or her distinct personality, preferences, and goals. This form of therapy may be conducted in meetings that include all members of the family (conjoint family therapy), with multiple families in one group (multifamily groups; Kiser, Donohue, Hodgkinson, Medoff, & Black, 2010) or with subgroups of individual family members (e.g., siblings in one meeting, parents in another; one or the other parent and one child together). Generally, it is most efficient and effective to involve family members simultaneously to foster cohesion. It also is essential to redefine therapeutic issues as a challenge that involves all members equally, to counteract the tendency in troubled families for some members to be viewed as the problem (the "identified patient") or the cause of the problem (the "scapegoat") who must be "fixed." Instead, family therapy defines the "problem" as one that belongs to all members who are having difficulties getting along with and supporting one another. All are helped to play a constructive role in dealing with this "shared problem". An exception to this occurs in some family approaches to incest, when the offender must take primary responsibility (Courtois, 2010).

The emphasis in family therapy on developing shared solutions for shared problems is particularly important when family member(s) have experienced complex trauma, because their posttraumatic symptoms can lead them to be blamed and marginalized or even attacked by others in the family. The following comments give a few examples: "His flashbacks/night terrors and irritability are problems for everybody. We tiptoe around and walk on eggshells to not upset him"; "He [or she] is so depressed all the time, not interested in anything we do or being with us as a family and staying in bed all the time"; "The drinking is really bad—anytime he [or she] gets triggered by something, we can count on it getting worse"; or "When she accused our grandfather of molesting her, it ruined his life and upset everyone else in the family. Now, nobody speaks to anyone else". Family therapy is designed to help members discover how they can break through impasses and contribute constructively to help others to recover from the fear, hurt, shame, and guilt caused by trauma, whether they were directly traumatized as victims or as witnesses or were indirectly affected by the traumas suffered by others in the family.

Family Therapy Vignette

The following simulated case vignette provides a sample of family therapy involving Sandra (who had a history of complex trauma from childhood and who had been retraumatized several times in her adult life), her mother, and her stepfather. Sandra's mother continued to be closely involved as a caregiver and *de facto* case manager for Sandra, who had persistent difficulty in keeping an independent residence or a job. Sandra and her mother met periodically with Sandra's individual therapist (as requested by both) to engage her mother in reinforcing the knowledge and skills that Sandra was learning in treatment. However, when Sandra experienced a crisis precipitated by an adverse reaction to a thyroid medication, she had to be hospitalized for several months for both medical and psychiatric care. She had been living in a group home for disabled adults, but the home's manager was unwilling to have Sandra return because he felt her symptoms were too unstable and severe for the staff to manage. This led to a family crisis, because the only alternatives appeared to be for Sandra to return to live with her parents or to be placed in a state psychiatric hospital for the chronically mentally ill. Sandra was unwilling to accept either alternative, having developed a delusional belief that her mother was trying to take her disability income and keep her a prisoner in the family's home and that going to the hospital would be a life sentence that would leave her with no choice but to kill herself. At the same time, Sandra's "voices" (a combination of auditory hallucinations and flashbacks) returned, forcefully telling her to cut or kill herself.

Sandra's mother was adamant that the only safe plan was for her daughter to return home. Her stepfather, however, was angry about Sandra's attitude toward her mother and burdened by what now appeared to be an endless prospect of having to put Sandra ahead of "having a life for ourselves." After many years of unwavering support for both, he now insisted that they had to stop "rescuing" Sandra. While hospitalized, Sandra initially refused to see her therapist or her parents, relenting only when her medicine and psychiatric treatment kicked in to help her think more rationally—at which point she was nearing discharge and crucial placement and care decisions had to be made.

THERAPIST: Good to see you again after such a stressful period for all of you.

MOTHER: (*Sighs, looks at Sandra smiling but tearfully.*) I really thought we'd lost Sandra when she got suicidal from taking that thyroid medicine and took the overdose. And then when she wouldn't have anything to do with us when she was in the hospital.

SANDRA: (*Looks intently at her mother.*) I'm sorry, mummy, I didn't know what I was saying. I didn't want to hurt you, I never want to lose you, you know that, don't you?

MOTHER: Of course I know. It just scared and hurt me that you didn't know me, and it seemed like after all the times you've been suicidal, that this time I'd lost you.

SANDRA: No! You'll never lose me, but I thought you were trying to control me and I couldn't trust you anymore. That was just the medicine, not really me. Don't be angry with me, I can't stand it if you are angry with me!

THERAPIST: (*turning to stepfather*) Mr. R, were you afraid of losing Sandra, too? [Helping the parents join together while defusing Sandra's intense focus on her mother]

STEPFATHER: I sure was, but it was worse for her mother, because she was right there and saw Sandra stop breathing until the paramedics did CPR. I don't want my wife to have to keep going through this. It's taking a toll on her health and on our relationship.

THERAPIST: So you're very concerned about both your wife and your daughter, you don't want to lose either of them.

STEPFATHER: It's been a strain on all of us. I want Sandra to be safe, but I don't think we can keep putting our lives on hold to take care of her. She has to live her own life.

MOTHER: You know I have to do whatever is needed to be sure Sandra is safe, Martin. I'm the only one who has kept her out of the hospital and alive for all these years, and I'm not going to stop just when she needs me most.

THERAPIST: You protected Sandra when she was just a little child and her biological father was drinking and violent, and you've never stopped working on ways to help Sandra have a good independent life, Mrs. R. Your commitment to and love for your daughter is unmistakable, and I see how much that means to Sandra. She cares deeply about you, but she can't be your support system because she's the daughter and you're the mother. It looks like, from what we've just heard from your husband, that he has recognized the importance of your care, and he's tried hard to be supportive to you. But it must be difficult, because you've all been caught in a vicious cycle when Sandra's symptoms get bad, and you can never be sure when or if this depression will return or whether it will improve over time and with more treatment. This has been a tremendous strain for all of you, and it's no one's fault, even though I heard you say, Sandra, that you're afraid your mother will be angry with you for this.

SANDRA: I know I've been a burden for them and they've done more for me than I can ever make up to them. I afraid I will lose her because I'm making her sick and because she is tired of me. She probably wouldn't have gotten the cancer. And if she dies, it's my fault, and I can't live without her.

MOTHER: You know I've recovered completely after the surgery and chemo, Sandra, and you were a big help to me and your stepfather when I was sick and in treatment. You didn't make me sick, and caring for you is important to me. I want you to have a good life and I'm going to keep supporting you. And I intend to live a long life and many more years!

THERAPIST: Sandra, do you trust what your mother is telling you? She is very certain that her relationship with you continues to be important to her, sometimes stressful, but not something that caused her cancer. Do you believe her?

SANDRA: I want to, and I know she means it, but I've been so mean to her and such a worry for her. And for my stepfather, who's always been there for me, too.

THERAPIST: Do you think they're here now because they identify you as a problem to them? When you look at how they look at you now, do you see frustration or anger, or something else?

SANDRA: They have a right to be angry and I think my stepfather is frustrated with me.

THERAPIST: (*turning to stepfather*) Are you angry at Sandra, Mr. R, or is it something else?

STEPFATHER: I'm frustrated, but it's because I love both of them, a lot.

THERAPIST: And don't want to lose either of them?

STEPFATHER: That's right, of course. (*Quickly wipes a tear from one eye.*) I don't know what I'd do without either of my girls.

THERAPIST: Is that the kind of emotional support that has helped you recover so well, not only from the cancer, but when you had the surgery on your back, Mrs. R?

MOTHER: That's exactly right. Martin has been a rock for me and for the whole family. I want him to be happy, too. He's had to put off a lot.

THERAPIST: What has it meant to you to be a coparent for Sandra, and also your stepson and other daughter, Mr. R?

STEPFATHER: It's meant a lot to me. I don't say it often, but I wouldn't trade being a dad for anything. Like the times when Sandra and I go and have a walk around the mall together and get a milk shake—which her mother says is too fattening, but it's our time together—that is something I never get tired of doing.

THERAPIST: Can you hear what you mean to your stepfather, Sandra, and see it on his face?

SANDRA: (*Looks anxiously, then with increasing calm, at her stepfather.*) I can.

THERAPIST: And would you agree with him that he and your mother also need to be sure to take care of themselves and have a good life as a couple? Not to go away from you, but exactly the opposite, to be able to be with you, while all of you build good lives for yourselves on your own and together as a family?

SANDRA: (*Looks anxiously at her mother.*) Does this mean that you don't want me to live with you, so you and daddy can stop taking care of me and have your own life?

MOTHER: That's not what Dr. F said, and no, it's not true. I just want you to be as happy and independent as possible, and I'm not going to stop doing what I can to make that possible. Daddy and I need time together, but it's not an either–or choice. Now that you're doing so much better, when you come home and are settled in, then you and your aunt can house-sit while we take the trip to Florida that we've been planning.

THERAPIST: So coming home can be the next step forward for everyone in this family, and you've all worked very hard to make this possible in spite of the recent setback.

Commentary

The therapist helps family members to establish (or regain) ways of interaction that promote a shared sense of security. Rather than supporting Sandra's stepfather in his view that she and her symptoms were the "problem," the therapist helped him experience their shared attachment as the basis for increasing her relational security, thus reducing her distress. This, in turn, allowed his wife some "down time" to plan some independent activities. This had the effect of reducing his frustration. The vignette also shows how, at times of crisis or when family bonds have become frayed or conflicted, family therapy can complement individual therapy and restore communication and relations when they are interrupted by traumatic stress symptoms. Family therapy did not completely resolve Sandra's difficulties with suicidality and self-harm. Thus the entire family gained a way to think about, prevent, and respond to symptoms that had previously seemed uncontrollable. Although other therapeutic interventions (e.g., pharmacotherapy, individual and group therapy) may be needed to comprehensively address severe psychiatric and medical symptoms such as Sandra's, trauma-informed family therapy can potentially make the symptoms more manageable by enlisting the whole family in developing more secure and emotionally regulated relationships.

CONCLUSION

Trauma has a "wake," as Figley (1985) so cogently noted. Not only is the individual victim affected, but his or her loved ones are as well. This fact has not been adequately recognized in the treatment of traumatized clients, a point made by Johnson (1989), who called for more attention to the client in relationship and the application of concurrent individual and couple counseling. Systemic therapies have a great deal to offer in the treatment of the relational effects of complex trauma. Gains in relationship development and the modification of attachment style can serve as models for changes in other significant relationships. The resolution of traumatic stress reactions in the survivor can have a major impact on his or her intimate relationship and on members of the entire family, and vice versa.

Models of systemic treatments of varying intensities and durations that parallel treatment tasks of the phase-oriented model for complex trauma have been presented. Many of these have been developed in recent years, and others are under development and outcome testing. Groups are now available in many different formats, and different types can be used in different phases of treatment. For example, structured, educational groups support the tasks of Phase 1 by providing information and skills-development groups offer opportunities for role playing with others and feedback. Couple and family treatment explicitly recognize the significance of the client's spouse or partner and other family members and the impact that traumatic stress reactions can have on them. These modalities can be implemented across all phases of treatment and can complement and enhance gains made in individual therapy.

Systemic treatments provide a unique forum for survivors of interpersonal trauma. Bloom (1997) called for "relational healing for relational injury," and therapy and other interpersonal treatment approaches provide a context within which to begin repair of the social contract (Scott, 1999). Systemic treatments provide the opportunity to examine attachment/relational styles and roles based on dysfunctional dynamics within past abusive or neglectful contexts and for experimenting with and replacing them with more mutual roles and interaction styles. All are in the interest of developing more self-referenced and satisfying present and future life choices.

PART III

ADVANCED TREATMENT CONSIDERATIONS AND RELATIONAL ISSUES

CHAPTER 8

Into the Breach

Voids, Absences, and the Posttraumatic/Dissociative Relational Field

In this and the following two chapters, we shift focus from the specific elements of the treatment to model some of the more nuanced and complicated issues in the treatment of complex trauma. These issues and elements are not typically found in the treatment of nontraumatized populations, and therapists not familiar with them may be caught unaware. We provide these chapters as information to therapists to help them anticipate these issues and provide suggestions for their management.

What do we mean by "into the breach"? Many clients with complex trauma histories describe feeling not just impaired but empty or absent. This is not the pleasant emptiness that occurs in meditation or the kind of absence that results from taking a break from life's hectic pace. Instead, as we have discussed at different points in this text, survivors describe a painful sense of not being able to find within themselves any emotions, thoughts, or sense of personal identity and of not feeling "real" in the world. In order to meet the client where she or he lives psychologically, therapists must recognize and enter this inner void, or the "breach." And this must be done with exquisite care so as not to add to the client's psychic pain by violating his or her innermost privacy. In this chapter, we discuss ways in which therapists meet their clients in their desolate or tumultuous inner psychological landscapes and how they help them to build or to retrieve and restore their missing sense of self, emotions, thoughts, and beliefs from the void. We also discuss the posttraumatic/dissociative relational field in which the treatment takes place.

THE INNER EMPTINESS AS DESCRIBED BY COMPLEX TRAUMA SURVIVORS

The Void of the Self

Many complex trauma clients feel unreachable because they perceive there is no one inside to reach, nothing human that could be saved, and no spirit that developed or that could ever be. Yet their descriptions of their personal and emotional emptiness suggest a vivid awareness that something is missing, rather than a factual description of an actual void. When the individual is truly not present, even on a transient but normal basis—such as when preoccupied with thoughts or daydreams or in tragic instances such as brain injuries or diseases that cause dementia—the person is not aware of his or her own emptiness. In fact, some complex trauma survivors are unaware of their own absence; more often however, they are acutely aware and feel tortured by this awareness even if they have become resigned to it. Thus most of them simultaneously feel absent, lost, invisible, or in an emotional void while being present enough psychologically to recognize this absence and to yearn (albeit often without real hope or understanding) to be able to somehow find the "me" who was long ago unrecognized by others and seems to have gone missing as a result. Howell (2005) described the dissociative mind in this way.

When therapists encounter the superficially matter-of-fact way that many trauma survivors describe their agonizing sense of emptiness, they can make the mistake of accepting it at face value. This can lead to misguided attempts to find and rescue the missing psyche, which tend to confirm the survivor's belief in his or her own absence and the impossibility of regaining a self. Or it can lead to a mistaken pessimism about accomplishing anything in therapy, based on the false assumption that the client lacks the capacity for self-development and related hope, motivation, insight, or even rational thought. In fact, the *client is **not** missing in action or AWOL in a permanent way*. In most cases, there is no actual deficit in the client's ability to feel, think, or be motivated—she or he is too busy experiencing and coping with ongoing stress reactions to be able to allocate the biological and cognitive resources needed for self-awareness (Lanius et al., 2010; Lanius & Freeven, 2013; Porges, 2013; Schore, 2003a). This client is overwhelmed and does not know how to see (or to be) beyond the turmoil and beliefs created by traumatic stress reactions to recognize that she or he can be emotionally alive. Moreover, the survivor usually operates from a deficit position due to lack of response by caregivers, interactions that were needed to support development of the self. The lack of attunement, response, and synchrony on the part of caregivers did not mirror or reflect the child back to him- or herself to encourage the development of identity, much less self-worth. The self-void results, in part, from this nonattunement and nonresponse. As several of our clients have asked, "How can I have a self, when no one saw me, cared about me, or all they wanted me to do was be quiet and not bother them?" "Can I still have a self if nothing is there?" "Nobody ever noticed me or helped me to be me." It is for reasons such as these that delayed and latent development needs to be addressed and resumed.

At the outset and during the course of therapy it is therefore important to carefully listen to how the client describes her or his sense of self, especially regarding inner emptiness. The unique words and phrases used by each individual offer essential clues to what is needed in order to regain a sense of self and a meaningful inner and outside life. Consider these typical statements and the direction they suggest for therapeutic exploration (for which we provide some exploratory prompts in italics):

- "I have a hole in my soul."—"*What do you feel in the rest of your soul that still remains?*"
- "Something essential is missing in me."—"*What would be different if you got that back?*"
- "I'm not the person I might have been."—"*Who have you hoped and dreamed of becoming?*"
- "This isn't the life I was meant to live; I feel like I'm living someone else's life."—"*How would your life be different if you were living your own life?*"
- "I don't know who I am"; "I'm constantly numb and I don't know what I feel."—"*Are there times when the numbness isn't so complete, or when you can see what's behind it even if you can't actually feel anything?*"
- "I can't keep track of myself; I lose time and have these huge gaps in what I can remember about my life every day."—"*What happens right before and after those gaps occur?*"
- "I'm broken into fragments."—"*Can you see or feel any of those fragments enough to describe them?*"
- "I'd be better off dead because I'm dead inside."—"*When did you first realize that you felt dead inside? What happened leading up to that? Are there any times you have felt alive? Where and when?*"
- "I'm only alive when I'm hurting myself or when someone else is hurting me."—"*What do you feel at those times? How do you acccount for this?*"
- "God has abandoned me."—"*What would it be like if you could feel God's presence? Maybe it's not as much about God as about other people?*"
- "I'm invisible, like a ghost walking through my life where no one ever sees me."—"*Who would they see if they could see you? Can you accept others seeing you?*"
- "Pain and rage are all I know; I'm incapable of any other feelings."—"*What are your pain and rage trying to communicate? What do they need you or someone to understand? It is doubtful that you are incapable of other feelings.*"

At times, the void manifests itself in a client's presentation of silence and near muteness. Such a stance can be enormously disconcerting and frustrating (even enraging) to therapists who try (sometimes valiantly and over a long period of time) to evoke communication and response. In such a case, it may be more helpful for the therapist to understand the silence as a paradoxical means of communication of the void and the related detachment and disconnection from others in the interest of self-protection. It may also be the way a client communicates what it was like during childhood or during or after the trauma.

The Emotion Void

Clients describe themselves as numb and many experience alexithymia, an absence of emotion or the ability to recognize feelings. They are devoid of being in touch with their feelings, thus missing a crucial mechanism of self and self-awareness. As discussed, this numbness can be offset with emotional flooding and dysregulation. Emotions are thus a source of distress rather than information about self. These issues are increasingly recognized and addressed in the developing field of the affective neurosciences.

The Somatic Void

Clients often describe themselves as depersonalized and outside of their bodies. Somatoform dissociation can be so pervasive that clients report feeling as though they have no body and being unable to experience physical sensations. They may also describe feeling totally unable to control what they and their bodies do, a phenomenon most evident in DID, when other parts of the self take over executive control. Clients may report things "happening to them from the inside" that make them feel like automatons, as though they were invaded by aliens and as being at the mercy of other parts-selves who want to punish or hurt them, sometimes in the interest of "shutting them up for talking." The essence of work with dissociation is for the client to get "back in touch" with him- or herself, a process that may only occur over time with specialized interventions and protocols and with great intentionality and perseverance on the part of both client and therapist (See Boon, Steele, & Van der Hart, 2011, for a most helpful client workbook in this regard).

The Void of Unfinished Business

Complex trauma can also leave another void: that of unfinished and unresolved emotional business that shows up in delayed form years and even decades later, long after the trauma itself has ceased. Survivors often report feeling flooded with overwhelming and fragmentary memories or diffuse and confusing emotional reactions and states that they experience as creating an unbridgeable distance between them and other people—and at times full detachment from themselves. The breach or gap between the survivor and self and then between everyone and everything else is expressed in many ways. Here again, the survivor's words can provide the beginning of a therapeutic dialogue if the therapist can hear the message of longing and determination, as well as the more obvious one of hopelessness:

- "I feel so separate from everyone and everything in my life that I could be on another planet."—"*What would happen if you were not so separate, if you could feel close to other people? Would that be a planet you want to live on or could live on safely?*"
- "I start to remember the abuse and then everything goes blank."—"*When you're ready, at any point in our work together but not necessarily now, you can tell me what you do remember before your mind and emotions go blank and we can figure out what you need to know or do to make that safe enough so your mind doesn't have to protect you by going blank. Until that time, your mind and emotions are doing their job to protect you.*"
- "I become that 5-year-old and I'm so cold and alone that I want to cry for help, but I know no one will help me because I'm so worthless and bad."—"*What is the help that that 5-year-old you needed—and still needs—in order to be able to feel supported and worthwhile?*"
- "I feel nothing when someone touches me or so much pain that I want to scream."—"*What do you need another person to understand and do so that you won't have to cope with being touched in hurtful ways and so that being touched will happen only with your consent and in ways that you feel are right for you?*"
- "I am so small and unimportant that no one knows I exist."—"*Actually, I know that you exist but understand that you feel invisible and worthless. Can you let this recognition in a bit? What would help you begin to be more visible to me and to others?*"

As illustrated by these poignant statements and the sample therapist responses, the sense of emptiness is not a true void within but rather the product of coping with overwhelming and trauma-induced distress and disregard, often alone and in isolation, without needed response, reflection, assistance, or explanation. The "breach" created by complex trauma is a combination of extreme emotional turmoil and a self-protective defense that involves shutting down of awareness of the turmoil in the absence of support and soothing from others. The "breach" in which therapists meet these survivor clients can be understood as emotion dysregulation managed by shutdown and dissociation, the only coping options that might have been available. Bollas (1987) and other analysts have talked about this void as "unformulated experience" and as involving implicitly encoded information that is outside of the individual's conscious awareness and that often forms gaps in awareness. Schore (2013) discussed the implicit self and means of making the implicit or potential self more explicit and conscious. This missing information can be retrieved and brought to conscious awareness in the interest of creating a more integrated and coherent sense of self and personal narrative.

Disconnection from Others

Many survivors describe painful disconnection and alienation from others. They often describe not being like other "more normal" people and as not fitting in with others, feelings that are bolstered by their low self-esteem and self-loathing. They may not have learned interpersonal or social skills in their families of origin (from which they might also be alienated or with which they might be engaged in ongoing and unsatisfactory interactions and unmet expectations), deficits that impact their ability to have relationships or to achieve intimacy with others. Though they want to fit in, they are plagued by the impact of past exploitation and betrayals and by neglect, bullying, and nonresponse. Some may be able to function in an "apparently normal" way and to be superficially compliant in their interactions with others, but underneath the facade, they may be highly mistrustful and have other emotions out of their awareness, such as anger and resentment. In some cases, they act out their anger in hostile and passive–aggressive behavior and the mistreatment or abuse of others. At times, disconnection from others is volitional, sometimes going to extremes. For example, some survivors are so relationally injured that they become recluses and hermits, often preferring the company of companion pets to that of other humans. They may interact with other human beings only to the degree that they must. Or they may be so disengaged and alienated that suicide becomes their primary option.

Understanding the Inner Void Caused by Complex Trauma

Shutting Down Feelings

Additionally, many survivors describe how, in the course of experiencing chronic traumatic exposure without needed response or intervention, they learned to *not feel* their emotions (alexithymia) or their physical reactions, both means of dissociation. Instead, they learned to fantasize alternative selves and scenarios (e.g., to deal with escalating domestic violence between his parents, a client described discovering that he could shut off his feelings and imagine himself as a superhero). This very common learned response may have initially been deliberate, intentional, and lifesaving; over time it became an automatic way to avoid or shut off emotional responses, especially those associated with painful traumatic episodes. Unfortunately, these shutdowns can later occur in sporadic and unpredictable ways that leave clients feeling at their mercy and out of personal control. At its extreme, some survivors feel as though they live life in solitary confinement, trying to understand what they did to deserve their fate and trying to make sense of their reactions. Some describe themselves as all alone and numb, with nothing but the occasional feeling of being haunted by nightmarish memories (or fragments thereof) that cannot be fully recalled but that never go away. They feel fragmented, shattered, and not whole, quite unlike their more normal and integrated counterparts in the world.

Splitting and Compartmentalization

Another type of breach involves splitting off and compartmentalizing the trauma and its cognitions, memories, and physical sensations. This type of dissociative coping often is obscured by compensatory skills and personal resources that the survivor has learned to rely on to "cover up" or "not know about" their profound distress:

- "I can't ever let myself know what really happened or I'd die from the horror."
- "I blank out any memory or feeling from the bad times, so they never really happened."
- "I immerse myself in work so that I don't have to feel or remember anything, and I don't stop working until I am so tired that sleep overtakes me and I escape into oblivion."
- "I devote myself to my wife and children so I never have to think about the horrible un-family that I grew up in."
- "I remember at age 8, it was so bad in my family that I just stopped feeling. I'd go into fantasy land and imagine that I was a superhero who could save everybody. I learned I didn't have to stay there if I didn't want to."
- "I learned how to stop the physical sensations. During the physical/sexual abuse, I learned not to feel anything. The abuser couldn't make me feel anything and that's how I got some control. It doesn't take much for me to totally shut down all physical reactions, and then I can shut my feelings off, too."
- "I just change the subject all the time, in conversations, at work, in life, so I never really have to feel anything and nobody gets to know the real me."

This breach between the survivor's conscious awareness and knowing or feeling anything related to traumatic memories or the emotions associated with them may additionally be achieved by rationalizing or minimizing the trauma or abuse and its effects:

- "I never thought about it; I just did what I needed to do."
- "The abuse challenged me—I grew from it and learned how to cope with hardship and to be successful."
- "I never looked back and just aimed for the future."

- "I never had a childhood—it's no big deal."
- "That's just the way it was. Everybody was bad off."
- "I primarily relied on myself because there was no one else who could guide me."
- "I trust no one but myself—why should I?"

Both types of posttraumatic responses (intrusive reexperiencing and numbing) involve experiential voids and may create opportunities for new ones to develop. Under these conditions, the "fight–flight" stress response takes the form of defensive action and running away, and the "freeze and immobility" response has the effect of blocking awareness of what is being felt and where the feelings are coming from. Survivors feel at the mercy of this cycle of response–shutdown that can occur totally out of their awareness and control. They respond by becoming hypervigilant to their environment and inner responses while striving to keep up appearances, to keep their "game face" on and to appear "apparently normal" when dealing with the outside world (Van der Hart et al., 2006).

We offer the following vignettes of individuals with complex trauma histories whose lives were overwhelmed or who were pushed to the very brink of their coping resources to illustrate how this sense of being empty and absent can ensue.

Janet

Janet left home at 16 to escape a violent and incestuous father and an alcoholic mother. By age 12, she had begun to emulate her mother by drinking to excess to block out the memories of the sexual attacks, her mother's absence, and her painful emotions. Once she left home, she was unable to keep a job due to her addiction that had grown to include street drugs. She went on welfare and resorted to occasional prostitution. By age 21, she had three children by three different men (all of whom had been violent and otherwise abusive to her and none of whom stayed in contact). When not living with a new man, she was at times homeless and on the streets, in temporary shelters, or living with her children in housing provided by a battered women's program. She had been able to achieve sobriety during her third pregnancy and was taking parenting courses and studying for her GED in programs provided by the shelter.

While in the shelter, she agreed to blood testing for AIDS in return for food coupons offered as part of a community program. Through the testing, she learned that she was HIV positive, a finding that plunged her into depression, back to her addictions, out of housing, and back to the streets. Her children were taken by Social Services and put into foster care, and she ultimately gave them up for adoption. Thereafter, the Health Department and Social Services lost contact with her, until several years later when she sought medical services after developing full-blown AIDS. Although in her late 20s, Janet was ravaged by the disease and looked much older. Her prognosis was dire, and she was admitted to a community hospice program, where she died shortly thereafter.

MICHELLE

She sought treatment in her early 40s after a life in and out of hospital and residential programs. Michelle had recurrent major depressive episodes with psychotic features for which she had been treated with multiple concurrent psychotropic medications and electroconvulsive therapy (ECT), all with limited success. She also carried a host of other diagnoses, including anxiety disorders, personality disorders, and schizophrenia. She was brought to the community mental health center by a friend who was concerned about a recent decline in her mood and in her ability to maintain herself physically. She was obviously very depressed, unkempt and unwashed, and showed signs of psychomotor retardation. She was hopeless and wanted to kill herself to escape her emotional pain, but she complained of not even having enough energy to "successfully pull it off." She was afraid that if she made a suicide attempt she would botch it and have to live with the results. An inpatient hospitalization was required for preliminary stabilization before she was discharged to an intensive aftercare program. There she received intensive treatment for her refractory depression. She disclosed a history of a violent gang rape when she was an adolescent and the subsequent mistreatment that she had received from police after she reported it. She had not previously divulged this history to anyone, except to one friend, who had told her to "put it behind her and get over it." She had tried to do just that but couldn't.

At the other end of the spectrum are those clients whose survivor skills were compensatory and resulted in their being extremely successful and self-sufficient. These skills and adaptations may have led to considerable life achievement, especially according to such external standards as job success, social standing, financial resources, and so on. A tendency to overwork as a main coping mechanism has been identified by many therapists who treat this population. "Workaholism" may operate in tandem with other addictions (such as alcoholism and addictions to sex, eating, shopping, and so on) or may develop after the individual is in the process of recovery from another addiction. Overwork simultaneously allows the individual to suppress and defensively avoid painful emotions by keeping overly busy or by collecting accomplishments and related acceptance and acclamation from others. This pattern frequently leads to success in careers and other life spheres, achievements that establish financial independence and means while bolstering self-esteem and feelings of competence. However, as is discussed in the remainder of the chapter such success may be the proverbial "house built on sand" without the adequate foundation of an integrated inner life. Survivors with a history of unacknowledged and unaddressed trauma remain susceptible to having a range of psychophysiological reactions triggered in quite disparate ways that are not always explicitly evident; that is, they have unfinished emotional business that has been dormant but that resurfaces, as the cases following illustrate:

Jeffrey

Jeffrey, a highly successful mental health professional, sought treatment after being confronted by his wife about a number of credit card charges for paid sexual encounters. What had begun as exclusively online activity had, in recent months, escalated to real-life sexual encounters with individuals he met online. These had escalated in frequency and intensity, taking up more and more of his time, attention, and energy, resulting in changes in his normal behavior and style that had made his wife question what was going on. His sexual interactions were with both men and women, causing his wife to confront him about being bisexual or gay. Jeffrey was mortified that his porn use and activity with prostitutes had come to light. He was shocked that he was so out of control and that he had so seriously betrayed his wife and undermined their marriage. He professed to deeply love his wife and family.

A review of his history revealed him to be a "wounded healer" who had never dealt with his own past. For most of his childhood and adolescence, he had been physically abused and belittled by his mother, an out-of-control alcoholic, and not protected by his absent father (who avoided being with his mother yet never confronted her alcoholism). During high school, he had been sexually abused by a female teacher and had bragged to his male friends about the joys of being seduced and indoctrinated into sex by an older woman. The sexual contact had ended abruptly when his teacher suddenly and without much notice moved out of state and shortly thereafter married her childhood sweetheart. Jeffrey had missed her profoundly, was confused and embarrassed by her abrupt abandonment of their relationship (which he had internalized as "true love"), felt enormously rejected, and never told anyone else of the seduction and abuse, including his wife. He married in his 20s and by all accounts had had a happy marriage, had been a successful parent of two children now grown and on their own, and had established a large and lucrative group psychotherapy practice.

Over the course of the past year, his mother (who continued to drink heavily and to be verbally disparaging) had died after a prolonged bout with ovarian and breast cancer, and his father had been diagnosed with Alzheimer's disease. Jeffrey and his siblings had rallied to care for their mother over her years of illness and now, instead of gaining a needed respite, were being called on to provide financial support and other forms of care for their father. In addition to the stress of caring for his parents, Jeffrey had recently assessed a female client who reminded him of his high school teacher and what had transpired between them. Jeffrey still viewed that relationship in romanticized and idealized ways and found himself longing for her and the comfort and refuge she had provided him during high school, when things were especially bad at home.

When Jeffrey sought treatment, his marriage was "barely alive," and his wife—who was devastated by his betrayal and the extent and seriousness of it—insisted on treatment as a condition of her not leaving him immediately. Jeffrey knew "there had to be a connection" between past and present and reluctantly agreed to begin psychotherapy (something he had previously avoided even during his clinical training, always professing to be "too busy" for the time that a personal therapy would take and claiming that he had analyzed himself enough to know what he needed to know to be a successful therapist). He also agreed to have a program installed on all of his computers and phones that would block his access to his usual porn and other sexual sites, to give his wife access to and permission to monitor his communications (except those to and from patients), his credit cards, finances, and his schedule, and to regularly attend 12-step Sex and Love Addicts Anonymous (SLAA), Adult Children of Alcoholics (ACOA), and Al-Anon meetings. He also agreed that, if he could not control his sexual compulsions and relapsed, if he developed co-addictions, or if his wife insisted (due to what she perceived as lack of progress and in consultation with his therapist), he would enter a more intensive, specialized, month-long residential treatment program.

Julie

Julie was the married mother of two who sought therapy for "feeling like she was going crazy" and not knowing why. A careful intake determined that she had developed a host of depressive and posttraumatic symptoms soon after the recent death of her maternal grandfather who had sexually and physically abused her for a number of years. She never told anyone about the abuse at the time of its occurrence in order to protect her mother. She had determined to forget it and get on with her life. Subsequently, she had mostly forgotten it and had never disclosed it to anyone, including her husband, whom she had married because he was "nice, predictable, and very loyal," although not very emotionally open or available. They had married right after college, had their children soon after and had been successful as parents.

Julie had been a stay-at-home mother who had loved the experience and who only began work when her sons were in high school. Her depression had started after they left for college, a normal life transition, yet one that left her feeling bereft and without purpose. She questioned her marriage and felt highly estranged from her husband. When her grandfather died, her depression intensified inexplicably—she became extremely despondent to the point of becoming suicidal. When her husband tried to encourage her to "pull yourself together, you and your grandfather never got along anyway," she became enraged. Subsequently, she began to drink to excess and to cut herself in order to stop the symptoms and the feelings she was having. She was overwhelmed, confused, and hopeless at the point she sought treatment, as were her family and friends.

As can be seen, hard work and concentration, workaholism or other externalizing behaviors, extreme self-sufficiency, and defensive avoidance and sequestering can carry a high price tag for previously traumatized individuals, and these predominant defenses can break down during times of life stress when triggered in some way. What constitutes a specific trigger at a particular time is highly unpredictable and can be quite spontaneous. The avoidant or detached client is especially at risk for this type of breakdown. As an example, consider Hector, who certainly exemplifies this coping pattern.

Hector

Hector had unknowingly exceeded his strongly honed self-reliance and coping abilities when his unit deployed to the war zone. Soon after arriving, he was caught in a fire fight in which he believes he killed several enemy combatants and he saw some of his buddies killed or seriously injured. While on a reconnaissance mission in a military vehicle, he was subjected to an improvised explosive device (IED) blast that had been triggered by an adolescent (causing him to be increasingly mistrustful of local children and adolescents, whom he had previously sought to befriend) that caused him unspecified injury, and was also exposed to a number of atrocities, including the rape of a local woman by a soldier.

Several months later, when on a break from the front lines, he heard news about the priest abuse scandal that was unfolding in Europe and the suggestion of Pope Benedict's implication for having reassigned abusive priests to new parishes while a bishop in Germany. Hector was profoundly disturbed by this because he had always revered the pope as God's representative on earth. He found it hard to believe that the pope could be so callous and nonprotective of children. News of the European clergy abuse scandal was a secondary trigger that caused the emergence of previously suppressed and inaccessible memories of his own abuse by his parish priest. He became flooded with unwanted images of the priest, along with the details of the abuse, and felt disgust with himself that "he had let it go on for so long and that he had been so stupid." He felt that he must have deserved or liked it and that it meant that he really was gay—or worse, in his words, "a pervert" who seduced the priest into molesting him. He began to experience nightmares and night terrors about the sexual activities with the priest that disturbed what little sleep he was able to manage in the war zone. He became increasingly out of control and angry and, at that time, turned his rage toward the enemy. When his tour ended and he returned to the states, he continued to experience major symptoms and distress for which he had few emotional or social resources to cope. His anger and violence toward others continued, as did his use of drugs and alcohol and his intention to commit suicide.

These cases illustrate the varied kinds of dissociative breaches in awareness and integration of memory and emotions that must be dealt with directly and sensitively in order for psychotherapy to be effective. The fundamental goal is to help clients to identify and work through memories or emotions and associated beliefs and behavior patterns that they had shut down. Dissociation can provide a kind of repository for disavowed or intensely conflicted posttraumatic memories and symptoms, painful emotions, trauma-distorted beliefs and cognitions, and compulsive and impulsive behavioral strategies for enacting these memories, feelings, and beliefs. *The psychotherapeutic alternative to dissociative compartmentalization and breaches is the development of self-regulation skills that, over time and with repeated exposure and increased tolerance, allow the reintegration of what had previously been cut off in the interest of coping and survival* (Ford et al., 2005), as discussed in Chapters 5 and 6. Until self-regulation abilities are developed and clients are able to self-modulate, they are without needed personal resources especially when faced with accumulated life stressors, lack of external emotional support, reminders of trauma, and disruptions of the dissociation that had maintained previously. Severe dissociation presents several challenges beyond those described here; this is the focus of the remainder of this chapter.

UNRESOLVED TRAUMA AND LOSS: DISSOCIATION AS DISCONTINUITY OF SELF, AWARENESS, EXPERIENCE, AND KNOWLEDGE

According to *Webster's Dictionary*, the prefix *dis-* refers to "doing the opposite of; be free of; deprivation of/removal from; exclude or expel from; opposite or absence of; not." Psychiatrist and dissociation authority Richard Chefetz (personal communication, 2009) creatively coined the phrase "diss-ing of the self" to describe the process by which these clients dealt with their ongoing *dis*tress by, *dis*sociating or using other forms of *dis*avowal, *dis*owning, *dis*integration, and *dis*simulation and through personal *dis*respect and *dis*empowerment. The ability to dissociate has been found to be more pronounced during childhood and adolescence, making it a primary means of coping and self-protection, especially in the absence of response or help. It is both a process and a defense resulting in a rupture of the self that is especially available in situations of entrapment, in which repetitive exposure to abuse and trauma are the norm and appropriate response and protection are lacking. When fight-or-flight defensive responses are impossible or ineffective, dissociative collapse and tonic immobilization occur to prepare the organism to contend with ongoing threat and related terror and to provide analgesia and anesthesia during physical attack. In situations of ongoing danger, children nonvolitionally and automatically go into these states of physical and emotional freeze and immobilization, extreme coping responses that protect them at the time but that become problems when they are overused and/or used out of context, as often happens when these children become adults (Putnam, 1989, 1997).

Major *dis*continuities and personal *dis*orientation characterize the lives of scores of these clients, many of whom, at one end of the continuum, are mildly dissociative or, at the other end, dissociate to such a degree that they meet criteria for dissociative disorders, including DID. Common personal discontinuities include gaps in or loss of personal awareness (including time loss and confusion as to time, place, behavior, and emotional state), personal history (including autobiographical as well as traumatic memories), basic knowledge and abilities, physical sensations and abilities—up to and including switches in self-state (perceived locus of executive function) and personality state.

Personal discontinuity is so common, in fact, that Lanius and colleagues

(2010, 2012), based on the findings of their neurological research studies regarding the extensive use of dissociation in some individuals with PTSD, have suggested a subtype of PTSD in which dissociation, more than other trauma symptoms, predominates. They have also noted the generally unrecognized amount of *dis*sociation that is included in criteria for the diagnosis of PTSD. In fact, the *alternation between intrusion and numbing symptoms*, the core dialectic of all traumatic stress disorders (Horowitz & Smit, 2008), has been identified as a *dissociative process* (Nijenhuis & Van der Hart, 2011), involving alternation between episodes of dyscontrol, as if the traumatic events were happening or about to happen, and emotional shutdown, a compulsion to avoid memories of the trauma. This is not just distressing but a clearly distinct state of mind for most people with complex trauma, as if their emotions, thoughts, and actions were those of very different persons from their normal selves. This process can be understood as dissociation of the ordinary self from the survivor self.

The French psychiatrist Pierre Janet was the most prominent clinical researcher of his time who developed detailed insights into dissociation as a means of coping with extreme experiences and losses that evoked "vehement emotions" that overwhelmed the individual's ability to cope psychically and to remain integrated. Janet (1889/1973) postulated that there was a "disaggrégation" of the personality into subsystems that divided up the responsibility for managing the overwhelming emotions. Janet believed that this prevented the person from being able to achieve a sense of ownership of the experience or what he called "personification" (e.g., "It happened to me"; "I can no longer maintain that it only affected that part of me") that, along with "presentification" (i.e., having the emotion in real time and associating it with its origin—"I'm having this reaction now because it is related to what happened to me and what I did not feel or process at the time; it is not happening in the present although it feels like it is"), characterizes how an integrated self responds (Van der Hart et al., 2006). Janet understood that in order to survive emotionally, the traumatized individual dissociated and, in the process, lost the ability to remain intact and integrated. The cost of this adaptation was not just a sense of feeling fragmented and out of touch with him- or herself but also being at the mercy of dissociated, out-of-control, and unpredictable intrusive and numbing posttraumatic symptoms managed by shifting from part-self to part-self.

Memory becomes correspondingly fragmented, with some knowledge accessible only to one or a few of the parts of the self, leading to major gaps that present difficulty for the survivor. This difficulty is ultimately shared by the therapist, who might not know what part of the client's self he or she is interacting with or "who" within the collection of disconnected part-selves will remember from session to session. The dissociative fragmentation of the self that developed as a means of surviving the distress evoked by trauma can become a kind of psychological black hole in which the therapist—and the client—often cannot "find" him or her. This is because the client is out of his or her awareness, that is, unintentionally only partially and temporarily psychologically present at any given moment. This is the "breach" within the self, what Bollas (1987) called "unformulated experience," and what Bromberg (2003) called "the spaces" in which dissociated clients live. Per Bromberg, therapists must "stand in the spaces" and help to make previously unmade connections between past and present in order for clients to internalize what was split off and, in the process, regain an integrated sense of self. Again we turn to Hector as an example of this process.

Hector

Hector's parents both had traumatic circumstances in their backgrounds. Hector's mother had been sexually abused by an uncle over the course of several years, something she had never revealed to anyone. His father had been raised in an intact and loving family, but he had been tortured for his political beliefs as a young adult. Although the move to the United States was planned and was a welcome escape from the politics of their country, Hector's parents were unprepared for the degree of change and the economic challenges that they faced when they emigrated. Both missed their families and familiar community contacts and supports. Together, they endured Mr. Alvarez's PTSD symptoms without understanding them and without seeking help, as that would involve "the authorities," something to be avoided at all costs. Mr. Alvarez increasingly turned to alcohol to cope and was violent toward his wife and young son. Mrs. Alvarez tolerated this additional abuse because she had no place to go and because she loved her husband and was loyal to him; yet she became increasingly depressed and withdrawn over time. She used her religious beliefs and her church attendance as her release. She was unable to do more than go to work and to church and left the bulk of caretaking and parenting to Hector.

From early on, Hector coped by dissociating: He described how he would daydream while at school and wish that he belonged to another family. He was mocked for his "spaciness" and his good-boy behavior by his peers, experiences that caused him to withdraw further into a fantasy world that was highly different from his normal life. Over time, it became evident that Hector's dissociative psychological fragmentation had reached a serious enough degree to meet criteria for DID. He experienced involuntary switches in executive functions between different "Hectors" (e.g., the invisible hiding boy; the happy, unconcerned free child; the rageful combatant with his aggressive father; the loving protector of his mother; the priest-abuser's "special friend"), each of which had no knowledge of the other (i.e., amnesia between different self-states). The major challenge for his therapist in the first phase of therapy was to help Hector recognize these different self-states and understand how they all were extensions of a single Hector who had needed to cope as a child by taking on different roles that become distinct part-selves.

It is helpful in dealing with the dissociative process in complex trauma survivors to look for times of "apparent normalcy." We have learned to look for and ask about how the client is "there and not there" simultaneously and about subtle signs of emotions that seem to be missing or that might be evident only through such interpersonal mechanisms as the transference–countertransference, enactments, and projective identification (as described in Chapters 9 and 10). That can mean the therapist identifying what he or she is feeling as the client is relating a traumatic scene without emotion and sharing these feelings in response. It also involves "nudging" the client to be more direct and specific, as the use of unclear referents may be quite common. A related therapeutic strategy is to create circumstances of emotional dissonance to encourage a greater range of responses and associations—for example:

"If what happened to you happened to someone you knew, how would you feel? How is it then that you can't allow that feeling for yourself?"
"Can you identify how you felt as a child?"
"You just said you would be afraid of doing 'it' to your own child—what is the 'it' you are referring to?"
"You are able to empathize with other members of this group whom you would never blame for their abuse, yet you can't let in the same feedback for yourself. What is that about?"

In essence, clients are encouraged to explore what has been avoided and is outside of conscious awareness by encouraging and engaging with the "learning brain" (Ford, 2009a), using the process of mentalization (Allen, 2012; Fonagy et al., 2002), strategic questioning (Kluft, 1999, 2000), and relationship (Howell, 2011). Clients can be invited (with support and encouragement) to feel what they normally do not feel and to allow themselves to observe and think about this process while it is happening. Observations about the use of dissociative language can be made, and clients can be invited to try more personalized and first-person language—for example:

"I just noticed that you referred to your body as '*the* body.' Can you acknowledge that the body you are describing is yours?"
"In referring to your mother, I can't help but notice that you identify her as *the* mother. Are you aware of this? Can we discuss why you refer to her in the third person?"
"You continuously change from the first to the second person in describing yourself and your reactions, almost as though they don't belong to you. Are you aware that you do this? What do you make of it? Can you own more of your reaction and feelings?"

Questions such as these are designed to chip away at the avoidance and dissimulation (in the process, disengaging the "survival brain" and reengaging the "learning brain"). They are designed to encourage clients to take more ownership (rather than disowning) by stating things from a first-person perspective rather than keeping them in the second or third person.

The client's security of attachment to the therapist along with encouragement and support provide the opportunity for personal exploration and ownership of emotions and information about which he or she had been unaware or had avoided. It is now believed that this process of reflective attunement literally reflects the client back to him- or herself, in the process building new neural networks that allow more energy and information flow across the brain and leading to greater neural and personal integration (i.e., building structure where there was fragmentation) and a related and integrated sense of self (Cozolino, 2002; Schore, 2003a; Seigel, 2007, 2012). As discussed previously, the "learning brain" (prefrontal and medial parts of the brain) develop in ways that down-regulate the "survival brain," or the limbic or emotional brain structures. Over time, the client is less likely to be physiologically and psychologically overtaken by traumatic stress responses related to an overactive survival brain and more able to respond to experiences with less reactivity and therefore with more control.

MAPPING THE TERRITORY: SEVERAL MODELS OF DISSOCIATION

The BASK Model

Braun (1988a, 1988b) conceptualized dissociation in keeping with Janet's early formulation and developed a model called BASK that describes how split-off emotional and somatic content might return in implicit Behavioral, Affective, Sensation, and Knowledge forms that convey information. When reconstructed and interpreted as to its origin or meaning, this material becomes explicitly known to the individual and others so that it can be integrated rather than remain separated. Significantly, the exploration, decoding, and interpretation of the meaning of the dissociated material is the client's to make and not for the therapist to either suppress or suggest (Courtois, 1999). The therapist's role is to support the client and provide sufficient reflection of behaviors, affects, and sensations to enable the client to increase his or her knowledge about what was previously emotionally and cognitively intolerable and held out of awareness. The therapist acts as a guide rather than as the meaning maker so as to not appropriate the client's autonomy and control.

Doris

We can apply the BASK model to the example of Doris and her early confusing reenactment with her therapist. The reader will recall that Doris was seemingly satisfied in the first session but that her *behavior* in the second session changed to an assertion that she must leave therapy due to the *affect* of disgust and anger and the physical *sensations* of feeling rigid and sick to her stomach. These reactions, which occurred implicitly outside of her awareness of their origin and meaning, could all be interpreted and made conscious by the therapist's reflecting her confusion back to Doris and asking her about previous similar *behavior* on her part and any *knowledge* of when it started, why it started, other occurrences, and so forth. Over time and with discussion, Doris began to allow herself to *know* and to discuss how her *feeling* of connection to others and being treated well by them (beginning with experiences with her mother) always resulted in her later being rejected and abandoned. She therefore had protectively learned not to trust anyone who was nice to her and was paradoxically *disgusted with herself* after positive interactions because she had allowed herself to be vulnerable to being hurt again. Thus her anger and disgust were preemptive emotions designed to protect her but, in the process, kept her from getting what she longed for and needed. This new perspective presented by the therapist led to new *knowledge* and self-understanding on Doris's part and a lessening over time of her defensive aggression and withdrawal.

Structural Dissociation

As discussed in the earlier chapters, Van der Hart et al. (2006) proposed three levels of dissociation of the personality, each associated with a greater degree of traumatization and correspondingly greater use of dissociation and each related to the client's attachment history and style. The first level involves a division in the normally integrated aspects of the self and personal experiences that create the "apparently normal personality" (ANP) that can function normally in a variety of life spheres and tasks as long as the traumatic emotions are avoided. These are held in one "emotional (or traumatized) personality" (EP), and this division is characteristic of PTSD. It is exemplified by **Mary Jane**, a woman with a secure attachment history, who was raped by an acquaintance in college and who in her embarrassment and self-blame for its occurrence never told anyone about it and immediately set out to live her life as though it never happened. She was fairly successful in doing so, although she sometimes felt mildly depressed and anxious for no reason she could identify. Her latent PTSD was dormant for years and emerged abruptly in delayed fashion during a sexual interaction that served as a reminder of the rape. She became highly symptomatic after this event and thought she was going crazy due to the intensity of her reactions.

The second level of structural dissociation, associated with complex PTSD, involves the development of an ANP that functions well (and sometimes in exemplary fashion) and more than one split-off EP. **Jeffrey** (introduced earlier) provides an example of this type. Despite a number of traumatizations in his formative years, he was able to carry on and succeed by blocking out the chaos of his family life (he maintained an estrangement with his parents for a number of years after he left home), "forgetting about" his high school teacher and becoming extremely detached from others and self-sufficient (avoidant/detached style). His workaholic lifestyle assisted him in this suppression and he was rewarded with professional status and economic success that shored up his self-esteem. Cracks began to appear in this carefully maintained exterior when he had to care for his cancer-ridden mother and later when she died. He found himself feeling a wide range of reactions, including resentment at her addiction and at not having had a carefree childhood, something he had been able to provide for his children despite his upbringing. He began to feel increasingly lethargic and depressed, feelings that increased when his father was diagnosed with early stage Alzheimer's, requiring intensified caretaking and monitoring. Jeffrey's occasional porn viewing began to change and increase during that time period. He rationalized that he needed a little distraction and relief to help him with the additional stresses he was facing. As the situation escalated and he was unable to deal with the plethora of feelings associated with his complicated bereavement, his retreat into porn increased as well. He shocked himself the first time he agreed to meet an online contact for a real-time sexual encounter. This began another escalation of his sexual behavior and he found that he was attracted to sex with men as well as with women. When his wife confronted him, he felt emotionally overwhelmed, out of control, and ashamed.

The third level of structural dissociation is associated with DID and involves a high degree of variability and floridity of presentation of more than one ANP and a number of EPs. This degree of dissociation can remain dormant and unseen for years or even decades, can emerge spontaneously during what Kluft (1995) identified as "windows of diagnosibility" that open after adequate triggering has occurred and then submerge or disappear again; alternatively, they may be a constant occurrence and in constant evidence whether accurately identified or not. Many family members describe the client with DID as moody or as different at different times (sometimes as "weird" and "crazy"), but they usually do not have information necessary to know what is happening.

Suzy is such a client. She had been sexually abused by an uncle. During adolescence she was raped on several different occasions, one a brutal gang rape. She was addicted to drugs and alcohol, had a major eating disorder, burned herself frequently, had made several low-level suicide attempts, and had been battered in several intimate relationships. She had been treated in a number of residential facilities for her assortment of disorders—she had been diagnosed as having borderline personality disorder, bipolar disorder, major depression (recurrent), anxiety disorder, substance abuse not otherwise specified (NOS), eating disorder NOS, and schizophrenia. She had been on many psychotropic medications, none of which worked for long. Although her trauma history was known, she was never asked about it and never assessed for PTSD or a dissociative disorder. Her dissociation began to emerge when she first got clean and sober. A therapist observed her switch into a child-like state and initiated an assessment for DD and DID. Suzy was found to have several primary ANPs: her "student self," "work self," and "the part who keeps therapy appointments." EPs were part-selves of different ages, emotional states, and functions: "the part who burns me to protect and/or punish me," the "little girl" (in describing this part-self, she spontaneously spoke of her in the third person and said "I hate her!—all of this is her fault"), the "angry adolescent," "the one who takes care of me," "the drinking me," "the one who likes sex and likes to control men," "the one who hates sex," and so on. While Suzy had been aware of "voices in my head" for quite some time, it was only at point of diagnosis that she was able to begin to identify them. As she explored them over time, she came to understand them as split-off parts of herself that held details of her experiences and her emotions. They had initially developed as self-protection in a context of ongoing physical and psychic danger.

Me–Not-Me

In recent years, Chefetz and Bromberg have developed a workshop on dialogues between "me–not-me" designed to illustrate the process of disowning and disavowal that characterizes the self of many of these clients (Chefetz & Bromberg, 2004). Their aim is to guide therapists in helping dissociative clients to move from a position of fragmentation of the self to a more integrated and functional self. These dialogues between the part-selves of "me–not-me" were developed to identify the disjuncture of self into disconnected and unrelated self-states (like the ANP and the EP of the structural dissociation model) that create a void in the individual that must be bridged emotionally and physiologically with the help of the therapist "standing in the spaces" (Bromberg, 1998). In neurodevelopmental terms, the process of brain neuroplasticity and the development of new neuronal networks created by this bridging allow integration (i.e., healing) to occur. Schwartz (2000), in his book *Dialogues with Forgotten Voices*, describes dissociation as follows:

> Dissociation is a desperate effort to preserve life and sanity by constructing an identity to manage (for example, disown, compartmentalize, diffuse) pain, anxiety, terror, and shame. It involves the creation of self- and other-representations rooted in psychic exclusions (*Not me/Not him/Not happen*). . . . During and after the trauma, the child imitates, pretends, distracts him/herself, enters altered states of consciousness; later in life, dissociative survival has to be bolstered continually by an arsenal of avoidance, addiction, and camouflage strategies. (p. 5; author's italics)

Schwartz presents therapy as an intersubjective process that encourages the client to explore and find what is missing and what has been discredited and disowned in order to restore and integrate it (also described by others such as Howell, 2008, 2011; Kinsler, 1992; Kohlenberg & Tsai, 1998). He describes a process of "losing and finding the self," the loss through the process of dissociation necessitated by the trauma and the recovery based on a reflective presence (provided by the therapist, peer group, significant others) that encourages a continuity of self and experience. As we noted earlier regarding the lack of expectable reactions and feelings, the reflective therapist must be attuned to both what is *in* the room and what is *not in* the room, that is, what has been excluded and kept out as much as what is presented by the client. The therapist must be ever mindful of the common use of disavowal and discrediting of self and experience that are common survival mechanisms and the displacement of emotion. We sometimes ask a question such as, "What has been left out?" or "What is not here today?" and have sometimes been surprised at the answers.

Summary and Synthesis: Dissociation as a Form of Coping with Emotion Dysregulation

A common thread running through these formulations of posttraumatic dissociation is that it is an overlearned and largely involuntary form of coping with extreme emotions and physiological responses. As described by Ford (2009a):

> *Extreme emotional reactivity* and *disorganized attachment* alter the interaction between working memory and episodic/autobiographical memory . . . ; this alteration manifests itself as structural dissociation. Extreme emotional reactivity may result from significant stressors and/or certain personality dispositions (e.g., irritability, inhibition, or anxiety sensitivity . . .). Emotional reactivity alone does not lead to dissociation; and it may, instead, lead to suicidality, emotional numbing, rage without fugue, depersonalization, or a sense of being quite different from one's usual self. Similarly, confusion about or difficulty in sustaining trust, intimacy, and mutuality in close relationships can occur as the result of major disruptions in primary relationships . . . but severe relational problems do not, alone, lead to dissociation.
>
> On the other hand, when a person experiences emotions and primary relationships as extreme, unpredictable and unmanageable, then this individual is likely to have great difficulty in sustaining a consistent organized sense of self. Extreme emotions can cause a person to feel so changeably different from moment to moment that it may seem that there is no consistent "me." Or, there might be several "me's" whose emotions are so different that they seem not to be the same person. Persons with disorganized attachment may perceive others as constantly and unpredictably changing. When this happens, relationships become a source of conflict and distress, rather than security or succorance. This leaves the person with no external framework to help to regulate affect (e.g., to feel soothed by contact with others). . . .
>
> When extreme emotional reactivity and disorganized attachment occur, *I postulate that dissociation develops as an automatic (versus consciously instigated and controlled) attempt to reinstate bodily integrity by shifting the body's dominant mode of operation from self-regulation to self-preservation.* (p. 472; author's italics)

In recent years, researchers have discussed how largely automatic processes of *self-preservation* ordinarily assist the development of integrative self-regulation capacities and a coherent sense of self—that is, sensorimotor bodily awareness—and meta-cognitive monitoring (by which the individual observes and revises her or his thoughts and modes of thinking). These processes of self-preservation are both implicit/somatic and mental (e.g., expectancies, appraisals, motivations). When extreme affect dysregulation and attachment disorganization make self-regulatory processes insufficient to restore bodily integrity, dissociation occurs in a defensive attempt to prevent further psychobiological disintegration. When this occurs, the integrated functioning of self-preservation and self-regulation is abandoned in the interest of bodily integrity. Consequently, the dissociative split separates the preconscious/automatic modes of self-preservation from the conscious modes of self-regulation, in the service of psychobiological survival.

From this perspective, the treatment challenge is for the client to regain "integrated functioning of self-preservation and self-regulation," in order to increase tolerance of the emotions, thoughts, and memories that were previously intolerable. Thus addressing posttraumatic dissociation involves much more than simply enhancing a client's anxiety management skills or educating the client about the usefulness and importance of healthy emotions. It also involves more than reworking traumatic memories, because dissociation is a protection against the sine qua non of trauma-memory-processing therapies, namely, knowing about the memories and their meaning and feeling their full emotional impact. Addressing posttraumatic dissociation requires the reinstatement—or creation anew—of the capacity to experience and modulate extreme emotion states. We now discuss the relational field in which this work occurs.

WORKING IN THE BREACH: THE POSTTRAUMATIC AND DISSOCIATIVE FIELD

In the first section of this book and throughout, in our case descriptions and clinical vignettes, we have sought to describe some of the typical and the more idiosyncratic and personalized posttraumatic, dissociative, and developmental reactions and adaptations to complex trauma. Thus far, we have focused on dissociative phenomena in particular and disconnections in self and experience. Even the most experienced therapists feel overwhelmed when faced with clients who are in the throes of dysregulated posttraumatic responses and behaviors and who have a limited sense of self and a limited ability to quell or manage their reactions. It is easy to lose one's bearings when with a client who is experiencing a florid flashback of a painful traumatic episode; one who is glazed and dazed-looking and totally unresponsive in the moment; one who dramatically changes in demeanor, use of language, and apparent age; one who is detached and highly contemptuous of the therapist's efforts; one whose perceptions are highly distorted and who is reexperiencing trauma responses out of context; one who is reenacting traumatic experiences or responses in some way; or one who is so preoccupied with not losing the relationship that the therapist feels smothered and trapped. Loewenstein (1993) published an important chapter on the topic of the posttraumatic and dissociative aspects of transference and countertransference in the treatment of DID that is highly pertinent to our discussion here. Although transference and countertransference are presented more formally in Chapter 10, we introduce Loewenstein's concepts of the *dissociative/posttraumatic transference relational field (or matrix)* within which the therapy takes place. Quoting him:

> Abuse-related and trance-based phenomena are ubiquitous [in this relational field]. . . . I will focus on transference "field effects." . . . For simplicity, dissociative and posttraumatic aspects of the transference field will be discussed separately. In actuality, *these processes are simultaneous and interactive in the treatment situation and are blended with more classical forms of transference*. . . . For the most part, these transference/countertransference difficulties are unavoidable. It is the *more-or-less successful management* of them that leads to their eventual resolution over the long term. (1993, p. 62; italics added in phrase; author's italics in the last sentence)

Posttraumatic Themes That Arise in Treatment

Loewenstein (1993) identified five major *posttraumatic themes* recurrent in the treatment of abused and traumatized clients that provoke response in therapists: (1) management of boundaries and limit setting; (2) the wish for a cure through love and nurturance; (3) overt and covert flashbacks in the transference; (4) lack of trust and the expectation of abusive intent; and (5) reactivity and impulsiveness. To make the relational field even more complicated and daunting, these five themes are entwined with those that are more related to the dissociative process, some of which are described here. They also occur in tandem with other, less trauma-based or more subjective, transference themes (as described further in Chapter 10). Although these themes and challenges have been presented at different points in this book, they are discussed here in a different way, as part of the *relational matrix* in which the treatment takes place and as "field challenges" associated with that matrix. Their identification and management are highly significant to successful treatment.

Boundary Management and Limit Setting

An aspect of the relationship that continually requires monitoring is the maintenance of appropriate boundaries, especially important for those clients whose boundaries were routinely disregarded, crossed, or blurred. In consequence, clients show one or more of the following adaptations and patterns regarding internal and external boundaries that can make the establishment and maintenance of therapeutic boundaries particularly difficult. In one, the client develops *excessively rigid internal boundaries as self-protection* against either overly loose boundaries between and among family members that resulted in dual relationships, including physical and sexual abuse and other forms of personal intrusion; rigid and punitive family interactions; or both. In another, the client *lacks internal boundaries and has little or no external demarcation between self and others.*

This pattern typically developed in a family in which differentiation and individuation were not fostered and generational role reversal and "negotiable," dual, and blurred boundaries were the norm. The client who is used to warding off additional abuse and trauma through rigid hypervigilance, control of self and others, and self-sufficiency or those who seek to meet attachment needs by caretaking and being vigilant and attentive to the needs of others will unconsciously seek the same roles in therapy. For both types, therapeutic boundaries, no matter how well defined and articulated, may feel quite foreign. For the overly controlled, self-sufficient client, the invitation to be more engaged and less self-protectively ensconced may be threatening, at least initially. For the client unused to boundaries between self and others, therapist limitations may feel punitive, unfair, or painful. This client might feel rejected or threatened by a therapist who is differentiated and self-sufficient and who therefore does not have a need for caretaking and who is unwilling to be a friend outside of the treatment context (and, in this regard, is quite different from other, more dependent or demanding caregivers and others). Therapists must have the ability to keep their boundaries but to have some flexibility in their application. Gaining the ability to assertively negotiate needs (personal empowerment) and to maintain personal boundaries are goals of this treatment, so client requests should be given consideration and discussion; however, the establishment and maintenance of suitable boundaries and privacy are essential for self-development. It is these differences in style and expectations that challenge the client to experiment with different roles and modes of interaction.

Wish for a Cure through Love and Nurturance

Clients with preoccupied and disorganized styles, in particular, may engage in a variety of behaviors to ensure the therapist's special attention and caring, what Chefetz (n.d.) and others have labeled the "erotized transference" and the "erotized maternal transference." Clients may challenge whether and how the therapist cares. They may either seek out extra attention from the therapist that proves their specialness or they may provoke the therapist to behave as others have by trying to seduce him or her (with gifts, offers of services, or frank sexual approaches). In these ways, they may seek to shore up their negative self-esteem from the outside and through the therapist's overinvolvement or rescuing. This behavior may have a less obvious but common motive involving hostility toward the original withholding or abusive primary attachment figures played out with the therapist, who is coercively invited into the role of the all-providing "good mother or father." In this way, clients attempt to avoid dealing with past losses or, alternatively, seek to replicate the special status they gained in past abusive and exploitive relationships by reenacting dual roles, including, in some cases, becoming sexually involved as the "price" of being in a relationship.

The therapist should anticipate such issues and begin treatment with the communication of clearly demarcated boundaries and limits that can be returned to when breakdowns or challenges occur (e.g., the client asking for touches or hugs during sessions or for personal disclosure, special favors, or extended sessions; requesting a friendship outside of therapy; overusing phone or e-mail contacts; repeatedly canceling or treating the therapist with hostility and the therapy with contempt; or offering special favors or gifts or seeking to be sexually involved with the therapist; see Chapters 3, 9, and 10 for further discussion). Again, it is the frustration of these expectations through use of a different attachment style that is not exploitive and that focuses on the safety and needs of the client that demonstrates the trustworthiness of the therapist.

Overt and Covert Flashbacks in the Transference

Spontaneous flashback phenomena (conscious and unconscious) that occur both within and outside of sessions can severely interrupt the process and relational field. These can be fear inducing and disconcerting for both client and therapist. Skill building in emotion regulation and grounding techniques are effective as antidotes to these experiences over time and with practice. Here we offer two vignettes of the occurrence of flashbacks during sessions.

Lily

Lily had been in therapy for several months seeking to recover from her history of child sexual abuse and two rapes in adulthood. She arrived for her session, entered the therapy room, looked at her therapist, who had a new haircut, and began to back away, shaking, and saying: "Get away from me, get away from me." Lily closed her eyes and was breathing shallowly and she moved to the couch where she began to thrash and moan and was now pleading, "Don't, please don't." Needless to say, her therapist was taken aback and had no clue to what had prompted this behavior which he quickly identified as a flashback. He responded by having Lily reconnect with the present by opening her eyes, deepening her breathing, scanning and identifying colors in the room, and slowly allowing herself to make eye contact with him, while he told her in a firm but calm tone that she was safe, she was in the office, and she was having a flashback of what had occurred previously but was not occurring at present. After a while, Lily settled down and was able to sit up and talk about what had happened. It turned out that the trigger was the therapist's new haircut and his jacket which resembled one worn by one of her abusers.

Jeffrey (*Continued*)

Jeffrey's female client reminded him of his high school teacher with whom he had been sexually involved. After a session with the client, he unconsciously reenacted that trauma when he sought sex from a woman online who looked like his old teacher. He was seeking the nurturance and approval he had previously gained from their relationship at a time when his life was highly stressed by family events and parental responsibilities. Although this was problematic coping, he could have instead attempted to seduce and sexually engage his client. In this instance, he had enough control to go elsewhere. It was in a therapy session, when his therapist inquired about any antecedents of his behavior, that he was able to put the pieces together and to make conscious his desire for the comforting he had experienced as part of the sexual abuse.

Lack of Trust and the Expectation of Abusive Intent

The posttraumatic transference field is also characterized by fear of the therapist and expectation of being misused, mistreated, exploited, or disregarded in reenactment of past experiences, especially those with caregivers and authority figures. Some of these fears and expectations are expressed in subtle ways and play more to the client's unassertive and victimized self, and some are blatantly aggressive and controlling in intent, as the following vignette shows. Therapists must achieve some degree of desensitization to these negative expectations and to the possibility that they will be acted out behaviorally, in order not to respond with reprisal and hostility. Instead, in some cases, they must consider their ability to continue the treatment under the circumstances and must establish workable boundaries while encouraging the client to become consciously aware of his or her motivations and behavior.

Franco

Franco arrived for his therapy session with his pants unzipped and a glazed look in his eyes. He sat on the couch and spread his legs so the therapist could see his partially erect penis. Although the therapist was aware of feeling stunned and unsure of what to do, he quietly asked Franco to zip his pants, which he did, and then asked him what he thought was happening. He replied that "it" was going to happen anyway so they might just get it over with. Every other teacher or counselor had "f---d" him, so what made this therapist different? The therapist reaffirmed that sex had no place in their relationship and that he would not be sexual in any way with Franco, who stormed out of the room yet returned for his next scheduled session, looking sheepish and expressing relief that the therapist had both morals and boundaries. The therapist, who had been unsure that Franco would return, learned that he had experienced the refusal to be sexual with him as a corrective experience and as one that built his trust in their relationship. He and Franco frequently returned to discussion of this incident and how he had been revictimized so often that it was an anticipated event whose occurrence he was attempting to control. The therapist helped him develop assertiveness skills to refuse unwanted or coercive sexual contacts.

Reactivity and Impulsiveness

This vignette illustrates another aspect of the posttraumatic relational field, that of reactivity and impulsivity rather than forethought, caution, and planning on the one hand and/or passivity and the ability to be assertive of personal rights and preferences on the other. The inability to manage personal boundaries and emotion dysregulation are at the root of either the impulsivity/recklessness or passivity/submissiveness that is often implicated in revictimization. **Doris** gives an example of a client who operates in reactive and impulsive ways. Therapy that helps clients to separate feelings from automatic behaviors and to anticipate the consequences of behavior before acting and that teaches assertiveness regarding needs and preferences is of particular importance when emotion dysregulation leads to irresponsible or compliant behavior that may be endangering. The process is also changing brain functioning from the limbic to the prefrontal part, enabling more thoughtfulness, preparation, and awareness of consequences of behavior.

Dissociative Themes That Arise in Treatment

According to Loewenstein (1993),

> dissociative aspects of the transference field have characteristics associated with hypnotic phenomena, including (1) absorption and focused attention; (2) amnesia and hypermnesia; (3) incoherence of self and personal discourse; (4) altered perceptions and trancelike phenomena, including "entrancement" of the therapist; and (5) cognitive distortions such as literalness and tolerance and rationalization of illogic and contradiction [also known as trance logic]. (p. 62)

Unless he or she is working with someone who is highly hypnotizable or who is high in the quality of absorption, a therapist is unlikely to see characteristics similar to those in nontraumatized or nondissociative clients. Dissociative aspects and themes can be disorienting in their own right but are especially so when combined and intertwined with some of the posttraumatic reactions just discussed.

Focused Attention

Clients with dissociation are, by definition, avoidant and selectively attentive. They can focus their attention in ways that attend to certain aspects of experience as they simultaneously do not attend to others (e.g., "knowing and not knowing" something; being hypervigilant to danger in situations that are safe, while being hypovigilant and passive in situations that are rife with danger and risk). Behavior such as this is quite paradoxical. It can totally mystify therapists who are unaware of this dynamic and process (and even therapists who are!) and can easily ensnare or entrance them in the process of the "illogical logic" of trance. When working in this relational field, therapists themselves may feel disoriented, scared, confused, and "deskilled," as well as dissociative. They may feel a great deal of irritation and anger at the client for "doing this to them" and must counter it with the recognition that the client has not done so with any intent; rather, through the transference and relational field, they have been "invited or entranced into" the client's world, a process that, when identified, can assist them in understanding what their client's world is like and in empathizing. Therapists who understand this process are less likely to be upset when it happens and to recover more quickly by getting regrounded and staying emotionally regulated. They should use it as information about the client. Although avoidance may be commendable in not wanting to cause the client more pain, it is not necessarily therapeutic. Avoidance on the part of the therapist may stem from the therapist's not wanting to experience the client's world and the pain of the client's story or hear any more about it, as the following case vignette illustrates.

Bonnie

Bonnie had a history of revictimization despite being hypervigilant in the therapy sessions regarding her safety and the therapist's trustworthiness. As she reported on her social and dating activities, it was obvious to the therapist that she was lacking in appropriate cautions and was lax regarding her personal safety. She socialized in unsavory locations, where she drank too much and flirted continuously. She routinely left these locations with men she had just met and had frequent unsafe sexual encounters about which she later expressed shame and regret. When the therapist attempted to discuss Bonnie's unsafe behavior with her, she shrilly accused him of blaming her for her victimization, for intensifying her shame, for being a prude, and for not wanting her to have sex. In one response scenario, he backed off, fearful of upsetting her further. She stormed out of the office and slammed the door. Consider, though, an alternative ending to this scene: The therapist held firm in stating his concern for her and told her he refused to be a "passive bystander" while she endangered herself. He could see that she was upset with her behavior and he wanted to help her to develop other ways to have social contacts and to maintain her safety. When he said that, she softened and began to cry, saying that no one in her family had ever paid attention to her safety.

Amnesia and Hypermnesia

Therapists can find themselves lulled into their client's amnesia or hypermnesia. They may experience amnesia when they fail to remember what the client reported from session to session, when they forget other important clinical material or to do something they said they would do (e.g., make a scheduled outside phone contact when a client is in distress), or when they feel completely without their normal therapeutic skills. Hypermnesia and absorption may be discerned by therapists when they realize they are fully engrossed in their clients' memories and experiences, even outside the context of the treatment, and when they have difficulties maintaining psychic and emotional boundaries between themselves and their client. The following vignette illustrates this pattern.

BONNIE (*Continued*)

The therapist found that he was continuously worried about Bonnie between therapy sessions and checked for text or phone messages from her, especially on Friday and Saturday nights when she socialized. He had suggested that she contact him if she were feeling uncomfortable or threatened, and she often did so on weekends. He would "coach her" on how to get out of bad situations and how to get home safely. In sessions, they would replay the incidents, often to the exclusion of other pertinent issues. Over time, the therapist became aware of dreading Friday and Saturday nights and of feeling trapped in the role of unwitting "chaperone". Bonnie increasingly relied on him to rescue her when she ended up in an endangered situation that he came to realize could have been avoided. He sought consultation that allowed him to reset boundaries and to engage Bonnie in developing a safety plan that put the responsibility on *her* for maintaining her safety. He no longer was as available for her messages and used every opportunity to reinforce her when she applied her plan.

Incoherence of Self and Personal Discourse

Clients who are highly dissociative and who have a disorganized/disoriented attachment style are frequently incoherent or dysfluent in their self-presentation, their ability to recount autobiographical information and in their transference responses (Crittenden & Landini, 2011; Main & Hesse, 1990). Therapists will find themselves confused as they listen to the client, losing the thread of what is being said, or being led into different story lines by deflections and displacements. For example, a question about a painful event might result in incongruent laughter and body language (e.g., a smile when discussing abuse or pain), as well as multiple changes of topics and reference points. Asking about feelings might bring about a change of topic or scenario and a shift into intellectualized discussion devoid of any emotion. A reference to something the client previously discussed might or might not be remembered. Incoherence, along with the push–pulls of relational attachment and distancing on the part of the disorganized/dissociative client, is disorienting for the therapist who must struggle to remain responsive and "steady state" and to be able to point out the client's disjunctures and dissimulations in order to bring them to conscious awareness and ownership. The goal is integration that allows a more complete narrative to develop (White, 2011).

Jerry

Whenever Jerry discussed something unpleasant, he grinned. As he became more aware of this pattern with the therapist's feedback, he would say "I must be feeling something, because I'm smiling and it's not funny." Over time and with practice, he was able to become much more facially congruent with the painful emotions he was feeling (as one client said, "My face caught up with the rest of me"). Once, the therapist noticed that Jerry had tears in his eyes and looked sad. When he made these observations to him, Jerry denied being tearful, saying he had something in his eye that was causing it to "leak water." He later admitted that he had been terrified of showing his tears because his father often threatened to "give him something to cry about" and he had vowed he would never show the weakness he associated with crying ever again, no matter what. (In this example, notice the dissociative language: Jerry was not crying. It was his eye that was leaking water).

Monique

When she first started treatment, the therapist realized that as he listened to Monique, who was speaking English (her first language), he often could not follow her and had no idea what she was communicating. She was highly digressive and protected herself with a "wall of words." This became quite disconcerting for the therapist until he thought of the word "incoherent." Thereafter, he was not so thrown by how Monique presented herself and was able to slow her down and give her feedback about how she skipped from topic to topic in seemingly random fashion and to help her to more coherently organize her discourse. This pattern is exemplified in the ongoing case of **Doris**.

Altered Perceptions and Trance-Like Phenomena, Including "Entrancement" of the Therapist

Another aspect of the dissociative transference field having to do with altered perceptions and trance-like phenomena includes hallucinations or pseudo-hallucinations. Of course, these are also foreign and disconcerting to the therapist, who might diagnose or treat the client as psychotic or react in ways that involve fascination or repulsion, depending on what the client is expressing and how, and also the therapist's own history and capacity. For example, a client who is having flashbacks that involve graphic depictions of sexual activity could provide a turn-on for some therapists and repulse others. Or a client who perceives himself to be the devil incarnate and screams at the therapist to "let him (the client) go and to let him (the devil) have the client's soul to himself to further despoil him" would likely be highly upsetting but could be fascinating as well.

Clients can dissociate (or hallucinate) in *positive* psychoform or somatoform manifestations, i.e., those that involve intrusions and additions (s) of what are often implicit (out of the client's conscious awareness and stemming from the existence of different parts) in terms of content, emotion, physical sensations, and behaviors. An example is of that of **Anne**, who began writhing in her seat and later on the office floor while screaming about the searing pain in her groin. She was also screaming for her assailant to get off of her and was pushing and kicking while yelling for others to help her. This was the way she began to recall multiple rapes by her brother and his friends. Another example involves **Suzy** (a client with DID), who, after being invited to think about something that had been prohibited by her abuser, began to hold and rub her abdomen. She later told her therapist that she was being "kicked from the inside by those who sided with her abuser and who were angry with her for 'breaking the rules' and talking."

The opposite pattern of *negative* forms of dissociation or hallucination, involves extractions, removals, and the loss of content, emotion, behavior, and sensation that were previously available in both psychoform and somatoform manifestations. As an example, **Anne** was amnestic in the session following the one previously described. When the therapist referred to content from the prior session, Anne looked shocked and asked her what she was talking about (making the therapist question her own memory and sanity—she was being "entranced into not knowing"). The return of what had been dissociated was again remembered, and the therapist's inquiry was disturbing the homeostasis of "not knowing" that Anne had returned to between sessions. As the therapist continued to talk about the events of the previous session, the client looked at her and said "you must be saying something important, because I can't hear you." Her not remembering and not hearing are examples of psychoform and somatoform dissociation. Experiences such as these are disorienting and disconcerting to the therapist.

Cognitive Distortions

The following quote by Schwartz (2000) is quite descriptive of what it can be like for both therapist and dissociative client to work with cognitive distortions:

> The dissociative system is like a labyrinth of mirrors and trapdoors, and the dissociative process the ultimate intrapsychic trickster. It reverses cause and effect and self and other configurations, and obscures (or lies about) the individual's connections to his/her history. Lost in time, fragmented in identity, hypervigilant to the possibility of exposure while ostensibly guarding against all manner of other catastrophes, and truly confused in all relationships though pretending not to be, dissociative survivors become the victims of their own dissociative roller coasters. Tragically, the vicious cycles involving

> impression-management and avoidance of feelings, memories, and detection frequently cause people (professionals included) to doubt and distrust everything severely dissociative trauma survivors have to say. And that leads to further rounds of self-doubt and invalidation for the survivors. (p. 17)

As noted earlier, therapists need their own grounding and ability to maintain equanimity when in this relational field with all of its contradictions and logical inconsistencies.

Flashbacks

Flashbacks are inherently dissociative, as well as posttraumatic. Here are three more illustrations of their manifestation in therapy sessions.

Lu-li

When she was quite young Lu-li had been sexually abused by her maternal grandfather, who had threatened her with death if she ever told anyone. She had kept the secret since that time. Her grandfather was now dead and she sought help for her various symptoms. She disclosed the abuse to the therapist in considerable detail during the first session. Afterwards, Lu-li's eyes rolled back, her eyelids fluttered, and she became mute and unresponsive. She had moved into a terror state involving immobilization. The therapist had to ground her and interrupt her unconscious flashback, all the while feeling uncertain about what to do and terrified that the client was highly damaged by her disclosure.

Pierre

When the therapist went to the waiting room to greet Pierre for his session, she found him huddled into a corner, rocking back and forth, and sucking his thumb with his eyes closed. Needless to say, other clients in the waiting room were relieved when she arrived. Pierre remained unresponsive for a good 15 minutes, during which time the therapist worked to bring him back to the present, before he was able to reorient in time and place and walk into her office. He reported that he had been frightened by an unexpected phone call from his older brother, who had violently sexually abused him and with whom he had cut off contact. Their mother had given his brother his phone number because he was coming to town for a visit and wanted to stay with Pierre. Pierre had received the phone call while in the waiting room where he had reverted to a terrified child.

Myrium

As a devout Muslim woman, Myrium wore a headscarf for modesty and prayed five times a day. Although her work office was required to accommodate her, some of her office mates were intolerant and would taunt and berate her. While describing this to the therapist, she had a flashback of an episode of taunting by a group of soldiers in her hometown when she was a teenager and had narrowly escaped being gang-raped. She gasped, collapsed on the floor, and began to beg that she not be hurt. She later said it felt like it was happening again.

Impact on the Therapist

Therapists faced with these types of posttraumatic and dissociative behaviors in the therapeutic relational field (along with transference–countertransference and enactments and reenactments, described further in the next two chapters) frequently report feeling confused, scared, and unsettled in response. They feel as if they are being drawn into the world of the posttraumatic/dissociative client, an experience of extreme personal disorientation along with a host of other strong feelings and reactions. Furthermore, they report feeling disempowered and fragmented, "deskilled" by their experiences with these clients, often uncertain of what they are dealing with, doing, and why. Yet, viewed from another perspective, such immersion in this world provides a unique, firsthand, *in vivo* opportunity for therapists to gain important information and opportunities to identify with, understand, and empathize with clients' past and current experiences. As they are enjoined with their clients in this particular and foreign relational field, therapists have the difficult task of remaining physically and emotionally grounded and regulated while simultaneously attuning to and responding. *It is through this process that therapists present the client with a different and corrective relational and response experience that encourages integration rather than disintegration and dissociation.* Bromberg wrote that the therapist "stands in the spaces" of what has been defensively split off and what returned in dissociative and posttraumatic symptoms to help the client identify and assimilate this material in the interest of wholeness and continuity.

Therapists are assisted in staying grounded and responsive in this challenging relational field by many factors: their knowledge base, experience level, and skills; their own mental health; the structure and sequencing of treatment; and ongoing attention to elements of the treatment frame and the principles of treatment. As discussed, these serve as foundations to return to when confused and overwhelmed by the enormity of a client's distress or by a client's relational challenges. Additionally, regular opportunities for trauma-referenced consultation and supervision help therapists to explore and discuss their disoriented and disorganized experiences with clients (including their countertransference and vicarious trauma reactions) and help them to maintain (or regain) their perspective and their therapeutic footing (more on this in the next two chapters).

CONCLUSION

Therapists working with complex traumatic stress disorders must literally work with "what is there" as well as "what is not there" in both the client and the relational field they both occupy. Paradoxically, they must enter the voids of the client's self and experience by approaching rather than supporting the client's stance of "a-void-ance." They must enter the breach, but when they do, they enter a relational matrix that is rife with posttraumatic and dissociative themes and challenges: invitations to take on roles from the past, trance and hypnoid states, conscious and unconscious flashbacks, invitations to rescue, the holding of "logical illogic," or trance logic and entrancements and other processes of which the client is largely unconscious and unaware. The therapist's job is to hold steady-state in his or her reality and ability to self-regulate, and to stay present for the client, inviting him or her to know and feel what was protectively avoided or dissociated from a stance of inquiry and support and grounding the client in the reality of the present. Through this containment in secure attachment and responsiveness on the part of the therapist, the client has the opportunity to identify and integrate disintegrated and disowned parts of self and experience, contributing to healing.

CHAPTER 9

Walking the Walk

The Therapeutic Relationship

One outcome of increased study of psychological trauma and its treatment over the past several decades has been the heightened recognition that traumatic stress often has adverse effects not only on victims and survivors but also on family members, friends, colleagues, coworkers, and professional helpers whose exposure is secondhand rather than direct (Devilly, Wright, & Varker, 2009; Jenkins & Baird, 2002; Way, VanDeusen, & Cottrell, 2007; Way, Van Deusen, Martin, Applegate, & Jandle, 2004). Therapists working with traumatized clients hear about terrifying, horrific events and experiences that likely fall outside the scope and purview of anything they ever experienced or possibly ever imagined was possible. They are routinely exposed to the clients' traumatic experience(s) and their initial and long-term impact (including secondary elaborations), in words (sometimes involving very graphic depictions of gruesome events and atrocities), in somatic reactions and behaviors, and in the relational matrix involving interaction patterns, such as reenactments within and outside of the psychotherapy. These trauma-influenced relational patterns and expectations can be unrelenting to the point of trying the patience of even the most dedicated and composed therapist, in the process causing the loss of personal and professional bearings.

In this chapter, we discuss relational challenges and the opportunities they present that are in addition to the particular challenges presented by the posttraumatic and dissociative states and the relational matrix (Chapter 8). When challenges and potential pitfalls are known ahead of time, they can be anticipated and planned for (Chu, 1988) and they might even be sidestepped altogether. We begin by considering the impact on the therapist of hearing and feeling the emotional distress that clients suffer due to having experienced complex trauma—this has been labeled *vicarious trauma, secondary trauma*, or *compassion fatigue*. We then discuss the *therapist's use of self*, stressing yet again the importance of balancing authenticity with clear professional boundaries. The use of self involves a willingness to connect with the traumatized client, that is, not to just "talk the talk" but to actually "walk the walk." As discussed in the previous chapter, this relational matrix contains many dissociative and posttraumatic minefields that can confuse, perplex, and exasperate therapists. These can dramatically alter the treatment trajectory and its success or failure (Loewenstein, 1993).

"Risking Connection" is both the name of a trauma-informed services curriculum developed by Saakvitne, Pearlman, and colleagues (Saakvitne, Gamble, Pearlman, & Lev, 2000; *www.riskingconnection.com*) and an apt description of the double-edged sword of relational engagement in the treatment of or provision of social and human services to the victimized. "Risking connection" *refers both to the traumatized client and to the professional helper: Both personally take a risk when they form a relationship (connection) that aims to help the client to overcome the terror, helplessness, and horror of surviving traumatic events and their aftermath*. As we discuss this personal impact, we emphasize the need for therapists to attend to their own mental and physical health through active and ongoing self-care strategies, including engagement with colleagues, connections with family and friends, adequate time to destress, and attention to personal needs. "Helper, first heal thyself" (and keep thyself healthy) is the applicable guideline here.

In the final section of this chapter, we discuss client attachment styles and the challenges they present. It is as important for therapists to attend to the "fit" (or lack of fit) between their own attachment styles and those of their clients as it is for them to be aware of the clients' styles. Because attachment working models of complex trauma survivors tend to be insecure, they are likely to fluctuate when clients encounter stressful challenges either in their lives or in psychotherapy. As a result, the fit between the attachment styles of client and therapist may vary at different points. In order to ensure the client's safety and progress, a therapist must therefore be prepared to flexibly adjust his or her stance or the intensity of the treatment when either the client's attachment style or the client–therapist fit becomes disorganized.

VICARIOUS TRAUMA AND PROFESSIONAL GROWTH

Vicarious trauma was first described and defined as therapists' posttraumatic stress reactions resulting from hearing their clients' stories and learning about their posttraumatic reactions and impairments and from interacting with the traumatized (McCann & Pearlman, 1990; Pearlman & MacIan, 1995; Pearlman & Saakvitne, 1995). Several related terms have been used to describe the psychological impact of the treatment of trauma survivors, including *compassion fatigue* (Figley, 1995, 2002b), *secondary trauma* (Elwood, Mott, Lohr, & Galovski, 2011), and *empathic strain* (Berger, 1984; Wilson & Lindy, 1994). Each term, though slightly different in focus, refers to the *process of change or transformation* (personal as well as professional) *in the helper* as a result of relational engagement with and provision of services to survivors of trauma. Pearlman and Saakvitne (1995) viewed the transformation as inevitable. Other writers and researchers, however, are not as definite in taking this position. In fact, a recent review of the construct and the empirical literature (Elwood et al., 2011) showed mixed results. Therapists reported not frequently experiencing "clinically significant" levels of symptoms uniquely associated with trauma-focused treatment.

Whatever their perspective on its inevitability, virtually all clinical experts have opined that vicarious trauma reactions—when they occur in the course of a therapist's career—can result in substantial distress to the therapist and that they should therefore be anticipated and prepared for. If not identified and managed, vicarious trauma has been found to impair professional judgment and ability to function effectively, and it can be detrimental to personal mental health and health status and to personal relationships. Trauma can be compared to a toxic substance. It requires the mindful application of methods to limit and contain exposure and toxicity so that it does not cause additional damage.

It is important for therapists to be aware that clients do *not* deliberately "traumatize" or otherwise cause them to have reactions of this sort (Pearlman & Saakvitne, 1995) and that experiences of vicarious trauma do not necessarily compromise either the therapy or the therapist's (or client's) well-being. We prefer to frame the experiencing of palpable emotional reactions that result from empathic engagement as a positive challenge for therapists to proactively manage, rather than something to fear or avoid. To keep things in perspective, it is worth recalling that vicarious trauma is less daunting than the incapacitating posttraumatic distress faced by clients. Nevertheless, careful attention is required so that vicarious traumatic reactions do not compromise either therapists' ability to provide sensitive and effective treatment or the quality of their personal lives. The seriousness of this caveat is underlined by the fact that, in some instances, unmanaged vicarious traumatic stress reactions can result in full-blown secondary PTSD *in the therapist*, causing impairment that can then derail the treatment.

Vicarious traumatization is best understood within the context of the essential relational nature of psychotherapy. As we have discussed, these clients bring their "lessons of abuse" and their learned cognitions and beliefs (schemas) about self and others (described in Chapters 5 and 10) into the transference (known as "traumatic transference") and "invite" their therapists (with conscious intention or not) into complementary or contrasting countertransference positions and into enactments. Much of the communication is implicit and coded and thus not always in verbal form, so therapists must get to know the client well enough over time to be able to interpret and learn the client's indirect communications. At times, this can be frustrating and exhausting, particularly taxing therapists' ability to maintain compassion (hence the term "compassion fatigue"). For example, **Hector**'s therapist learned that when Hector asked for help when he felt isolated or alone, he communicated this indirectly (and quite paradoxically!) by reverting to an old habit of avoiding appointments (using excuses such as "forgetting" or having no transportation). When avoidance became more the rule than the exception, the therapist began to feel annoyed and came to doubt Hector's commitment and willingness to stick with the treatment and his honesty. He was able to regain a therapeutic perspective and approach the problem calmly by reframing the dilemma as a reenactment of Hector's known way of coping—that is, rather than asking for what he needed, he self-protectively pushed away from others due to his fear of being rejected and abandoned.

The Other Side of Vicarious Traumatization: Posttraumatic Resilience

Although complex trauma treatment has many trials and "treatment traps" (Chu, 1988, 1998, 1999, 2011) and has been aptly described by Chu (1992) as "the therapeutic roller coaster," it can also offer great rewards for the therapist. These include both the sense of connection and accomplishment that come from learning the client's unique personal language and perspective on the world and the satisfaction of witnessing the healing power of the therapeutic dialogue and its growth potential. Decoding clients' communications can be exhilarating and rewarding when the client indicates that he or she has been understood and when personal development results. The compassion that motivates a therapist to persist in "entering the void" and forging a genuine relationship can be a source of renewal and reengagement that counterbalances the inevitable times of discouragement and fatigue.

Just as survivors can grow and develop in the aftermath of trauma, a process that has been labeled *posttraumatic growth* (Joseph, 2011; Joseph & Linley, 2008; Tedeschi & Calhoun, 1995; Werdel & Wicks, 2012), so too can professionals who work with them (Sanness, 2011). Therapists and others describe a sense of awe and inspiration gained from working with their clients and the resilience they displayed at the time of the trauma and subsequently. Many further note their awe regarding clients' sense of morality and ability to empathize with others, qualities that are in stark contrast to how they were treated.

The term "posttraumatic resilience" was coined to describe the potential benefits to the professional of experiencing vicarious trauma of this type (Hernandez, Gangsei, & Engstrom, 2007). These benefits include feeling better able to face and overcome both personal and professional problems and increased hope for and trust in the potential goodness of people and the world. Thus, responses to trauma, including resoluteness and morality in the face of malice, can temper the therapist, change his or her perspective on the world, and increase personal resilience, as well as humility. These provide vital counterbalances to the stresses of this work.

Implications for Professional Training and Helping Systems

As discussed at other points in this book, training programs have not consistently included trauma in their curricula nor conveyed to trainees that, in the course of their work, they can be adversely affected. Psychotherapy, counseling, social work, and other social and human services, by their very nature, have many characteristics that create strain and risk for the professional that can accumulate over time, creating disillusionment and even indifference to the plight of the clients, leading to professional hopelessness and burnout. When the challenge of recovering from traumatic stress reactions in the helper complicates the services, *professional burnout* may be exacerbated by secondary or vicarious trauma reactions (Adams, Boscarino, & Figley, 2006). Fortunately, quite a few books have been published in recent years on the topic of professional self-care as an ethical imperative when providing psychotherapy in general and especially to traumatized clients (Baker, 2003; Cozolino, 2004; Norcross & Guy, 2007; Perlman, 1999; Rothschild, 2006; Saakvitne et al., 2000; Saakvitne & Pearlman, 1996; Weiss, 2004; Wicks, 2008).

It is not just the client–professional relationship that engenders compassion fatigue and secondary or vicarious trauma. A perspective broader than the individual professional is needed to identify the stressors created by organizational, bureaucratic, and economic pressures in helping systems (Bloom, 1997, 2010; Bloom & Farragher, 2010; Harris & Fallot, 2001). Over the past several decades (with a dramatic acceleration in the economic recession these past few years), there has been a disconcerting trend involving diminished funding and reimbursement constraints, staffing cuts, increased managed care documentation requirements, and restrictions on insurance coverage causing organizations and practitioners to reduce the services offered while increasing the demands (e.g., size and complexity of caseloads documentation) on the service provider. This is essentially a recipe for burnout.

In a recent book, Bloom and Farragher (2010) document these systemic changes and call for a radical change in the medical/mental health/social services system as a whole to combat or prevent these additional strains from compromising not only the services provided to clients but also the health and effectiveness of professionals who are "on the line and in the trenches." Ample evidence documents incidents of accidental or intentional physical and psychological harm that occur within the very organizations (and by helping professionals within them) that are supposed to prevent or ameliorate the harm that clients have experienced. With depressing regularity, the systemic problem (such as policies and procedures that permit or even encourage careless, insensitive, disrespectful, or inadequate treatment of clients not only by professionals but also by line staff and administrators) exacerbates traumatic stress symptoms. In addition to advocating for increasing the extent to which entire helping organizations are trauma-informed (Adults Surviving Child Abuse, 2012; Fallot & Harris, 2008; Harris & Fallot, 2001; Saakvitne et al., 2000), the sanctuary model (Bloom, 1997; Bloom & Farragher, 2010) and related approaches call for additional efforts on the part of educators to adequately prepare students by including information on trauma and the need for ongoing self-care efforts in their training. These proposals have been made with the intention of *protecting both the client (especially one with a complex trauma history) and the therapist or other helper.*

THE THERAPIST'S USE OF SELF: PSYCHIC AND SOMATIC DIMENSIONS

In virtually all schools of psychotherapy, the relationship between therapist and client has the greatest degree of endorsement as an empirically supported treatment strategy, and "a deep synergy between treatment methods and the therapeutic relationship" is acknowledged (Norcross & Lambert, 2011, p. 5). (See Vol. 48, Nos. 1 and 4 [2011] of the journal *Psychotherapy* for a series of articles on evidence-based psychotherapy relationships.) Across the board in research studies, elements of the relationship constitute factors that potentiate other treatment techniques and interventions. This is especially likely to be the case with interpersonally traumatized clients, as research by Cloitre and her colleagues has demonstrated (Cloitre, Stovall-McClough, Miranda, & Chemtob, 2004). Specific *personal dimensions* of the relationship and *mindfulness* on the part of the therapist are especially important (Fosha, Siegel, & Solomon, 2009). Recently, *somatic dimensions* involving mindfulness and specific body-based therapist awareness of self and client have been encouraged (Ogden et al., 2006; Ogden & Fisher, 2009, 2012; Rothschild, 2006; Schore, 2003b; Siegel, 2010, 2012a, 2012b) as means of opening new avenues to the client's personal development, leading to a changed capacity for attachment and emotions and a changed experience and consideration of self (Cozolino, 2004; Siegel, 2007, 2012; Schore, 2003b).

Understanding the "Self" of the Therapist

A Secure Base

The therapist is called on to provide the complex trauma survivor with an alternative attachment model (Farber, Lippert, & Nevas, 1995). This is similar to, but also differs in important ways from, the client's actual relationships with parents or other caregivers. Quoting Dozier and Tyrrell (1997) on this matter:

> From an attachment theory perspective, the therapist's work with a client is similar to, yet more difficult than, the mother's with her infant. In either case, a primary task is to provide a secure base that promotes safe exploration. The mother's task is easier than the therapist's because she need not compensate for the failures of other attachment figures. . . . The task for therapy is often made more difficult because of the client's previous experiences with unavailable or rejecting caregivers. Clients' working models frequently lead to expectations that are rigid and inconsistent with reality, as when an available, empathic therapist is perceived as judgmental and rejecting. The client must rework the model so as to be able to establish the therapist as a secure base. Thus, exploration of prior working models cannot wait until after a secure base is established; rather, the processes occur in tandem. According to Bowlby (1988), the client's exploration of his or her model of the therapist is a critical task of therapy. . . . We suggest that change in the client's working model of the therapist, of attachment figures, and of specific others in his or her work are prerequisites to more fundamental change in working models of the generalized self and others. (p. 222)

Attachment issues and styles are described at greater length subsequently. Suffice it to say that it is not enough for therapists to simply encourage their clients to trust them and feel secure in the therapeutic relationship. In order for therapy to provide a genuinely secure emotional base, the therapist must have a personal working model of relationships that is secure and a related ability to emotionally self-regulate. *This does not require that the therapist must be perfect or be free from insecurity.* Rather, it is the therapist's ego strength and self-capacities that undergird the ability to recognize and deal with personal insecurities and to weather the ups and downs of all relationships (including that with the client) that offer the opportunity for the client to revise his or her insecure working model to one that is more secure. In turn, this promotes identity and self-development.

Use of Self to Mirror the Client: Empathic Mindfulness and Mentalizing

Therapists who work with this population are particularly called on to *use themselves as the means of recognizing and reflecting their clients back to them* through attunement, resonance, and synchrony (both emotional and physical; Allen, 2012; Schore, 1993b). At the most basic level, therapists must bring their humanness to this endeavor and strive to connect on a human-to-human basis with individuals who are likely to mistrust and resist them (Pearlman & Courtois, 2005; Kinsler et al., 2009). Recent neuroscience research findings—particularly the mother–infant developmental and affective neuroscience research—support the significance of human connection and empathic personal mirroring to human emotional growth (Schore, 2003a, 2003b; Siegel, 2012) and to social development (Fosha et al., 2009).

Thus disconnection from others and self must be replaced with connection that provides positive reflection and opportunity for expanded awareness to counter construction and expanded personal and interpersonal options (Miller & Stiver, 1997). Mindfulness (Fosha et al., 2009) or mentalizing (Allen, 2012; Allen, Fonagy, & Bateman, 2008) on the part of the therapist promotes the process of relationship-based development in the client. The mindful therapist (Siegel, 2010) is one who is engaged, committed, and caring and who is aware of him- or herself and how that self relates to the client to potentiate healing interactions. The therapist must be attentive to the possible meaning inherent in nonverbal and verbal communication to and from the client. In addition, as the therapist mentalizes (or engages in metaprocessing about interactions with the client), he or she formulates and tests hypotheses about the potential meanings. This *dual awareness* permits the clients not only to feel understood and valued but to have a role model and coach as they learn to mentalize (Allen, 2012). In his book *The Mindful Therapist,* Siegel discusses the therapist's use of self and knowledge of brain functions to help in the design and implementation of treatment strategies (Siegel, 2010).

This process of empathic mirroring and modeling of mentalizing replicates the developmental processes involved in the formation of secure inner working models by children in their relationships with caregivers in the first years of life (Schore, 2003a). As a result, even when attachment working models are profoundly disorganized, clients are able to gradually (although not without expectable setbacks, regressions, challenges, and resistances) take in the empathic mirroring provided by the therapist. Over time, this response and attunement help in developing a sense of self and of personal worth and, correspondingly, a capacity for healthier and more responsive relationships. This shift from insecure to secure patterns of attachment (identified as "earned secure" style) has been documented as occurring in meaningful, respectful adult relationships, including therapy (Dozier & Tyrell, 1997; Main & Goldwyn, 1994; Travis, Binder, Bliwise, & Horne-Moyer, 2001). Therapists can best help their clients to make this developmental shift if they themselves operate from a secure/autonomous or "earned secure" attachment style that reflects a positive sense of self, self-esteem, and a capacity to relate with others in healthy ways. This style allows them to stay balanced and emotionally regulated in their interactions. In addition to the benefit this can have for the client, there is no better prophylaxis for vicarious traumatization and compassion fatigue than using mindfulness and mentalizing both during therapy sessions and when reviewing and debriefing past sessions or planning upcoming ones. Consistent with this view, a recent study found that therapists' self-reported empathy and personal and professional growth were positively correlated and that those with higher levels of empathy also reported less adverse effects of vicarious trauma on their sense of growth (Elwood et al., 2011). The extent to which the therapists felt supported by their organizations in dealing with the impact of vicarious trauma was unrelated to self-reported personal growth, suggesting that the internal resource of empathy may be more important in dealing with vicarious trauma than external support (yet external support is also crucial) (Bloom & Farragher, 2010; Harris & Fallot, 2011; Saakvitne et al., 2000).

The lack of trauma-specific education and training notwithstanding, not all therapists (due to their own temperaments, emotional capacity and tolerance, interest, and personal history) can or want to work with this population. Among those who do, not all possess the ability and willingness to do the hard and never-ending work of mindfulness in relation to both clients and themselves. Therapists are obliged to engage in self-assessment regarding their practice and areas of expertise and should ethically remove themselves from the treatment of patients they are not temperamentally or otherwise suited (or trained) to treat. Furthermore, there may come a time when the therapist no longer wants to work with a specific population for any number of reasons, including the desire for a less demanding caseload, the presence of high life stress, or impending retirement.

Therapist as Human and Humble

Therapists must also approach their work from a position of humanness and have a degree of humility (Kinsler et al., 2009; Pearlman & Caringi, 2009; Pearlman & Courtois, 2005). Although the therapist is professionally responsible for the management of the overall treatment, it is best not to approach the client from a position of being the "authority on high" who has all the answers or who will provide for all of the client's needs. Similarly, a narcissistic, self-important therapist style involving the expectation that the client meet the needs of the therapist—rather than the other way around—is a misguided one, in general but particularly with this population. It repeats what many have already experienced in primary relationships and continues the pattern of externalization and meeting the needs of others.

This psychotherapy is a joint endeavor, an unfolding process in which self-exploration can take place with the therapist in the position of supporter and guide who does not have all of the answers but who is attuned and who intentionally applies specialized knowledge and strategies. The relationship and process are co-created over time in ways that may seem "messy" because they often are nonlinear, noncausal, and unpredictable in the immediacy of the here-and-now of the session (Boston Change Process Study Group, 2010). Yet it is in the thick of this process that the development of new and expanded "ways of being" takes place. From this perspective, *it is the client who makes sense and meaning of his or her own experience*, with the therapist as facilitator but not dictator or controller. Thus interest in exploring the client's personal experience takes the place of interpreting his or her psyche or controlling behavior by someone on the outside, shifting the client's locus of control from external to internal.

Active Stance and Intentionality

The inactive therapist who remains silent or who waits passively for the client to engage will more than likely be experienced as invalidating and unwelcoming or will cause the client to work hard to capture the therapist's attention and approval. This stance places the therapist in a role of "passive or disinterested bystander" or even "victimizer" and the client into the role of either "victim" or "rescuer." For this reason, it is contraindicated in the treatment of this population in particular. The therapist must be willing to engage and be active in encouraging what is often a fearful (or even terrified), mistrustful, and avoidant client and must have patience and "staying power" whether the presentation is reluctant, resistant, evasive, or fearful/avoidant when the client shifts back and forth between being connected and disconnected (i.e., attached and detached, or when flooding the therapist with information or when witholding). Attachment is both longed for and dreaded. Relationship closeness becomes the paradoxical trigger for danger, causing protective and proactive detachment that can upset and confuse the therapist, who thinks the relationship is going well (it likely is!) but who is unaware of the defensive use of disengagement. This relational cycle continues until it is identified and resolved over time in a relationship that is responsive and trustworthy (but not perfect!) in an ongoing way.

In order to do this work, therapists must learn about relational dynamics associated with different attachment styles and to track their emergence in treatment. In terms of the attachment styles of therapist and client, contrary to what might be expected (i.e., that clients would be best matched with someone with their same or a similar attachment style), the findings of a number of treatment outcome studies suggest the need for the therapist to approach the client from a different style, that of secure attachment, to make possible the adoption of a more secure inner working model. The development of a therapeutic alliance and bond is one that takes time and effort (Bernier & Dozier, 2002; Farber et al., 1995; Kinsler, 1992; Obegi, 2008).

Although this point seems self-evident, it is advisable for therapists to understand their personal motives for having chosen psychotherapy as their profession as well as their reasons for choosing to work with traumatized individuals. This is done in anticipation of clients who question or challenge the therapist's explanations or commitment and who project their hostility, shame, and self-contempt onto others, anticipating and expecting that others feel the same way about them as they do about themselves. This is a recurring position and a means of self-protection. It may take a long time and much effort for clients who lead with this projection to let down their guard enough to let in a caring rather than a critical response and to come to the point of trusting the therapist and his or her motives and intentions.

Hector

As discussed in previous chapters, Hector's mistrust was palpable. He began therapy by challenging the therapist at every opportunity. He questioned the therapist's motivation and was hostile in response to the most innocuous and circumspect inquiries. He was obviously uncomfortable and continuously taunted the therapist about what he wanted from him (Hector) and whether he was going to assault and abuse him as other men had done. The therapist found it exhausting to be with Hector until he was able to understand and empathize with how terrified he was under all of his bravado and invective. This understanding allowed him to respond to Hector with interest and concern rather than from a position of defensiveness. Hector was taken aback by this and by the therapist's support of what he understood to be Hector's understandable fears ("realistic paranoia"), his strengths, and his need for self-protective mechanisms.

Psychologist Philip Bromberg captured this process in the following quote: "The ability of an individual to allow his self-truth to be altered by the impact of an 'other' . . . depends on the existence of a relationship in which the other can be experienced as someone who, paradoxically, both accepts the validity of the patient's inner reality and participates in the here-and-now act of constructing a negotiated reality discrepant with it" (Bromberg, 1993, p. 160).

The Uniqueness of Each Relationship: The Intersubjective Perspective

This perspective was discussed in Chapter 3 as concerns the uniqueness of each client and the necessity for the therapist to be open and responsive to this singularity. It is helpful for the therapist to consider that each treatment dyad as one of a kind, co-created by its two unique participants over its course. In other words, no two treatment relationships are the same. The therapist makes adjustments reflexively but must also bring reflection to bear in attempting to relate in a "good-enough" way to the needs of each client. Rather than operating from a rigid and rule-bound stance, therapists must maintain a degree of flexibility and must utilize (and model) skills of collaboration and problem solving, customizing the treatment to the client's needs and context, all within established professional boundaries and limits (Briere & Lanitree, 2011; McConkin, Newman, Fogler, & Keane, 2012). A more permissive and flexible outlook and style of interaction is usually in direct contrast to what the client had previously experienced.

At times, consideration must be given to operating outside of established limits and boundaries, usually on a time-limited basis and due to something out of the ordinary. As noted by Gutheil and Brodsky (2008), boundary crossings are not the same as boundary transgressions. A boundary might be crossed in psychotherapy for many reasons, hopefully after deliberation and consultation. Any out-of-the-ordinary modification to standard procedure should be noted in the patient's chart, along with the rationale for it and its consequences. For example, one of us (C.C.), over the span of a 30-year clinical career, on two occasions with two different clients has attended gynecological examinations, sitting behind the client and offering support. In one case, the client had an unremitting phobia that prevented examination for severe and potentially life-threatening hemorrhaging and the second required a feared examination in the immediate aftermath of a violent current rape by the original perpetrator that left her vaginally and anally injured. In both cases of what would be identified as an unorthodox (and infrequent) type of intervention, these clients reported feeling relieved and safe. The therapeutic relationship subsequently was strengthened.

Advances in technology (such as e-mail, texting, and Skype) and telehealth approaches to treatment are also pushing boundaries and establishing new ways of providing therapeutic services. All of the major professional organizations are now developing guidance for therapists working within these modalities and outside normal parameters.

Empathic Attunement

A psychotherapist must have the capacity to empathize. This involves extending one's personal perspective to understand that of the client, even when he or she interacts in ways that are challenging, confusing, erratic, or emotionally shut down. The capacity to "walk in the shoes of the other" is very helpful to understanding and involves mindfulness and mentalizing on the part of the therapist. Wilson and Thomas (2004), in their book *Empathy in the Treatment of Trauma and PTSD*, wrote:

> Trauma work requires the therapist's immersion into the phenomenal reality and ego-space of the person suffering from PTSD. *Empathic attunement* is the capacity to resonate efficiently and accurately to another's state of being; to match self–other understanding; to have knowledge of the internal psychological ego states of another who has suffered a trauma; and to understand the unique internal working model/schema of their trauma experience. Empathic capacity is the aptitude for empathic attunement and varies greatly among therapists working with PTSD patients (Dalenberg, 2000). Effective posttraumatic therapy rests on the cornerstone of empathic ability and the facility to sustain empathic attunement. (p. 7; authors' italics)

They also wrote:

> Put another way, empathic attunement allows the therapist to decode what the client is transmitting about his/her experience and state of mind. In order to grasp the meaning of clients' often indirect or unconscious communications, therapists must carefully follow the dynamic flow of information provided by the client's: (1) words; (2) affects; (3) memories; (4) thoughts; (5) body postures; (6) voice modulations; (7) expressions of personality; and (8) " 'here and now' " ego state presentations of the saliency of integrative consciousness. (p. 10)

To these we would add the full array of somatosensory communications: not only body postures and voice modulations but also the range of visual (e.g., gaze, facial expression), kinesthetic (e.g., body motions and movement patterns), tactile (e.g., approach and avoidance of touch), and proprioceptive (body position) and interoceptive (body state; e.g., tension, warmth or coldness, tingling, dizziness) modalities, and attachment style/inner working model and relational capacity and self-development.

Empathy, however, must be tempered and modulated, as too little or too much can become the means by which therapists defend against their clients and their stories, in the process becoming problematic to the treatment. Wilson and Lindy (1994), in their pioneering book *Countertransference in the Treatment of PTSD*, articulated a dynamic model of empathy and what they identified as empathic strain, in which too little (Type I) or too much (Type II) results in therapeutic error and an interruption in what is most beneficial for the client. They wrote: "Empathic strain results from those interpersonal events in psychotherapy that weaken, injure, or force beyond reasonable limits a salutary therapeutic response to the client. Countertransference processes are only one source of empathic strain, yet we believe that in the treatment of PTSD, CTRs [countertransference responses] are perhaps the primary cause of treatment failure" (p. 15).

Empathic errors (i.e., misunderstanding or misinterpretation of the client's intended or actual communication) can occur as a result of countertransference—that is, from the therapist's own personal history, the nature of the client's trauma history, institutional factors (such as a lack of support or training), and specific aspects of the client's personality or life history that have particular personal meaning for the therapist (see Chapter 10 for more extensive discussion). Of particular concern, countertransference can lead a therapist to confuse empathy with sympathy, for example, by overidentifying with and attempting to rescue or becoming overinvolved with a corresponding loss of professional boundaries. Substituting sympathy for empathy tends to result in a reciprocal dependency by therapist and client based on the assumptions that the client is too damaged or fragile to be able to change or to heal and that the therapist must therefore rescue or provide. Too little empathy, in contrast, results in therapist disinterest, disengagement, distancing or withdrawal, nonresponse, evasion, and even aggression. This response may constitute a form of victim blaming or of using the client's weaknesses and vulnerabilities as indictments or entitlements.

The Distance–Closeness "Dance"

Psychotherapy involves a sensitive ongoing negotiation in the dyad, largely unspoken, in which both parties achieve an emotional distance that is "not too close or too distant." Baker (1997) wrote of this with regard to the dissociative client. Both client's and therapist's ability to tolerate closeness and connection are determinants of the relational distance that is most helpful for the client, and this will vary both within and across therapy sessions with the same client as his or her emotional state changes. This also varies between clients, with some needing more space and others less. Flexibility is required, as needs and trust levels change over time and boundaries and limits are subject to challenge and revision.

Restating the recommendation made previously, established and communicated boundaries and limits are needed, but the therapist must be aware that these will be questioned and tested, at times in subtle ways but sometimes in florid ways that are shocking. For example, consider these case examples that range from the more mundane and commonplace to the more shocking and uncommon: a client who asks the therapist for a hug at the end of every session; a client who wants to know why he and the therapist cannot be friends outside of therapy sessions; a client who cuts herself during or immediately after a therapy session and bleeds on the office carpet; a client who comments in a sexualized manner on the therapist's body or suggests having sex with the therapist; a client who sits so as to frequently "accidentally" bump into or touch the therapist physically; a client who asks repeatedly about details of the therapist's intimate relationships or close family members; a female client who arrives wearing no underwear or a male client who is "accidentally unzipped" and who expose themselves to the therapist; a client who hostilely inquires what the therapist gets out of working with trauma and why he or she doesn't just "f—off, die, and get it over with"; a client who repeatedly comes to session intoxicated or under the influence of drugs; or a client who produces a weapon or announces that he or she is carrying one and never goes anywhere—including therapy—without having it at hand.

It goes without saying that it is a challenge to respond therapeutically to situations such as these, knowing that they "go with the territory" of interpersonal violation and violence. Yet therapists must be capable of restating and maintaining boundaries and limits and of taking direct action, such as ending sessions, firmly but uncritically insisting that the client modify his or her exhibitionistic or adversarial behavior, calling for assistance, getting a restraining or peace order, or pressing charges, initiating hospitalization (voluntary or involuntary), making the continuation of therapy conditional on the client's getting specialized treatment or becoming involved in support groups for addictive behavior, or ending the therapy if the client refuses to or cannot adapt to the boundary conditions necessary for safety. The continuation of treatment might require additional precautions (e.g., keeping the office door open, audio- or videotaping sessions, having a third person attend, not having weapons either in session or accessible) that are removed only once the specific threat or circumstance diminishes or resolves. And yet on the nonthreatening end of the spectrum, it is helpful for the therapist to have some flexibility. For example, with a client who requests to be held or hugged, the therapist might agree to shake hands at the end of the session. Or he or she might agree to a hug only after discussing its meaning to the client, only after assessing personal comfort with offering or accepting a hug, and after discussing how often, how, and when it will be offered.

We turn once again to the case of Doris as an example of dealing with closeness and distance.

Doris

Several months after becoming a bit more settled into therapy, Doris began to ask her therapist to tell her that she loved her at the end of sessions as a means of reassuring her. When the therapist attempted to discuss this request with her, Doris became explosive and disparaging. She accused the therapist of being "cold and indifferent," an "ice queen" who cared only about herself and the payment she received. If the therapist refused to tell Doris that she loved her, it meant that she really despised her. The therapist responded calmly and asked whether Doris would be open to more discussion because, from her perspective, it didn't mean that at all. Doris calmed down and agreed and the therapist proceeded to explain her position vis à vis Doris's "request." The therapist assured Doris that she cared about her but that she would not be pressured into making statements of love or of any other feeling. Doris would have to determine based on the therapist's behavior toward her and treatment of her how the therapist might feel. They agreed that Doris would take a small transitional object from the office (a seashell) to signify the connection between them. When Doris needed reassurance of the therapist's regard for her, she could use the shell as a tangible reminder.

Documentation and Consultation

Whatever the boundary challenge or crossing, the therapist should make notice of it in session notes and, in particular, document the actions made in response. Therapists are prone to not wanting to document situations such as these, often due to shame or similar emotions or feeling that they somehow caused the situation or didn't manage it well. To the contrary, documentation provides the "therapist's shield" (Caudill, 1977) in the event that the situation escalates in some way. Documentation is proof of the therapist's actions and the reasoning behind it. It is also advisable for the therapist to seek consultation and support on the matter at hand in order to get an outside perspective. This might mean another therapist, the manager or administrator in charge, the owner or administrator, the outside consultant or formal supervisor, the liability insurance company's attorney or therapist, or a business attorney, among others. Seeking assistance demonstrates that the therapist is active in reviewing the actions taken and in implementing others, with the input of other professionals. The worst-case scenario is for the therapist to "go it alone" without outside guidance and support. The therapist is then isolated, with what is likely a limited perspective tinged with strong feelings and other reactions, such as fear and shame, compassion fatigue, countertransference, and vicarious trauma, and is thus more prone to make mistakes.

Relational Breaches and Repair

As in any relationship, there will be times of tension, miscommunication, missteps, and errors in treatment. Although these might be minor, complex trauma clients might experience them as catastrophic and as signaling rejection and the end of the relationship. Therapists who expect to make mistakes and who know that some clients will interpret them as relational "kisses of death" will paradoxically have an easier time working with these issues when they occur (Chu, 1988). A major justification for not assuming the position as an "authority on high" is to establish the expectation that the therapist is not perfect, nor working toward perfection, but rather working hard at being responsible and "good enough." Van der Kolk, in his introduction to the book on countertransference and PTSD authored by Wilson and Lindy (1994), famously noted that the professional training of therapists does not involve training in their becoming angels or saints, but they are often hard-pressed not to function in just those roles when working with highly traumatized and highly reactive clients. A perspective that relationship errors and missteps occur, are to be expected, are open to discussion, and frequently provide opportunities for growth (even as they *feel like* major crises) is a good starting point for therapists to take, but it is likely to be contrary to what the client has experienced previously and therefore to what is expected. Wallin (2007) encouraged therapists to actively initiate repair: "Such sequences of disruption and repair—particularly repair initiated by the therapist—strengthen the patient's confidence that the relationship can be relied on to contain difficult feelings and help resolve them. In the process, they build the patient's capacity to make use of interactive affect regulation, which is a forerunner of self-regulation" (p. 197).

Relational breaches occur on both sides of the dyad: At times, it will be the therapist's actions or communications, and at others, it will be the client's. Some involve both. Depending on the severity of the breach on the client's side, the therapist may have to practice "tough love" and insist on the maintenance of boundaries and other responsibilities in the treatment relationship as discussed above. If the therapist erred, he or she needs to honestly own the behavior and apologize for the mistake (however, not from a position of abject shame). A sincere acknowledgement and apology can go a long way in modeling a new way of "being in relationship," one that is based on communication and mutual respect. Further, an appropriate apology can preempt the escalation that sometimes occurs when clients take ethics, licensing, or legal action against therapists. It has been noted in the risk management literature that many of these client actions are undertaken on the basis of calling the therapist's behavior into question and his or her subsequent refusal to acknowledge the behavior or its impact or to offer an apology. These unfortunate circumstances are sometimes compounded by additional actions taken by therapists (such as abruptly ending treatment with seeming indifference or hostility and with inadequate preparation or communication) that are further damaging and that add insult to injury (Dalenberg, 2000).

Therapist Honesty and Transparency in the Moment

Dalenberg (2000) conducted a unique survey of clients with trauma histories who had completed treatment to determine what they viewed as most and least helpful. Respondents indicated that therapists who were non-self-disclosing were the most difficult to relate to. Interestingly, this did not refer to the therapist's privacy about his or her personal life (although that is sometimes at issue) but rather the therapist's discomfort *with disclosing feelings in the moment and in the relationship*, especially with regard to anger. Respondents gave many examples of how therapist's anger had been acted out in ways that were passive–aggressive and even hostile. In fact, abrupt terminations without adequate notice, explanation, problem solving, or working through that lead to abandonments and other unethical behaviors are often due to the therapist's unacknowledged anger and resentment that has built over time.

It may take considerable courage for a therapist to admit to anger, but doing so has a number of readily identifiable benefits: It teaches that anger is an emotion like any other that can be managed through assertion and communication, that it does not have to be explosive and harmful, and that its resolution means that it does not simmer and come out in passive–aggressive and displaced ways. Clients with complex trauma gain a new perspective on relationships when they learn firsthand that they can be *angry and still maintain attachment*, in contrast to many experiences of the past in which anger was scathing and a prompt for criticism and for relational cutoff.

Doris

At one point in treatment, Doris's therapist realized she was feeling increasingly annoyed and angry about Doris's ongoing demands, challenges, and neediness. They felt never ending and even felt like they were escalating. The therapist sought a trauma-informed consultation in which she was able to vent her feelings away from Doris and was further able to strategize an approach. She decided to be direct in letting Doris know that she could not meet all of her needs in the way that Doris wanted, but that she understood their origin and would help Doris find other sources of support. For her part, Doris was surprised to learn of her therapist's discomfort, having thought that therapists were *supposed* to always be available and to not have any feelings about it—after all, that's why they chose their career. She was initially upset and felt criticized for being too needy (and therefore bad) but was then able to hear that she was not being *personally judged* but was being asked to make some *modifications to her behavior.* At that point in treatment, she had enough trust and experience with her therapist and had learned to differentiate between the personal and the behavioral to be able to be more flexible in her responses.

This case demonstrates that it is not simply the therapist's willingness to communicate personal feelings that is therapeutic. Honesty and emotional authenticity require more than spontaneous identification and expression of emotion. Instead, the therapist must engage in what has been described in the developmental psychology literature as "scaffolding." This term refers to the process of upgrading the therapeutic dialogue to higher levels of complexity, awareness, and connection regarding the client's capacities for feeling, reflection, personal agency, motivation, and so on (Wallin, 2007). Through this process, the therapist engages the client in reflecting on his or her own experience and models the process of mentalization. At the same time, the therapist engages in a parallel process of personal reflection, primarily outside the therapy session (not "on the clock" but on his or her own time), in order to be aware of and mindful about emotional responses and the meaning they have personally as well as in relation to the client. Therapists can express curiosity and encourage clients in developing their own in order to expand their self-exploration and their options beyond where they have been. In the process, curiosity elicits and encourages the consideration and implementation of change.

WORKING WITH DIFFERENT ATTACHMENT STYLES (STATES OF MIND) AND ISSUES

We now shift to a discussion of the client's attachment style or state of mind as it affects the process and technical aspects of the treatment and the therapist. As described by Westen, Thomas, Nakash, and Bradley (2006), the relevance of attachment theory and research to clinical practice is increasingly clear and attachment history is ever more related to personality styles and disorders. We earlier described the four predominant attachment styles associated with the client's formative relational experiences (these also have subcategories that might call for technical modifications; these are not discussed here but can be found in some of the references included in this section). As discussed in Chapter 4, these are assessed primarily through the Adult Attachment Interview (AAI; George, Kaplan, & Main, 1996), a measure of emotional regulation and interpersonal processes or other related measures such as the Attachment History Questionnaire (Hazan & Shaver, 1987). Information on the clinical application of the AAI and other attachment-based strategies is increasingly available (Crittenden & Landini, 2011; Steele & Steele, 2008).

To review: the four major classifications are: (1) secure; (2) insecure–preoccupied; (3) insecure–detached/dismissive/avoidant; and (4) insecure–disorganized/unresolved/dissociative. Discussed here are ways that these styles come forward in the clinical presentation and treatment relationship and strategies for working with each. As noted earlier, wherever possible, the goal is to assist the client in developing an "earned secure" style by providing a "safe base" in the therapy from which to explore him- or herself and others. The *treatment relationship is at once technique*, relational bond, and container; it provides modeling of relational response and containment for the client that promotes an expanded repertoire of feelings and expression (Kinsler et al., 2009; Wachtel, 2008; Wallin, 2007). Alexander and Anderson (1994) were the first to depict how clients with complex trauma (in this case, incest survivors) would present in treatment according to their predominant attachment style, and they offered strategies for working with them according to their styles. Recent articles and books by Brisch (2002); Crittenden and Landini (2011); Dozier, 1990; Muller (2009, 2010); Obegi (2008); Sable (2000); Steele and Steele (2008); Wallin (2007); and Wilkinson (2009) offer expanded discussion of attachment styles as they emerge in therapy, suggested treatment strategies by style, and preliminary clinical research findings that support this approach.

Secure Attachment Style

Although it might seem counterintuitive, some clients with complex trauma histories had secure relational attachment in their formative years and developed a resultant secure internal working model (IWM) and state of mind. Others were able to develop what has been identified as an "earned secure" style or substyle through later relationships with others (e.g., other relative, teacher or mentor, friend, spouse or partner) who provided an experience of secure attachment (Alexander & Anderson, 1994; Travis et al., 2001; Wallin, 2007). Depending on the type of trauma they experienced or were exposed to and its timing, intensity, chronicity, and accretion, securely attached individuals tend to have fewer developmental deficits and more resources to bring to bear in psychotherapy than do their insecure and disorganized counterparts. For example, they are less immediately and globally mistrustful of others, have a relatively healthy family and support system, have a generally positive self-concept and sense of self-worth, tend to be aware of and in touch with their emotions, have access to positive and negative memories, and tend to have positive and straightforward views of caregivers and authority figures and to be able to relate fairly well to them. This includes the therapist. They may also have fewer secondary elaborations of their symptoms and less need for the extremes of self-soothing. Per Stovall-McClough, Cloitre, and McClough (2008). They are likely to approach the evaluation process and treatment with the most cooperation and the least amount of ambivalence and to evoke in the evaluator or therapist strong feelings of empathy and compassion and a desire to help.

The course of treatment for the client with a secure or "earned secure" attachment style may be shorter as "compared to those with insecure attachment states of mind, an adult with a secure attachment is more likely to use help *effectively*, that is, in a way that confirms his or her previous experience" (Stovall-McClough et al., 2008, p. 322; authors' italics). This client requires less by way of stabilization, skill building, and other resourcing. He or she will likely move more directly into trauma processing and have less difficulty, particularly concerning self-determination and building a life and a future.

Insecure–Preoccupied Attachment Style

As the name implies, clients with this style of attachment are anxious and have a compulsive need for attachment and reassurance. Their attachment style is *hyperactivated*, and they have exaggerated affect and neediness; may present in ways that are demanding, chaotic, hysterical, illogical, and helpless; are sometimes uncooperative, and put excessive expectations on the therapist whom they idealize. They are often in the throes of self-doubt and have "merger hunger" with others, along with enormous fears of abandonment. They may be very difficult to comfort or to "settle down." When disappointed by the therapist in some way, they may be enraged, spiteful, and hostile, feelings that are not endearing and that push away the very person they are seeking to merge with. They are characterized as being continuously on guard and alert for indications of inconsistency or disinterest from others and heighten their affect as a means of maintaining attention. The case of **Doris** exemplifies this attachment style.

Their desperation and excessive neediness, along with impulsivity, poor judgment, low self-confidence, and a tendency to adapt to the expectations of others, may make these individuals quite vulnerable to revictimization, including by unethical or exploitive therapists. Alexander and Anderson (1994) wrote:

> In addition to feeling suffocated by the client's adulation, dependency, and fears of abandonment, the therapist is likely to feel overwhelmed by the unremitting quantity of crises and lack of self-protection presented by the client from this classification. The danger . . . is that the therapist will overreact to this understandable concern through excessive and intrusive caretaking, then reenacting the parent's pattern of retreating and ridiculing out of frustration and then, perhaps out of guilt, reengaging in an overly involved manner. . . . The therapist thus needs to be clear and comfortable about his/her own boundaries, power, and responsibility in the relationship lest any expression of ambivalence reinforce the client's feelings of rejection. While the therapist must consider the client's high-risk behaviors in terms of danger to self or other, the therapist is not able to control the client's behavior. The eventual goal of this therapeutic stance is to help the client develop her own internalized self-protection. (p. 670)

Therapists working with the preoccupied client further find it advisable to have boundaries and limits in place to invoke when the client is overdemanding and overly taxing. These can be used to help keep the therapist from being worn out and worn down, so it is directly in the interest of maintaining the treatment. Therapists can also suggest to the client that he or she seek additional sources of support in order to not overrely on one person to meet his or her myriad needs. Additionally, due to their tendency to exhaust or alienate others, clients may need to find varied support resources and to "rotate" between them (e.g., attending 12-step meetings or other self-help groups in addition to relying on friends and family members). Over time, and with consistency of support and attention, the preoccupied client may develop what Wallin (2007) termed "a mind of one's own," in the process learning that independence and self-sufficiency are not mutually exclusive of closeness with others. This client must learn to modulate his or her attachment needs and strategies by deactivating hyperattachment over time and with testing. This was the case with Sandra (described in Chapter 7), who, after spending many largely isolated years living in her parents' home, was able to become involved in volunteer work, establish an independent residence in a supported living apartment, and develop a network of friends with whom she could socialize.

Many of these clients may have a previous or current diagnosis of borderline personality and may play out the familiar relational push–pull or fuse or lose patterns and the heightened need to be special to the therapist. These may be the most likely clients to engage in an erotic or erotized transference with the therapist (described in the next chapter), especially but not exclusively when the client is female and the therapist male. As noted earlier, the client's attachment style and longings can result in a variety of revictimizations and misadventures, including in the therapy relationship. For this reason, therapists must remain mindful of their own attachment style and needs and the quality of their own lives and primary attachments, lest they lose their way and become overinvolved to the point of infatuation and sexual involvement.

Insecure–Detached/Dismissive/Avoidant Attachment Style

These clients tend to devalue or downplay the importance of relationships and are compulsively self-reliant, a style honed in childhood with parents who responded positively to the child's autonomy but not to the child's neediness, especially the need for nurturance and support. Many of these parents can be described as emotionally negligent, disengaged, or neglectful. In consequence, their children learned to fend for themselves and to be uncomfortable with intimacy, creating distance when a certain degree of closeness is achieved (their attachment style can be said to be *hypoactivated*). As adults, they are easily frustrated in relationships, not confident in the availability or consistency of others, are often experienced by others as hostile and critical, are extremely self-reliant, and are quite contradictory in their presentation. They may actively avoid therapy until they are desperate and unable to cope with their symptoms and life stresses; nevertheless, they begin treatment by minimizing their needs, having all the answers before they start, and disparaging the usefulness of therapy, the profession, and the likely helpfulness of the therapist. They are "world-class minimizers," adept at simultaneously denying the seriousness of their problems (past and current) and actively conveying high degrees of anxiety and distress that are denied and disavowed (i.e., "I got whupped almost every day but it was OK—that's how my mother let me know she loved me"; "My parents were always out drinking and we kids were left to fend for ourselves. We didn't mind, that's just the way it was"; "I'm totally exhausted by the chemo, but I had to do what she wanted because what else was I going to do? I did hard physical work on the house all weekend"; "You're going away for a week to a conference? Don't worry about me, I'm *fine* and I can *take care of myself*"—this said even by a client in the midst of a severe crisis).

Detached/dismissive clients tend to gloss over a lot, including their trauma history. Typically, they minimize it and its impact because they "refuse to be a victim" or because admitting to having had reactions causes them to view themselves as pathetic and as losers. They continue to dismiss their needs (from which they are alienated) because having needs would indicate weakness. Furthermore, if they expressed needs and these were not responded to, they would be devastated and would blame themselves rather than the person who responded poorly and disappointed them (Muller, 2010). This is an extremely common and a preemptive pattern in this attachment style, exemplified by the case of **Hector**. Wallin (2007) described the push–pull of these clients as a "catch-22":

> More often than not, such a patient begins treatment behaving as if the therapist either has little to offer or represents a threat that must be kept at bay. The Catch-22 here is that the patient's barriers against feeling make it impossible for him to feel much for the therapist, while the therapist's relative insignificance to the patient reinforces the barriers against feeling. Of course, this is the essence of the dismissing adult's defensive strategy in the face of his broader life problem. The patient's self-protective constriction of feeling and avoidance of closeness generate the emotional and relational difficulties that typically bring the patient to therapy. (p. 212)

The research team of Stovall-McClough et al. (2008) found that detached/dismissive clients were the "easiest" to evaluate and treat because they were so superficial and emotionally distant in their presentation making them easy to dismiss. Therapists must slowly and carefully engage them lest they end up supporting their avoidance (in a mutual process) or rejecting them out of dislike or frustration, processes that repeat prior episodes of nonresponse and abandonment. Instead, they must see the hurt and vulnerable child or the suffering adult inside the shut down or hostile, entitled, demeaning client who has learned to deactivate attachment as a means of self-protection. Rather than avoiding engagement, therapists are advised to actively connect but from a position of relative neutrality (not letting the client "get under the therapist's skin" in a way that results in rejection), to avoid power struggles as much as possible (yet to understand these struggles as a client's typical way of interacting with others that often results in alienation) and from a position of curiosity and curious exploration of these patterns with the client. Linehan's strategy of up-ending the client with an unexpected comment or response can serve to startle and shift clients like these from their defensive and closed position.

Chu (1998, 2011) advises the use of empathy *and* confrontation and the therapist's attunement to his or her own subjective feelings. These are clients who will likely not be comfortable with conventional therapeutic empathy (i.e., supportive and validating comments) and might be more responsive when the therapist is active in providing feedback on their typical relational behaviors (e.g., devaluation, idealization, control) especially pertaining to their impact on others. Indeed, an empathic understanding of these clients would suggest that their frame of reference is more akin to the former President Harry Truman's "show me" approach, and they would feel misunderstood by a therapist who is too "touchy-feely." The reframing of detachment as a reasonable means of self-protection in response to not being reliably tended to offers such a client understanding rather than criticism. From this position, the therapist can purposefully invite and challenge the client to move out of detachment and isolation and to accept available response and help (thereby engaging the attachment system; Muller, 2009, 2010). Treatment is also designed to address affect phobia and to identify, regulate, tolerate, and integrate previously unacknowledged feelings, particularly loss, grief, and shame.

The neurobiological substrate to working with these clients must be taken into consideration, as we have previously discussed. Their affect and behavior is consistent with an overdeveloped left hemisphere of the brain (involving linear logic and language) and an underdeveloped right hemisphere (involving nonverbal and intuitive communication and relational connections). Schore's (2003b) perspective is to relate to the client through the use of right-brain-to-right-brain communication that is largely implicit and nonverbal but that is then put into words that are accessible to these clients and that enable them to gradually access emotion over the course of therapy. A therapeutic stance of mindful presence assists attunement to the client's implicit nonverbal communications.

Disorganized/Dissociative/Unresolved Attachment Style

Dissociation is more likely to be correlated with this attachment style than with other categories as a result of intergenerational family dynamics involving gross inconsistency of care and response and repeated betrayal and trauma (Barach, 1991; Liotti, 1992). The parents, by virtue of their own unresolved history of trauma or loss, behave in ways that are unpredictable and inconsistent, both frightened by their own children or frightening to them (Main & Hesse, 1990). Children are placed in an attachment "double bind": the parent is at once the source of needed attachment and the source of abuse and pain (creatively labeled as "attack-ment" by Chefetz, n.d.). These clients are the most highly physically and emotionally dysregulated of all and tend to meet criteria for dissociative and posttraumatic stress disorders (chronic form) and avoidant, borderline, and self-defeating personality disorders. They are shame bound, see themselves in highly negative ways, and sincerely believe they were deserving of the abuse and neglect they suffered.

This dysregulation and the client's disintegration are highly apparent in the therapy (as discussed in the previous chapter), with clients behaving in unpredictable ways and having heightened emotional responses and almost no capacity to tolerate their feelings or to self-soothe. They are the most prone to externalize their distress and to self-medicate through a variety of addictive substances and behaviors, many of which involve risk and self-harm. All of these may be associated with particular states of mind. In the client with DID, some self-states operate out of the awareness of others and take over executive control. Therapists may be able to identify the disorganized/dissociative style through the lapses in the client's reasoning and discourse when under stress or when asked to describe their history and upbringing. They may present themselves incoherently, with their "story line" and emotional response "out of synch" with each other and quite fragmented. As mentioned previously, when discussing something painful or stressful, they might laugh or abruptly change the subject. Or, they might be prone to dissociate (or to switch into different part-selves, if they have DID) as a means of detaching or disengaging. What is more, through various defensive operations, these clients may project their overwhelming feelings onto their therapist, who is left "holding the bag," so to speak, to help them identify, decode, metabolize, and contain them.

Therapists must have patience and expect these clients to vacillate in terms of their integrative capacity (which is generally quite low, given the high propensity to dissociate and to use "primitive" defenses such as splitting and black-or-white, all-or-nothing, either–or forms of thinking, feeling, and relating to others), their self-compartmentalization and varied states of mind and self-states, and their ability to self-modulate and to engage in the treatment relationship. Like their detached/dismissive counterparts, they are likely to distance when they get close as a means of self-protection. It is therefore advisable for therapists to go slowly (especially early in treatment, until some stability has been achieved and skills have been developed) with care so as not to overchallenge these clients, as they can easily decompensate.

The treatment of relational trauma is at root of the unresolved client's symptoms. For these clients, *the therapy relationship is the therapy* (Kinsler et al., 2009; Schore, 2003b; Wallin, 2007). Treatment of these clients is rarely easy as it involves repeated testing of the therapist through enactments, direct challenges (e.g., "Why can't I have my gun with me here in therapy?"; "I dare you to hospitalize me"; "I'm really suicidal but I'm not going to tell you about my plan"), repeated episodes of crisis and self-harm (some of which may require extra monitoring, intensive safety planning, and inpatient stays), unpredictability, unreliability, ongoing chaos, repeated engagement in victimizing relationships, repeated retraumatization, and so on. Therapist patience is also called for in terms of the pace of the treatment and the tendency for repeated rounds of attunement–misattunement and relational repair in order for trust to begin to develop. If all of this weren't enough, given the degree to which they are dissociated from their bodies and physical sensations and are prone to self-neglect and self-punishment, these clients are the most likely to have a variety of chronic-stress-based physical problems and medical conditions and the least able to engage in appropriate and nurturing self-care and preventive medical treatment.

These are also the clients most in need of the full three-phase treatment model (Loewenstein & Welzant, 2010; Van der Hart et al., 2006). They also often benefit from a pretreatment phase that teaches the "rules of the road" and "lay of the land" of psychotherapy and that builds motivation for treatment (see Linehan, 1993). Following that orientation phase, the major preliminary tasks are psychoeducation, motivation enhancement, and the related teaching of skills for emotional regulation and life stabilization. The maintenance of safety and building of a support network are also priorities. Exposure-based techniques after a period of stabilization (and imaginal exposure in particular, per the findings of Stovall-McClough et al., 2008) may be the most effective treatment to counter ingrained avoidance and dissimulation. Through their ability to provide containment and "hold affect" and ultimately to put the trauma into words to create a more cohesive personal narrative, therapists work against dissociation and discontinuities, in the process helping the client develop greater self-integration and improved self-worth. Successful processing, however it occurs, allows the experiencing of traumatic memories without reliving them or being retraumatized by them. Harvey's (1996) treatment goal of the client having authority over his or her memories of the trauma and of him- or herself via mindfulness and mentalization comes to mind in this respect.

As a caveat, it is worth noting that clients with any of the other insecure attachment working models can, when highly stressed or in crisis, shift to a more disorganized state in their relationships and relatedness. This was the case for **Doris** when she became terrified of abandonment early in therapy and several times thereafter when reminded of past losses or rejections and during an EMDR session. Thus it is important for therapists to be alert to shifts from insecure to frankly disorganized attachment in any client with a complex trauma history. They must be prepared to intervene with increased support for basic stabilization and safety, as well as titrating the amount and intensity of trauma or emotion processing when the shift occurs. In a related vein, therapists should be aware that different part-selves in DID may have different attachment styles, requiring flexible conterresponses on the part of the therapist.

Attachment Styles of Therapists and Clients

The therapist's attachment style is obviously significant to the treatment outcome for clients with complex trauma. As noted above, various writers have suggested that, in order to provide security of attachment, therapists who operate from a secure/autonomous state of mind or their own "earned secure" style will be the most successful (Dozier, Cue, & Barnett, 1994). A secure style allows them to function with flexibility and to behave in ways that are consistent, "steady-state," and predictable for the client but that are *noncomplementary* to the client's predominant attachment style. The therapist must resist the normal pull to respond to the client's style in ways that are complementary or consistent in order to provide a different model of relationship that begins to challenge the client's predominant IWM; however, the therapist must also match his or her responses to the client's style so the client can be understood and accommodated (Dolan, Arnkoff, & Glass, 1993).

It is for this reason that the initial approach must "match" the client's style but that later responses on the therapist's part must be from an unmatched style that challenges expectations and past experiences. This is a quintessential support-and-challenge strategy. The *noncomplementary style and response are critical.* Unless the client's predominant style and expectations about relationships are put to question through different interactional patterns and responses and through other forms of feedback on the part of the therapist, there is no impetus for change. The therapist challenges the client's beliefs and rigid expectations about relationships and provides an opportunity for a corrective emotional experience (Bernier & Dozier, 2002). Take, for example, the therapist's interactions with a detached/dismissive client. The therapist must resist responding with disregard or contempt (in a "tit for tat" or "in-kind" reaction to the client's verbalizations) or colluding with his or her avoidance but instead must stretch to understand the client. Dismissal or collusion on the therapist's part will likely result in the client's prematurely leaving therapy without having received help or having developed alternative ways of coping and relating to others. Instead, the client's self-reliance and detached/dismissive stance toward others will be reinforced.

To counter the client's predominant operating style, the therapist must gently (but sometimes very directly) and persistently challenge the defenses that undergird it, while encouraging less detachment and a deepening of emotional awareness through consistency and predictability of response. The therapist helps by not buying the client's "cover story" (often involving the ANP; Van der Hart et al., 2006) and by identifying and acknowledging emotions, especially emotional pain, but in ways that are supportive and modulated to the client's capacities and tolerance. In the cases of **Doris** and **Hector**, therapist responses that were contrary to those they were expecting caused them to have different relational experiences that "got their attention." Over time and with repeated experiencing of calm, steady, supportive responses and interest on the part of their therapists, Doris and Hector were able to begin to change not only their own reactions but their core beliefs about themselves and about trustworthy relationships (i.e., their attachment working models).

Dozier et al. (1994) found that a secure style on the part of the therapist is not without unique subjective elements or variations. They commented that the therapist's own secure style can vary significantly in terms of the dismissive-versus-preoccupied dimension. Some therapists operate from a predominant comfort zone of keeping more distance (more on the dismissive/detached end), and some develop more closeness with others, including clients (more on the preoccupied end). These dimensions can affect how the therapist responds and it is therefore good practice to have some awareness about his or her predominant propensity toward one substyle or another. If one of these is the therapist's actual attachment style, it becomes all the more important to monitor. For example, the therapist who is preoccupied runs the risk of being gratified by the preoccupied client and becoming overinvolved and providing too much, rather than encouraging the client's development and independence. Alternatively, the same therapist might be more irritated and quick to end treatment with the dismissive and unappreciative client, as this style is so ungratifying. The therapist who is dismissive, on the other hand, must be mindful regarding his or her response to the attachment needs of the preoccupied client. This client will be experienced as fawning and insatiable, resulting in a tendency to detach rather than remaining in closer proximity by the therapist who struggles to achieve his or her comfort zone. Engagement versus detachment opens the process to examination and discussion.

Many therapists have their own histories of trauma. This does not prevent them from professional effectiveness, but, in order to do so, their posttraumatic adaptations must have been resolved to a degree to which they are not vulnerable to vicarious trauma and to being continuously triggered by their clients (Briere, 1996; Courtois, 1988, 2010). However, some previously traumatized therapists have a predominantly preoccupied, dismissive attachment style, and others have a disorganized/dissociative/unresolved style, each of which undermines their capacity to offer effective and healthy relationship-based treatment. Those with disorganized relational working models especially will be hard-pressed to respond to their clients in ways that are consistent and reliable. They will be easily triggered, and their own symptoms will tend to emerge and interfere with their ability to achieve a balance of empathy and constructive challenging in therapy sessions. Their personal issues will tend to seep into or color their perceptions of and interactions with clients. These therapists and their trainers and supervisors have a special responsibility to ensure that they get the assistance they need to function competently. Personal psychotherapy and ongoing guidance from a therapist who serves as a mentor, consultant, or supervisor are important under these circumstances in order to help the therapist to monitor personal issues as they arise and to be selective in working with less challenging populations and issues. When the therapist's mental health issues or lack of skills or capacity interfere with emotional engagement and modeling of secure attachment working models, psychotherapy is likely to be ineffective—or even iatrogenic, especially for clients whose complex trauma histories have involved coping with emotionally compromised caregivers.

Finally, as discussed earlier, the disorganized/dissociative/unresolved client is likely to be the most challenging type for therapists of all attachment styles because both hypo- and hyperattachment strategies will be used, often chaotically in ways that are seemingly unpredictable. The ever-changing presentations will likely vex the therapist, who will additionally be challenged by the vagaries of the posttraumatic and dissociative relational matrix. The therapist's attention to remaining personally on an even keel in response to the client's changeability is recommended and therapist mindfulness can certainly help. Psychiatrist Richard Kluft's notable comment in this regard is that he tries to "bore his clients into health," not literally (!) but by remaining constant and unvarying in terms of schedule, routine, presentation, personal equanimity, and responsiveness.

CONCLUSION

The greatest challenge in psychotherapy with complex trauma survivors is not to deliver a specific evidence-based intervention—although that can be extremely important—but to develop an understanding and a way of communicating with each client that helps him or her feel secure enough to take on the challenges of self-examination and personal growth. To do this, therapists must empathically come to know their clients and themselves—and establish a therapeutic relationship that at once expresses and is grounded in this personal knowledge. Survivors are used to dealing with people who do not know them (or who are not emotionally intelligent or aware of their own inner lives), and who, as a result, are prone to be neglectful, abusive, or simply disorganized and who themselves are emotionally unavailable and needy. When a therapist is able to "walk the walk" (and dance the dance) of empathy and attachment security with a client for whom this behavior is radically unfamiliar, clients' paradigms for understanding people, the world, and themselves can change equally radically as can their ability to relate to others. This then infuses each phase of therapy with a degree of emotional impact and security that makes it possible for even profoundly psychically injured individuals to stabilize and function safely and more effectively, and meaningfully process trauma-related memories and emotions, and begin to build satisfying lives.

CHAPTER 10

Transference and Countertransference in Complex Trauma Treatment

In this final chapter, we address in more detail how psychic and interpersonal dynamics associated with victimization and resultant reactions additionally affect the treatment relationship and what therapists can do to handle these issues effectively. We describe how complex trauma can be reenacted in the *transference and countertransference* and how therapists can be drawn into a number of common trauma-related countertransference positions and roles that are complementary to their clients' transference reactions. We use the concept of *projective identification* to describe how therapists can understand and respond to posttraumatic reenactments using their own (emotional and somatic) feeling states as guides. None of these reactions and processes is "bad" or problematic per se but rather serve as useful (albeit implicit and thus coded) information that may be the client's best way of communicating. In the final section, we describe various role enactments engaged in by therapist and client that are common in the treatment of complex trauma and offer ways to understand and to use them productively.

The therapist's attitude, as well as his or her own history of attachment and other forms of trauma and the degree to which they have been resolved, play a major role in the ability to successfully treat complex trauma. Although societal attitudes are slowly shifting with increased knowledge and recognition, they unfortunately remain largely disparaging and negative. Therapists are subject to the same stereotypes and biases and are thus influenced by the cultural surround and organizational culture in addition to their more personal reactions. Other challenges arise when therapists are castigated by peers for having empathy for and treating these clients (especially those who carry a borderline personality diagnosis or who are highly dissociative). Simultaneously and in apparent contradiction to this disparagement, they may find that all cases of trauma in their agency or community are assigned to them, a practice that can result in their becoming overloaded, exhausted, resentful, and angry (in addition to being vicariously traumatized by their clients' stories and their peers' behaviors). Identifying trauma-informed colleagues for consultation and emotional support is especially important in such a circumstance, as is the move toward trauma-informed services (Bloom & Farragher, 2010; Harris & Fallot, 2001).

TRANSFERENCE THEMES, ISSUES, AND REACTIONS

Gartner (1999) offered this succinct definition: "*Transference* . . . refers to all feelings and reactions to the therapist, conscious and unconscious, enacted or not, reality- or fantasy-based, that originate in and are *located in the patient*" (p. 234; italics added). Concerning transference and attachment styles, Brisch (2002) added: "Bowlby proceeded from the assumption that early-childhood representation of self and parents with their corresponding attachment and exploratory strategies are reactivated in the transference" (p. 79); this is a stance found in object relations theory as well (Fonagy et al., 2002). Transference issues are seen as arising from personal reactions of the individual that originate in his or her formative relational experiences with caretakers that have been internalized. Although clients with complex trauma are aware of many feelings and issues in their current lives, the fact that these feelings and associated beliefs are "transferred" from relational dilemmas that occurred implicitly earlier in life is largely outside of their awareness. It is usually obvious to therapists that something more is troubling these clients than can be accounted for by current life circumstances and relationships. So part of the therapeutic challenge is determining what is being "transferred" and how best to help clients recognize what is disconnected. When complex trauma is in the picture, this challenge includes determining how to help clients to distinguish trauma-infused beliefs and body and emotion states from the beliefs and feelings they experience when not in a posttraumatic or dissociative condition. This then involves the process of identifying and modifying their ways of thinking and feeling about themselves, other people, and the world through the use of cognitive-behavioral and affect-based therapeutic strategies, their physical and visceral sensations through experiential and sensorimotor therapies, and their relationships through interpersonal approaches to individual treatment and group, couple, and family modalities.

Just as transference reactions may be the best way the client can cope with and implicitly communicate about extremely threatening and distressing past experiences and current states of body and mind, countertransference responses may be the therapist's best way of understanding the client's dilemmas and countercommunicating. "Counter" transference, as the name implies, is the therapist's own transference reactions to those of the client. If unrecognized and unexamined, countertransference can lead to nontherapeutic or even harmful iatrogenic actions by therapists based on their own emotional biases, conflicts, or attachment or trauma history (Greenson, 1967). The problem of hurtful or even harmful countertransference-based actions by therapists is even more acute when clients' transference involves intense posttraumatic distress, such as feelings of rage, disgust, or hate (Winnicott, 1963). However, when therapists take steps to be aware of their countertransference issues and to regulate the strong emotional reactions that accompany their activation, these can be invaluable sources of information and lead them to an empathy with and understanding of their clients.

Traumatic Transference

According to Spiegel (1986), *traumatic transference* occurs when "the patient unconsciously expects that the therapist, despite overt helpfulness and concern, will covertly exploit the patient for his or her own narcissistic gratification" (p. 72) in much the same way parent(s) or other abusers did. Per Chefetz (1997), traumatic transference "is a given in the therapeutic situation of persons with post-traumatic disorders" (p. 259). Through this transference, the traumatized client communicates his or her fears and expectations of being revictimized and used by the therapist in some way. This is a difficult transference for therapists to accept and to tolerate. Another aspect of traumatic transference has to do with the treatment process itself. Although intended to provide help and relief, it might be experienced instead as abuse or pain that is being deliberately inflicted by the uncaring and even sadistic therapist. This, too, may elicit strong response in the therapist, whose objective is to provide help. Treatment must be undertaken with due consideration for the significance of issues such as these. They should not be minimized or dismissed but rather should be used to elicit more about the client's past experiences that would result in such negative expectations of others. A major challenge is for the therapist to understand how the treatment context and his or her role (as a stand-in for parents and other authority figures who were absent or abusive) might feel dangerous and hostile while he or she is concurrently working to create a safe enough environment for the material to come forward for identification and discussion.

Hypervigilance in relationships with others (including the therapist) is therefore to be expected, as these clients characteristically are on the lookout for ways that someone might take advantage of them. Chefetz (1997) noted how this can result in the therapist getting caught in the countertransference trap of proving him- or herself "better than" abusive and neglectful others and, in the process, avoiding negative emotions. It behooves the therapist to acknowledge base emotions and motives, the "shadow" (Kopp, 1980) and the related potential of all humans to have these emotions and to be exploitive and abusive. It is ironic but understandable that when therapists are able to accept and acknowledge such feelings, clients may experience them as more real and therefore more trustworthy. Therapists are also less prone to act on their feelings when they have identified and even embraced them.

Traumatic transference reactions may emerge in indirect or paradoxical ways. The client with complex trauma who seems only to have a positive transference and who idealizes the therapist as "the best" may be superficially compliant, eager to please and not alienate the therapist. This may, however, be a disguised traumatic transference in which the therapist is reacted to as a perpetrator who must be catered to, excused, and protected in order to avoid eliciting a wrathful reprisal if normal feelings of disappointment, fear, hurt, or anger are felt and (indirectly or directly) expressed. Defenses such as denial, repression, or reaction formation may be employed to avoid recognizing previously forbidden negative feelings. The therapist who can appropriately (i.e., without any direct or indirect blame, criticism, or retaliation) acknowledge negative or other thorny feelings as they emerge in the transference and countertransference and who communicates to the client that any and all feelings are acceptable and expectable provides a valuable model and a responsive context. As noted in the previous chapter, learning that individuals can be angry (or can have any other emotion) with one another and remain in a relationship is often eye-opening and growth-producing for survivor clients. It is a clear counter to the relational lessons from insecure/disorganized and otherwise abusive backgrounds in which disparagement, invalidation, and emotional and relational cutoffs were the norm rather than respect, encouragement, and discussion, resolution, and repair.

In a similar vein, the therapist should expect to be drawn into posttraumatic and related abandonment and rejection reenactments. For example, as noted at different points throughout this book, clients who were taken advantage of when an offender used a relationship against them (the process of "attack-ment" described by Chefetz, n.d.) may experience the therapist's empathy as dangerous rather than comforting. Quite ironically, it is at the moment of increased attachment and vulnerability that the relationship is most fraught with associations of abuse, causing clients to self-protectively disengage, a process that may be so automatic as to be outside of conscious awareness. At those points in therapy, the most accurately empathic communication by a therapist is a frank acknowledgement that the client's past experiences understandably have made kindness or compassion seem to be dangerous or deceptive. This can be followed by a clarification that one goal of treatment is to understand these reactions and their origin and another is to assist the client in developing knowledge and skills to make fully informed choices about whom to trust. The client's reactions are not perceived as threats to the therapy, a personal affront to the therapist, or a source of conflict between them, but as a first step in learning to differentiate safe, reliable, and trustworthy others from those who are not.

Detachment and withdrawal through emotional shutdown and through other interruptions, such as missing appointments and nonpayment of fees, might signal the client's self-protection in the face of perceived danger rather than noncompliance and hostility (although these, too, are possible responses). The therapist must have sufficient maturity and emotional resources to experience these disruptions and their associated negative transference reactions with some degree of composure and not make assumptions about them before bringing them to the client's attention for discussion and for the reestablishment of boundaries. This approach usually helps the therapist in not taking reactions personally or in retaliating in response.

In yet another difficult relational transfer, the surfacing and discussion of painful emotional material might cause the client to suspect that the therapist's interest is feigned and that, in fact, he or she is gratified by causing the client emotional pain. The identification of this type of transference must be made with sensitivity to its origin and again without the therapist taking it personally or striking back. Rather, the therapist is again called on to be self-possessed and to demonstrate to the client (often repeatedly), through his or her actions and reactions, empathic attunement to the pain rather than gratification in causing it. Thus the therapist walks a fine line in needing to approach traumatic or otherwise emotionally painful material (in some detail and not colluding in its avoidance) while respecting the emotional toll the process takes on the client. This calls for sensitivity to the range of the client's emotional capacities and pacing of the treatment.

Erotic Transference

Transference love (or friendly or affectionate feelings toward the therapist) was initially regarded as positive and can be seen as a precursor concept to erotic transference. Erotic as used here connotes *desire* and the *need to be special* rather than its sexual counterpart (although it can certainly be sexualized). Clients with complex trauma understandably long for something most did not have: to be seen as special and to be treated in kind. Quoting Chefetz (1997): "The erotic transference may be experienced as an intense, relentless demand to change the therapeutic relationship in response to the patient's special need" (p. 256). It manifests when the therapist feels "coaxed, enticed, lured, tempted, attracted, persuaded, charmed, corrupted or fascinated" (p. 256) by the client, resulting in shifts in the treatment frame in order to meet the client's longings and needs. It may only be identified once the therapist "comes to" and realizes that this client is being treated differently from others, sometimes after boundaries have been crossed and/or after identification in consultation or supervision. Gradual identification and verbalization of the client's need may be very helpful for the client, who can then own it and its legitimacy and resultant feelings (often grief and loss at not having been treated as special or with respect), while the therapist pulls back into the established treatment frame. It is not the therapist's job to make up for past losses but to help the client own and grieve them (Calof, 1987; Courtois, 1988, 2010).

When the transference is eroticized in the form of more direct sexual intention and behavior by the client, this sexualization may be a reenactment of sexual abuse or it may be an extension of the longing to be loved, prized, and admired as special, to give the therapist a unique gift of self, or to be in a special relationship. Conversely, a sexualized transference may have less to do with love and affection than with power and dominance as a manifestation of the client's history of relationships with caregivers or authority figures in which sexual activity and involvement played a prominent role. Thus, being dominated by the therapist and being in a dual sexual relationship might be expected as the price of attention or because it is an expectable aspect of any relationship. Sexualized transference may be a way for the client to induce the therapist to view him or her unconditionally available and/or as defiled or degraded. Attempts at sexualization may be the best way to test the therapist's trustworthiness and integrity, as we discuss next. The universal proscription against therapists reciprocating any sexual advances by a client or initiating such advances is a crucial boundary protecting the client from betrayal and violation.

Betrayal, Disillusionment, and Mistrust

Interpersonal betrayal and exploitation in the most significant attachment relationships adversely influences the ability to trust and creates enormous disillusionment in complex trauma survivors. It is for these reasons that the therapist can never take trust for granted, even that of the idealizing, dependent/preoccupied, or compliant client who professes unconditional trust or even after therapy has been ongoing for a period of time and a high degree of trust has developed. In order to be appropriately vigilant about trust, the therapist should be especially attentive to any aspect of the therapy that raises questions about his or her intentions and integrity and should make every attempt to be emotionally transparent in the moment and scrupulously honest.

Throughout the course of therapy, the client may consciously or unconsciously test the therapist in attempts to reinforce the belief that no one really cares or is truly trustworthy. While simultaneously craving it, the typical client with complex trauma fears the therapist's caring due to his or her predominantly negative self-perceptions and fears increased vulnerability to possible judgment and criticism, ultimately leading to abandonment, rejection, and reprisal. Such a relational trajectory may be seen as inevitable to the client who fears being seen as the client judges him or herself as rotten at the core and then as secrets related to the past are disclosed. Clients who have been repeatedly subjected to double-bind communication tend to place therapists in double binds that replicate those from their own troubled childhoods. Having had to defend themselves psychically against betrayal and abandonment from an early age, these clients are acutely perceptive about other people's points of psychic weakness, conflict, or pain. Thus, in their own repetition of "attack-ment" (Chefetz, n.d.), it is not uncommon for them to "zero in" on their therapist's most vulnerable personal issues when testing his or her ability to maintain integrity in the face of either opportunities to be seduced or exploited (e.g., when a client makes provocative erotic innuendos or direct sexual invitations) or assaults on personal and professional integrity, competence, and worth (e.g., interrogations by a client regarding the therapist's financial or ethical practices). Therapists, for their part, must do their best not to personalize this testing, even when it includes vitriolic and apparently irrational *ad hominem* accusations. Although the emotional turmoil engendered by these types of "tests" can challenge any therapist's poise and focus, the transference can be used to better understand the client's schemas about self and others.

As the therapy progresses and the client delves more deeply into salient relational issues or as crises develop inside or outside of therapy, transferential testing and resultant crises in trust should be expected to intensify or resurface. *Crises, by definition, are times when the need for proximity to the caregiver or attachment figure is greatest.* Anxiety develops concerning abandonment and being let down, which would replicate past experience. A crisis can provide the therapist with a singular opportunity to demonstrate trustworthiness by remaining responsive, available, and consistent. This presents the client with a relational experience opposite from what has been previously experienced and therefore expected. This has great potential to challenge and disrupt ongoing relational assumptions and schemas and to replace them with new ones.

An even greater trust problem for clients with complex trauma is trusting themselves, their own perceptions and reality, behaving in ways that are trustworthy and then believing that they are trustworthy. They often live with the expectation that others will hold them in the same contempt in which they hold themselves and, as a result, will treat them poorly and with disregard. Feeling undeserving of positive attention, they fear that sooner or later the therapist will discover their essential badness. They further expect a reenactment of any nonprotection, blame, or disparagement they previously experienced. *Because of who they are*, they fear that the therapist will shun and castigate them.

The disconfirmation of self and the restructuring of reality that are hallmarks of interpersonal trauma are reflected in the therapy, with the client constantly second-guessing his or her memories and emotions, all the while questioning personal sanity. The therapist's task is to assist in re-contextualizing these profound self-doubts and self-accusations in light of the exploitation, abandonment, coercion, and losses of the past. This approach supports the client by helping her or him to recognize that the intensity of current distress is understandable as a posttraumatic reaction or adaptation, in the process encouraging the identification and development of the client's self through the expression and reintegration of what was previously split off and through direct emotional spport.

Interpersonal and Intimacy Difficulties

Difficulties developing satisfactory and nurturing relationships can be a lifelong issue. Some clients (especially those with a detached/dismissive style) defend against the possibility of any more hurt or betrayal by cutting themselves off through hypoattachment. Their attitude may be expressed as "nobody/nothing will hurt me because I'm not going to put myself in the position of allowing anyone in. I can take care of myself. I'm fine, I don't need anybody." These self-sufficient individuals are typically isolated and withdrawn and might be indifferent to others or aggressive and abrasive in their interactions. It may be difficult, if not impossible, for them to accept positive regard when it is forthcoming from anyone, much less the therapist. These clients may do everything in their power to sabotage the feedback or relationship, reverse it, or flee from it. The therapist must maintain an awareness of engaging with a relationally injured and betrayed individual who is fearful (and even terrified) of engagement with anyone, especially an authority figure (and much less in a confined private setting in which self-disclosure is expected to occur) and must gradually encourage engagement without reinforcing fear of the disengagement/flight response.

To manage the anxiety of waiting for the "bad" to happen, some clients make it happen by engaging in self-defeating behavior, behaving aggressively, or otherwise manipulating the situation to bring about the expected response: "If it's going to happen anyway, I might as well make it happen so that I'm in control and I get it over with"; "If I'm going to be left anyway, I'll leave first; that way, I'll have control and it won't hurt as much." Self-sabotage can occur in many areas of life, in relationships with family members and friends, in school or work settings, as a way of defending against the anxiety associated with doing well or as a contradictory means of maintaining control and thereby maintaining safety. Even when they are obviously successful, these clients tend to disavow their own accomplishments and abilities and describe themselves as imposters. Furthermore, they discount the positive and seek ways (often unconsciously) to reverse it. Due to ingrained negative self-beliefs or the fear of being seen as selfish, the client may additionally disallow or renounce any needs or desires and respond to compliments and other positive feedback with anxiety, guilt, and consternation. He or she may diminish or externalize credit for all accomplishments in order not to draw attention from others (another way not to be selfish).

Another complication is that many of these clients have learned to present a false self (ANP) to the world as a means of avoiding distressing emotions and memories (EP). The client may appear to be engaged in the treatment when, in fact, he or she is only working on surface issues without internalizing them or actually making changes. Dissociative clients, in particular, describe not being able to remember what was said from session to session, keeping information out of awareness as a way of protecting themselves, and rejecting the possibility that they can establish and maintain personal control. In such cases, it is important for the therapist to serve as an "auxiliary ego" and "memory trace" early in treatment, to assist the client in activating her or his own working memory and long-term memory retrieval capacities, which have been taken "off line" by dissociation and avoidance. This does *not* mean encouraging clients to try to remember traumatic or other formative events from earlier in life in order to "restore" their memories or to regain "lost" or "repressed" memories. It is not the content of memories that is the issue, but instead the ability to retrieve and retain pertinent autobiographical information in order to become "known" to the self and more cohesive. Retrieving distant memories becomes increasingly possible as the client is able to engage in here-and-now memory processes that support increased self-awareness.

An opposite style is evident in some clients who inflate their abilities and sense of self with exaggerated competence, entitlement, and grandiosity to counter their feelings of depression, powerlessness, and "badness." Some may express anger and bitterness that their skills and talents have not been recognized or nurtured and may even use this fact to rationalize any lack of success or ability to achieve personal goals. A narcissistically inflated sense of self further defends against fear associated with being put to the test and developing relationships with others, as a type of self-fulfilling prophecy. Grandiosity and entitlement can be used to set the self apart in a superior way that alienates or intimidates others, including the therapist, in the interest of reinforcing a sense of being different, usually with the unintended effect of intensifying loneliness and isolation.

Interaction patterns such as these make clients needy of affection, nurturance, and attention, hungry for emotional resources that are viewed as available only from outside. The therapist is challenged with a client who does not trust or feel deserving of a good relationship and who unconsciously sabotages one as it develops and yet needs (and paradoxically actually expects to receive) exactly the nurturance that is most feared. Additionally, the intensity and sometimes the instability of the client's engagement can provoke strong counterreactions. The client is faced with a painful dilemma, one that the therapist must work at understanding and empathically reflect back. In order to recover from the traumatic psychic injury, the client must tolerate and allow the development of a reparative human relationship. Complicating the dynamic further is that many clients are exquisitely attuned to the reactions and feelings of others. Some describe themselves as radars and chameleons, constantly scanning for problems and changing behavior to accommodate the needs of others or to escape perceived danger and interpersonal conflict. Minor mood or behavioral changes in others are registered, often unconsciously, resulting in an instantaneous shift in response. Moreover, changes in others (which in reality may have nothing to do with the client) may be personalized or misattributed. With honest feedback from the therapist about his or her reactions and responses, the client has the opportunity to become aware of biased perceptions and appraisals and to change them.

Guilt, Complicity, and Responsibility

Many clients do not realize the extent to which they make themselves the guilty one, usually the *only* guilty one, and confound their guilt with their very identity and existence. They may continuously apologize for themselves and take a deferential stance with others, including the therapist. Many blame themselves for not having been able to say no or otherwise not having prevented their mistreatment or that of others. Their guilt also results from having been blamed and made a scapegoat and from the internalization of what they were told. Guilt may be the cover emotion that masks other associated emotions, such as sadness, shame, anger, and grief. Finally, they might be carrying guilt for what they did, as well as what they did not do, and for how they coped, especially with such issues as substance abuse, self-harm, harm of others, and suicidal gestures and attempts.

The survivor client may feel a combination of love (trauma bonding), unrequited loyalty, and hate toward the abuser(s) or involved others and may fear losing the good parts of the relationship if responsibility for abuse is directed at the guilty party. A client's protectiveness of the perpetrator may also be due to role reversal or "parentification," coupled with an overdeveloped sense of responsibility and misguided loyalty. The client may experience anxiety and a sense of being disloyal when giving up the role of "protector of the family or community and of its secrets." In discussing these issues, the therapist must not scapegoat the abuser or others even while not condoning abusive behavior, remaining mindful of the strength of trauma bonding and the pull of ambivalent attachment and loyalty (even when undeserved and unrequited).

Secondary Secrets

A particular transference may be most related to sexual victimization. Further confusion about feelings of guilt and responsibility develop in the child or adolescent who experienced *sexual pleasure*, *personal power*, or other reactions as part of the abuse and/or who sought revenge or to hurt others by seeking out contact and "willingly" engaging in the abuse with perpetrators or by perpetrating against others. These issues are the *secondary secrets* or "*secrets within the trauma secret*" (Courtois, 1988, 2010) that can have a very powerful hold. By virtue of strong feelings of shame associated with them, they might only be disclosed late in treatment. Their identification is essential in order both to lift the "veil of secrecy" that can stalemate therapeutic progress and to empower the client to reconsider beliefs about her- or himself that have been locked in by the combination of abuse and keeping secrets. When these issues finally emerge, clients may spontaneously disclose that these were their most closely shielded feelings and issues. Their exposure and resolution are therefore exquisitely sensitive.

Issues of Sexual Pleasure and Other Sexual Responses

Some abusers take great pleasure in the victim's sexual response, orgasm, and ejaculation. These may be used to support the rationalization that the victim enjoyed the abuse and as a means of coercion by inducing self-doubt, self-blame, or confusion. As a result, sexually abused clients may bring into the therapeutic relationship the belief that they must use sexuality as a way of gratifying or acquiescing to the needs of caregivers. Alternatively, they may believe that sexual behavior can or should be used to achieve power in relationships. They may interact in a sexualized manner in therapy as a conscious or unconscious abuse reenactment intended to reduce their emotional vulnerability.

The therapist who is unaware of this possibility or insensitive to its meaning may make the mistake of interpreting sexualization as seduction and attempt to deal with it simply by insisting that the client dress or act "more appropriately." Yet, the psychic and relational dilemma(s) that led the client to behave in a sexualized way should be the therapeutic focus. Just as it is essential for the therapist to insist on appropriate behavior on the part of the client, so too must he or she be scrupulous in maintaining appropriate therapeutic boundaries and roles. Judith Herman (1992b) counseled therapists to "respectfully refuse the client's invitation to become another sadistic abuser." *The responsibility for proper boundary management rests entirely with the therapist*, who has the ethical and professional duty to not exploit the client in any way, to protect the client's welfare, and to help him or her to develop the capacity and confidence to do so by recognizing traumatic reenactments. A protective, nonexploitive, and awareness-enhancing therapeutic environment is imperative for the client to experience how it is possible to be in a relationship not based on sexual interaction, sexual favors, or coercion. This foundation provides a basis for the client to recognize and choose intimate personal relationships in which feelings of sexual attraction and longing can be explored and safely experienced.

Hyperresilience and Parentified Caretaking

Some clients appear to be virtually invulnerable (i.e., superman or superwoman) and to be all things to all people, while juggling multiple roles and responsibilities and continuing to be self-effacing and deferential. Through hyperattunement to the needs of others, they care for and protect other, less functional or more vulnerable people. The outward indomitability tends to be an authentic (and admirable) positive quality rather than simply a facade, yet these individuals often tend to harbor (and fear acknowledging) deep feelings of guilt, shame, and inadequacy despite their, at times, remarkable ability to overcome many kinds of adversity. They often drastically underestimate their actual ability to maintain control, coming to view their abilities and personal worth either as a burden that they are fated to bear or as a sham and a mere defense against an ever-present and inevitable descent back into the chaos experienced earlier in their lives. Their caretaking may mask other and less positive feelings (such as rage and hostility), keep feelings of depression at bay, or may be due to their close identification with the underdog and the desire to provide others with better than they received. What they did not receive may make them exquisitely attuned to the needs of others.

Selfless (or self-sacrificing) caretaking of others can likewise serve as an overlearned way to manage and limit intimacy by preventing anyone from getting close. It is fairly typical for these clients to become involved with dependent, immature individuals who want someone to take care of them (at one end of the spectrum) or those who are cold, indifferent, dismissive, and/or abusive and who take much but give little in return (at the other). Whatever the style, reciprocity is lacking, and clients' needs are neither acknowledged nor met (by themselves as well as by others). These clients may seek help only when totally overwhelmed and desperate, usually when faced with multiple crises. They tend to be embarrassed and ashamed when seeking treatment because they feel they have failed. Indeed, seeking help puts them in an unaccustomed and even terrifying position that they interpret as meaning that "everything is falling apart" or "my true incompetence or worthlessness has finally been exposed."

It is left for the therapist to suggest a middle ground between these diametrically opposite views of self (i.e., as invincible and irreproachable vs. as powerless and reprehensible) and others. The therapist must take care not to be lulled by the client's presentation of being high functioning, pleasant, acquiescent, and caring at all times. Although these attributes are real and should not be dismissed as mere cover-ups or manipulations, they nevertheless *do* cover up emotions, beliefs, and tendencies that might be frightening, disorganizing, and appalling to the client. He or she can be extremely charming and convincing in manipulating others to overlook personal foibles and instead to be experienced as "all good." The cost to the client of using these real personal strengths to cover up doubts, fear, hurt, anger, and shame is a critical therapeutic focus. However, because therapy in this sense is akin to a public unveiling of the Wizard of Oz, it is important to help clients gradually recognize and accept their troubling feelings, thoughts, and impulses as real but manageable and not as a complete undoing of their self-worth or their overly positive persona. This is another reworking of the ANP (Van der Hart et al., 2006) in which the client's posttraumatic adaptation is recognized but is also dismantled in a way that allows him or her to control actions and interactions rather than to continue being compulsively driven by avoidance.

Another example of this transference pattern occurs when the client (usually one who is insecure or preoccupied) idealizes the therapist as the all-good and all-knowing authority figure. The therapist is put on a pedestal and treated with "kid gloves" and with undue deference. The client feels unworthy of attention, caring, or help from a person as exalted as the therapist and believes that the therapist's needs must be given priority with little or no regard to what the client might really feel or need. Although it can be helpful for a client to see the therapist as a role model, healthy feelings on the negative end of the spectrum and negative transference reactions that are problematic but important to address in therapy might go unrecognized and unexpressed by the client who believes that having or expressing such feelings threatens the relationship. In a contradictory fashion, beliefs such as these may be maintained by a client's implicit view of the therapist as too fickle, selfish, or withholding to tolerate the client's expression of her or his own feelings, thoughts, or needs, all the while treating the therapist as all powerful and potentially rejecting. In a variant of this presentation, clients may be frankly dismissive of the therapist and therapy, denying having any needs or perceiving the therapist as inadequate to meet them. Through such counterdependence the client devalues the therapist as a means of avoiding or defending against becoming aware of his or her fear of rejection and betrayal by anyone who is entrusted with his or her well-being.

In order to address these idealizing or devaluing transferences, the therapist must help the client to recognize and express feelings and perceptions that are based on legitimate grievances associated with his or her relational slips and missteps (i.e., the "empathic failures" that are committed by every therapist, no matter how experienced or skilled; Kohut & Wolf, 1978). Equally important, the client must be helped to safely acknowledge and express feelings based on a variety of real and perceived personality traits, professional status, and other life advantages attributed to the therapist. When the overidealization can be dismantled without harm or retaliation, it demonstrates that emotional expression is not only allowed but actually enhances the security and responsiveness of healthy relationships. This is in direct contradiction to the rigidity and punitive orientation that characterize unstable and one-sided abusive relationships.

Anger, Rage, and Outrage

Many clients with complex trauma are adept at disowning their feelings of anger, displacing and expressing them in disguised forms (e.g., through passive–aggressive behavior, manipulation, somatic complaints, self-blame, and self-injurious and suicidal behavior). The suppression or misdirection of these feelings is primarily due to fears of their explosive and uncontrolled discharge and inexperience with more modulated means of expression. The enraged client can be frightening for the therapist, who might self-protectively distance. If danger is not imminent, a more therapeutic strategy is first to accept and legitimize the anger (often this type of response is "settling" to the client, who experiences relief at having it recognized and at not being stigmatized or chastised) and then to assist in establishing boundaries, regaining control, and finding modulated means of expression and discharge. The application of skills for self-regulation supports the toleration and management of emotions without their being indiscriminately discharged against self or others (including the therapist). (See works on anger management in Self-Help Resources and Workbooks [in the online supplement to this book].)

Loss and Grief

As discussed previously, the client grieves for past and present losses, fears of losing significant relationships, including with the therapist, can intensify. Unfortunately, some of those fears may come true. As clients become healthier, stronger, and more assertive, they may become more autonomous or detached from abusive or neglectful others who, in response to being threatened by the changes, want them to "change back." Sadly, personal growth might come at the expense of long-term relationships that end up faltering or ending. Reliance on the therapist and supportive others may be particularly needed during these relational losses and transitions.

Within the therapy, separations for any reason (e.g., professional conferences, vacations, holidays, illness, childbirth, emergency, or crisis) or the impending end of treatment should be announced and prepared for well in advance whenever possible. Many clients need repeated encouragement to identify and express feelings about therapist unavailability, whatever the reason, to counter the tendency to be overly understanding and disowning of any negative feelings or neediness. If and when these feelings do surface, they might be dismissed by the client as childlike and uncalled for (e.g., "I feel like a crybaby when I feel like this and I can't stand it! I'm just being ridiculous to let myself be upset that you will be away"). The client clearly needs support and validation for whatever emotions emerge, especially anger and fear, which are so easily denied or displaced. In the event that the client holds faulty assumptions and misattributions about separations, if it seems appropriate, the therapist might be factual about the reasons for an absence ("All of us need to take breaks and vacations; I find they help me maintain the energy and focus I need to do this work") and sharing his or her emotions about the separation ("I will miss you and our time together"; "I will not forget you while I am gone, nor will you forget me; we'll keep each other in our minds"; "I hope you can use me as a model to allow yourself to take some time off"). Clients frequently benefit from knowing that the therapist's absence does not mean a cessation of caring, disregard, or forgetting or an abandonment (although it might feel like one), nor is it due to personal dislike or hostility.

Clients' fears are sometimes reflected in extreme concern for the therapist's safety during a separation. They might be highly superstitious that something bad will befall him or her as punishment. An accident or mishap would conclusively "prove" the client's malignant power and repeat the losses experienced in other significant relationships. Exploration and exposure of the faulty beliefs are warranted. The therapist can offer reassurance about intending to return and can further note that if something beyond his or her control were to happen, it would not be the client's fault, nor would it be personal punishment. The therapist should not make promises that are unrealistic, cannot be guaranteed, and are not under personal control (e.g., "I promise I will never leave you; I will always be available to you, no matter what." "Don't worry, nothing bad will happen to me.").

In keeping with the philosophy of individualized treatment, individualized plans for separations might be required. Yet the therapist must steer clear of overly solicitous and rescuing behaviors that convey that clients are helpless and unable to develop or rely on other sources of support. Clients (especially those whose attachment style is anxiously preoccupied or disorganized) should, in most cases and in accordance with clearly delineated boundaries regarding the therapist's availability and personal time, be encouraged to be more independent and to rely on others besides the therapist. On the other hand, the stress associated with separations should not be minimized or ignored and dependency not considered a weakness or a sign of pathology. In fact, building healthy dependency and interdependence based on secure attachment is a goal of treatment (Steele et al., 2001). Actions must be selected in response to client needs and after discussion about strategies and options that would be helpful. On occasion, separations are so difficult that hospitalization or participation in a partial hospital or other recovery program is necessary. Although not necessarily the treatment of choice, these options need to be considered for the client who lacks a support system, cannot tolerate the therapist's absence and felt support without decompensation, and cannot function or abide by the terms of an established safety plan.

Summary

This is but an abbreviated list of the possible transference reactions associated with complex interpersonal victimization. There are innumerable variations that emerge according to the client's unique experience and character that should be expected and welcomed as important communication and addressed individually. In the course of treatment, when therapeutic interventions enable clients to recognize rather than simply repeat posttraumatic transference dilemmas, they become more aware of the costs of both their victimization and the adaptations they have made to carry on in life despite abuse, betrayal, abandonment, or exploitation. At this point, clients often feel overwhelmed or frightened by the depth and breadth of their unmet needs and furious or despondent about the harm done and the opportunities missed as a result of having had to focus their lives on survival. These existential issues arise when complex trauma survivors become able to fully and accurately understand the traumatic challenges they have faced and the alterations that they had to make in their life paths and ways of living. These can be very poignant times in the treatment where the empathy of the therapist is especially important.

Awareness and acceptance of trauma-related transference issues need to be addressed gradually and in doses. It is essential that therapists help clients to recognize not only what has been lost or damaged by trauma but also what remains intact or can develop in themselves, their relationships, and their lives. Where warranted, the imbalance in past and current relationships needs to be analyzed and changed. Some relationships will no longer be acceptable or satisfactory, primarily those that were based on traumatic reenactments or beliefs about self and others that were shaped by trauma but do not reflect the client's (or their significant others') true self or best interests. Thus, crucial therapeutic gains in awareness can sometimes place clients at a crossroads in their personal relationships, feeling alone and unsupported just when they are genuinely most able to recognize and benefit from support. Clients are apt to be very dependent on therapy during this time (which most often occurs during the transition from Phase 2 to the application of therapeutic gains to present-day life in Phase 3) until more equitable and mutually satisfying relationships develop. Those family members and friends with whom supportive, trustworthy, and meaningful relationships are possible should be mobilized. A therapy group or self-help group may be useful at this difficult juncture as well to provide another source of growth and support.

Countertransference responses are the next challenge for the therapist working with clients with complex trauma histories. As with transference dilemmas, countertransference must be assessed and analyzed based on the information it can provide, as well as to determine by what means it can best be managed so that it does not interrupt or derail the treatment.

COUNTERTRANSFERENCE THEMES, ISSUES, AND REACTIONS

As observed earlier, professionals have no immunity from the dominant societal attitudes toward interpersonal victimization and trauma (Kluft, 1990b), nor do they necessarily have knowledge of or training for various extreme types of interpersonal trauma (e.g., incest: Courtois, 2010;

the Holocaust and other genocides: Danieli, 1984; political repression and torture: Fischman, 1991; child sex rings and prostitution: Lanning & Burgess, 1984; Farley, 2003; sexual and other forms of human trafficking and other forms of organized abuse, including clergy abuse and abuse within the military ranks. Therefore, professional training that prepares them to identify and manage their strong affective reactions is needed even as it is lacking. Learning how human beings (some of whom are health professionals) can systematically mistreat and abuse others, how parents can exploit and neglect rather than nurture their offspring, and hearing about it in detail can be enormously disconcerting and horrifying. Personal reactions, whether positive or negative, may be projected onto the client and into the therapeutic process. In this section, countertransference reactions are detailed, along with therapeutic and nontherapeutic behaviors that flow from them. These reactions are drawn from major themes found in the clinical literature, especially those that have been published in the past two decades on countertransference and trauma and PTSD (Dalenberg, 2000; Danieli, 1984; Wilson & Lindy, 1994); dissociation (Baker, 1997; Bromberg, 1995; Chefetz, 1997; Howell, 2011; Kluft & Fine, 1993; Perlman, 1999; Schwartz, 2000); and incestuous abuse (Courtois, 1988, 2010; Kluft, 1990a, 1990b, 2011; Pearlman, 1999; Pearlman & Saakvitne, 1995).

Gartner (1999) described *countertransference* as "all feelings and reactions to the patient, conscious and unconscious, enacted or not, reality- or fantasy-based, that originate and are located *in the therapist*" (p. 234, italics added). Pearlman and Saakvitne (1995) added another dimension, namely, the therapist's *feelings about his or her feelings and reactions*. Gabbard's definition adds yet another: "*a joint creation*, in which both therapist's past conflicts and the patient's projected aspects create specific patterns of interaction within the therapeutic process" (Gabbard, 1993, p. 13, italics added). According to Bromberg (1995) (quoted in Gartner, 1999), countertransference provides the therapist with "a powerful ongoing source of data—a forced invitation into the patient's world." The transference and countertransference occur in juxtaposition with and in response to each other in the context of the therapeutic relationship. It is in the immediacy and security of the present relationship that the client enacts with the therapist issues and relational patterns from the past, in the process allowing them to be identified and restructured.

Betan, Heim, Conklin, and Westen (2005) reported on an empirical study of countertransference phenomena as related to personality type. Their analysis yielded eight clinically and conceptually coherent factors independent of clinician's theoretical orientation, associated in predictable ways with DSM Axis II pathology. These are reflected in the following categories: (1) overwhelmed/disorganized; (2) helpless/inadequate; (3) positive; (4) special/overinvolved; (5) sexualized; (6) disengaged; (7) parental/protective; and (8) criticized/mistreated. The authors noted that therapists can make diagnostic and therapeutic use of their own responses to the patient when they aware of these typologies as related to the client's presentation and personality style (to this we would again add the client's attachment style, as well). This is especially needed for trainees and novice therapists (Neumann & Gamble, 1995).

In an early contribution to the literature on widespread countertransference reactions in response to incest (a prototype of complex trauma), Renshaw (1982) categorized them as connoting avoidance, attraction, and attack, labels useful in identifying and addressing them. *Avoidance* refers to the desire to deny, escape from, or not see the situation as it really is. Trauma avoidance is generally based on such emotions as anxiety, discomfort, repugnance, dread, and horror. *Attraction* connotes a moving toward, a voyeurism, fascination, a rescuing or overinvolvement, or arousal/stimulation. *Attack* is usually motivated by anger, disgust, blame, and condemnation of the trauma and its symptoms that are projected onto to those involved in it, including the client. The two problematic therapist positions having to do with empathic strain, identified by Wilson and Lindy (1994) and described earlier in this chapter, resemble Renshaw's categories: in one position the therapist avoids, disengages, and sets overly rigid boundaries, thereby abandoning the client and not providing needed response and support; in the other, the therapist is attracted and stimulated by the needs of the client or the particulars of his or her story or both, resulting in overinvolvement and blurred boundaries, sometimes including sexual contact. Both positions can involve aggression and power dynamics and can lead to boundary violations and revictimization. All of the countertransference responses described next fit into one or more of these categories.

Dread and Horror Leading to Denial and Avoidance

Therapists can be horrified when hearing a history of cumulative interpersonal victimization and subsequent revictimization and reenactments. Horror can lead to dread and fear and subsequently to defensive behaviors, such as the therapist's denying that the situation could have been that bad (even though doing so contradicts the therapist's emotional response), never bringing it up, refusing to discuss it, changing the subject, and encouraging the client to put it in the past to get on with his or her life. Although such reactions may be motivated by the therapist's and the client's understandable fear of making things worse or of the client's going crazy, they typically result in increasing the patient's isolation and despair. Circumstances such as these call for specialized supervision and consultation and for personal psychotherapy in some cases. When the therapist cannot get his or her negative reactions neutralized or under control, is unwilling to get consultation or training, or has other personal reasons not to be able to engage in the treatment, referral is indicated.

Shame, Pity, and Disgust

Horror and denial can lead to related emotions of shame, pity, and disgust that get projected onto the client and his or her behaviors, characteristics, or symptoms, thereby contributing to and reinforcing negative self-perceptions and feelings. From this position, the therapist might (advertently or inadvertently) convey that the client is irreparably damaged, corrupted or unlovable, a view that substantiates rather than changes the viewpoint already held by the client. Shame in the therapist is contrary to a positive sense of self and feelings of competence. Because shame involves internal representation of being devalued, therapists can develop concordant or complementary countertransference identifications with their shamed clients based on their own susceptibility to shame (Hahn, 2000). Their own shame can be activated, or they can internalize the projected shame of the client. Clients may defend against their feelings through avoidance, withdrawal, narcissistic entitlement, and even attacks on the therapist, who, in turn, may feel additionally incompetent, inadequate, and worthless. Mindfulness regarding personal feelings of shame and devaluation on the part of the therapist is necessary; if this is not adequate, consultation, supervision, and therapy are advisable.

Therapists who were never traumatized (or not as severely as their clients) and who had reasonably happy, nonabusive childhoods and "good enough" parents may be prone to feelings of guilt when they hear about the client's experiences and their aftereffects. In an attempt to protect the client against further pain and to relieve guilt, the therapist might discourage discussion of the trauma or be oversolicitous. In this latter circumstance, the client is treated as fragile and exceptional and as needing constant special arrangements, labeled "vicarious indulgence" by Turkus (personal communication, 2008). Two major problems are typical of guilt- or fascination-induced overresponse and rescuing: The client comes to expect it and may even want more, and the therapist begins to resent the rising expectations, demands, and neediness. If unrecognized and unaddressed, in cyclical fashion, feelings of resentment and anger fuel more therapist guilt, leading either to additional overindulgence or to acts of hostility.

Disgust is a powerful emotion that conveys revulsion and aversion. The expression of disgust is highly damaging, but it might be the best way the therapist has to protect him- or herself from other powerful feelings, including fear, helplessness, incompetence, and shame. Active antipathy on the part of the therapist may also be a way to manage his or her own unacknowledged sadism. Therapist and client may shift positions as abuser and abused, in the process playing out sadistic–masochistic roles with one another, or mutual torture, per Chefetz (1997). Both client and therapist are demeaned, as roles are played out rather than identified and changed. Obviously, this is a very charged situation that requires intervention to get the treatment back on track. It would even be better to end the treatment than to continue one of ongoing and unremitting sadistic–masochistic enactments without resolution.

Guilt and Associated Helplessness

Therapist guilt might also result from feeling helpless to undo the client's experience and from not having "magic powers" to make it all go away or make it stop hurting so much. The therapist might defend against this sense of helplessness by avoiding detailed discussion of the trauma, ostensibly to spare the client additional emotional pain. The therapist cannot undo the past or its effects but can accompany and support the client in identifying, accepting, and processing its repercussions, in the process, having a very different interpersonal experience. To do so, the therapist must learn about the trauma, no matter how horrific or gruesome, in sufficient detail to explore and understand it from the client's perspective; however, some techniques such as EMDR help the client to do so imaginally rather than verbally. As described in the earlier section on secondary secrets, it is sometimes the most closely guarded secrets or the most shameful aspects of the trauma that have the greatest impact; therefore, they need to be uncovered and become open to discussion or processing. The analogy of "cleaning out an infection" provides a rationale for the process that counterbalances the therapist's tendency to back away from details for fear of further injuring the client.

This said, and presented in Chapters 4 through 6, interventions must be carefully sequenced and paced when clients are asked to provide details and to approach and process the trauma. Per the phase-oriented model, factual information about the trauma is first requested during the assessment to provide a baseline of information. The facts and associated emotions are explored in more detail after the client has achieved a relative degree of safety and capacity for emotion regulation. The therapist's careful inquiry and ongoing support play major roles in allowing the story to be told and analyzed.

Rage

Trauma details can stimulate indignation and anger about the abuse and victimization and its various players and circumstances (such as the perpetrator(s), passive bystanders or colluders, "the system," cultural and ethnic beliefs and traditions, sexism and the status of women, religions that support rather than report abusive clergy, medical and insurance systems and procedures, colleagues who are not helpful or supportive, and so on). Quite illogically, these feelings can be displaced onto the client, who is viewed as somehow bringing on mistreatment and other victimization and because of his or her helplessness in the situation, but more specifically, because he or she exposes the therapist to it, causing him or her to feel emotional anguish. Although it can be therapeutic for the survivor to know that someone is angry about what happened, the therapist must exercise care in not dumping anger on the client (victim blaming), a very familiar societal response to the traumatized (the second injury: institutional trauma) that is wounding in its own right Therapists must own personal anger and pay attention to how the client responds to hearing that someone has angry feelings and outrage about his or her experience. Care is needed not to express it prematurely, before the client is capable of hearing and accepting it. When the feelings escalate to rage or become dysregulated, they are best dealt with outside of the therapy in consultation or supervision with professional colleagues or in personal psychotherapy.

Any projection of rage and other negative emotions onto the therapist, either through the transference or as a direct challenge to the therapist's caring as discussed in the Doris case, may elicit strong counterreactions, including complementary anger and retaliation. The therapist may experience rage at being identified as a potential abuser and compared to abusive others. The therapist might also feel anger after repeated and consistent but futile efforts (and possibly going the "extra mile") to prove trustworthiness. In some instances, the intensity of the survivor's rage may so overwhelm both parties that a therapeutic impasse results (Pearlman & Saakvitne, 1994). Because the therapist's inability to tolerate the client's projected rage and negative transference reactions or to understand and cope with his or her own countertransference rage can ultimately lead to a distancing from and rejection of the client and a premature termination of the therapy, the need for ongoing monitoring and consultation is underscored.

Grief and Mourning

Although the losses associated with complex trauma are not quantifiable, many therapists respond to them personally and grieve for what happened to the client and for all of the losses entailed (Boniello, 1990). This is the case in general, but therapists with their own trauma histories, histories of complicated bereavement or ambiguous loss, or those who have faced recent losses may be particularly affected. As with other emotions, clients can benefit when therapists share their grief and sadness about what happened to them. Responses such as these can provide support for clients' grieving, as there may be few other venues in which to mourn. However, grief and mourning reactions should be carefully monitored with attention to their not further burdening the client. As with other personal responses that might need airing outside of treatment, consultation, supervision, or therapy might be called for. Group therapy and other support groups are an additional context in which clients bereaved by their trauma-related losses might mourn in the company of others with similar experiences and reactions. As described in Chapter 6, ambiguous losses and complicated bereavement often lack a sharing context in which to receive acknowledgment and support.

Victim as Fragile; Survivor as Self-Sufficient

A perspective that exclusively views the client as victim usually results in overprotection or rescuing (in an attempt to compensate) while simultaneously conveying to the client that he or she is helpless and not capable. An overemphasis on the client's frailty ignores his or her strengths, resiliency, and capabilities in a way that short-circuits skill building, emotional processing, and trauma mastery.

From the opposite perspective, the client with complex trauma can be viewed as a "super-survivor," a hero or heroine who accomplished the extraordinary through superior resilience, intelligence, coping abilities, and self-sufficiency. This position is problematic due to its unrealistic glorification of the client's personal resilience and a related downplaying of what was endured and its associated suffering. It does not provide adequate recognition of the reasons that these capabilities developed nor the price paid for being so "brave" and "capable." The therapist with this perspective tends to reinforce defenses and self-sufficiency while discouraging emotional exploration and interdependence with trustworthy others.

Trauma Happens to Everyone

A related reaction minimizes or trivializes the client's unique experience by emphasizing that trauma is ubiquitous and that most adults and children have traumatic exposures or experiences. Although this might well be the case, this perspective assumes that all victimization experiences are the same or similar, ignoring essential differences in type, degree, severity, duration, subjective experiences and reactions, and so on. The therapist with such a priori views presumes to know about the survivor's experience and, on this basis, prematurely forecloses discussion of the details of the client's past or its individual meaning.

Language Use

Both therapist and client may defend against the reality of experiences of trauma by using muted, indirect, and inaccurate language. Such neutered terms as "contact," "sexual experience," "seduction," and "sexual affair" can minimize the coercion, abuse, assault, rape, violence and subjugation that the client reports. Some clients are unable to describe what happened to them with any directness or precision and resist using the word that is most accurate or descriptive (e.g., "rape," "incest"). It is advisable initially for the therapist to use the client's muted language but, over time, to encourage the use of more direct and accurate terminology.

A contrary situation arises with clients who are able to use direct words and wording (such as "rape" and "fuck" and accurate language for body parts) and those who are able to graphically describe what happened (sometimes this is an attempt to shock the therapist and to test his or her "staying power" and tolerance of the details). The therapist may find direct wording and graphic recounting so uncomfortable that language blunting is used to defend against it. The therapist does better to use the client's terms, as doing so indicates willingness not to shy away from the reality, details, and ugliness. It is better to share uncomfortable feelings or to ventilate those feelings outside of the session with supervisors and colleagues. At times, the therapist will be required to introduce accurate language or descriptions, especially with the client who routinely minimizes or disowns information.

Privileged Voyeurism

Privileged voyeurism refers to an excessive interest in and inquisitiveness about the details of victimization, especially those that are extreme, sexual, and that involve taboo activities. In its more general form, the therapist treats the client as an object of curiosity for having been involved in deviant, abnormal, or forbidden events and behaviors, making him or her feel even more like an aberration (often the case with incestuous abuse [Courtois, 2010]). In more specific form, the therapist focuses excessively (and sometimes exclusively) on the sexual aspects and details without similar attention to other issues. Clients who have experienced this response describe having felt pressured to detail the most intimate and the most humiliating and degrading sexual aspects and of being constantly redirected to them. The therapist comes across as spellbound or tantalized, causing the client to feel objectified and exploited and therefore revictimized. Responses such as these can remain hidden and not presented in supervision or consultation due to the therapist's secret gratification and related shame (or shamelessness). The therapist who admits to feeling overly stimulated or excessively curious (especially one without outside support or who practices in isolation or is in the throes of personal crisis) is in need of collegial consultation and supervision (and possibly personal psychotherapy). Keeping such responses hidden can lead to their reinforcement and, in the worst case, result in sexual transgressions and other actions that are coercive and violative.

Sexualization of the Relationship

As discussed in Chapter 2, adult survivors' sexual aftereffects range from a total blunting of sexual interest and response to indiscriminate and compulsive sexual behavior. At one end of the spectrum, some survivors are sexually naive, inexperienced, or shut down. At the other end, some are highly sexual and seductive and may be sexually addicted or may be conditioned to compulsive sexualization or to use sex to be powerful and in control, as a means of developing and maintaining relationships or of devaluing them, or to self-soothe or blunt ongoing distress. Unfortunately, both extremes can enthrall the therapist. The innocent, inexperienced, or "sexually anorexic" client may evoke protective and teaching tendencies in a therapist who may rationalize sexual contact as sex education and a positive learning experience (known in the literature as "the love cure"). The sexualized client who is sexually precocious, compulsive, and promiscuous, "leads with her/his sexuality," confuses sex with affection, power and control, or aggression, and eroticizes contacts with others, the therapist included, may be an enticing challenge to "fix" and to "satisfy." A more middle-ground but no less problematic situation develops when attraction develops between therapist and client that leads to infatuation and romantic and sexual feelings and longings. These may create difficulties for the dyad, but they are more easily disclosed and managed than those of the more extreme type.

The disclosure of experiences of sexual violation (especially those that are incestuous) in therapy can cause the therapist to view the client as sexually exciting and arousing by virtue of having been involved in taboo activity and, further, to view the client as the cause of the abuse ("he/she was so pleasing, sexy, or provocative as a child—who could have resisted?"), a stance found in the older professional literature (Courtois, 2010). The therapist might also view the client as "spoiled or damaged goods," as undeserving of respect and instead as deserving of abuse, a perspective that can be reinforced by any subsequent episodes of sexual revictimization or of sexual acting-out, promiscuity, prostitution, or other maladjustment that the client reports and/or plays out with the therapist or others. Learning about highly sexualized experiences, reenactments, and revictimizations and having them crop up in the treatment relationship can all play a role in the formation of therapist perceptions and expectations about the client and can wreak havoc if not thoughtfully addressed and managed and if boundaries are not established, maintained, and insisted upon.

Such thoughts, along with any personal problems and associated vulnerability or pathology on the part of the therapist, can unfortunately combine with the client's superficial compliance, learned helplessness, excessive dependence, dissociative style, compulsive sexualization, neediness, idealization (and even aggression or power), to make a "perfect storm." Without understanding and management of both the transference and countertransference, the relationship can easily become sexual, with the therapist developing rationalizations for its occurrence (e.g., "A sexual encounter facilitates the therapy"; "Sexual intercourse is a corrective emotional experience because it demonstrates love and tenderness on the part of the therapist rather than abuse"; "Sexual intercourse with the therapist constitutes *in vivo* sex therapy"; "The client is in need of good attention"; "The client wants a sexual encounter because he or she engages in behavior and dresses in seductive ways"). All of these rationalizations can be found in the literature on therapists (and other professionals who abuse) and in the documents related to lawsuits and board complaints.

Regrettably, sexual involvement in psychotherapy occurs quite regularly, despite the fact that it constitutes a serious ethical and professional violation. Research has established that female incest survivors are sexually abused in therapy in numbers disproportionate to those for other female clients by male therapists (Armsworth, 1989; De Young, 1981; Kluft, 1990a, 1990b). Less commonly recognized is sex between same-sex clients and therapists yet such contact does occur in numbers that are not yet determined. By virtue of the power differential involved and the violation of trust inherent in such a relationship (among other prominent dynamics), *sexual abuse by a therapist recapitulates the original transgression trauma as it counters trust and safety and trauma mastery, the goal of treatment.* The client suffers another significant relational betrayal-trauma and receives additional proof of the untrustworthiness and venality of authority figures as well as his or her own "evil eroticism." Chefetz (1997) observed an underrecognized dimension of erotic transference and countertransference: that it can be highly sadomasochistic when it involves power and control. In this scenario, therapist and client may reciprocally play out power dynamics and each alternately take on the role of victimizer or victim. This is discussed more in the next section on role enactments in transference and countertransference.

Therapists who are secure in their sexuality and who address and work through attraction and power issues can then identify with the victimized client and model appropriate behavior. With them, the survivor client has the opportunity to experience a caring relationship in which appropriate sexual boundaries are maintained and sex can be distinguished from affection and from aggression. Much information is now available on the dynamics of sexual abuse of clients by therapists, a major ethical violation in all mental health and medical professions and a crime in ever more jurisdictions. Bridges (1994), Gabbard (1989), Pope (1990, 1994), and Pope and Bouhoutsos (1986), among other researchers, have found that most mental health training does not attend to issues of therapist–client attraction, including sexual attraction. Trainees and therapists are therefore often on their own in determining how to respond to their own attraction to the client, to the client's expressions of love and attraction to the therapist, or to either the client's or therapist's frank propositioning or seduction of each other. Pope (1994) wrote the book *Sexual Involvement with Therapists* and, he and his colleagues wrote the book *Sexual Feelings in Psychotherapy* (Pope, Sonne, & Holroyd, 1993) to address this oversight and to provide needed training and discussion. A training videotape on the topic of sexual feelings in psychotherapy is available from the American Psychological Association that provides stimulus clinical vignettes for the viewer to watch and respond to. It also provides opportunities for discussion by providing stimulus questions.

PROJECTIVE IDENTIFICATION, ENACTMENT, AND COMMON TRANSFERENCE–COUNTERTRANSFERENCE ROLES AND POSITIONS

Projective Identification

Projective identification is another way in which the client communicates. Through this implicit or unconscious process, he or she projects disowned aspects of him- or herself and personal experience onto the therapist, who becomes the "emotional load-bearer" and can learn much about the client through his or her own feeling states and reactions as well as physical responses. As discussed previously, therapists can become entranced within their client's experience, actually feeling the feelings that the client does not recognize or routinely disowns, displaces, or disavows. Although it can be disconcerting for the therapist, it is yet another relational process by which the client can come to be "known" by what has been projected onto the therapist.

Enactment

How does the therapist understand and make best use of the unconscious communications of dissociative and posttraumatic clients that are contained within the projective identification, enactments, and transference–countertransference? Quoting Baker (1997), who analogized the process to a dance in which both partners learn steps and movements that, over time, become attuned and automatic:

> How alike this is to the therapy process. It is what we, as therapists, strive for, those aspects of the interaction which are beyond words and cognition, where therapist and patient may attain new levels of understanding through "the dance." This is the realm of knowing without saying, that which takes place in the countertransference through the experiencing and later understanding of projective identifications and enactments. Although enactments can be destructive (frequently the beginning therapist is admonished to beware of enactments), I propose that many are not only constructive, but vital to be able to be with the patient in her world. (p. 214)

Baker further proposed that the therapist understand enactments as inevitable and as explanatory of the client, who communicates authentically but implicitly and in primitive somatosensory ways as a result of having been harmed so early in the developmental process. Traumatization left the client with somatic imprints in his or her "right mind," but in conditions of speechless terror and without the words to describe or formulate experiences and feelings. Enactments put these internal experiences into actions. Wallin (2007) described enactments as involving

> *behavior*—including verbal as well as nonverbal behavior. But even when enactments are played out in speech (as they often are in therapy) their essential meaning lies not in the words that are spoken but, rather, in the nonverbal subtext generated by what the words actually do.
>
> In an enactment of transference–countertransference, what is enacted, verbally and nonverbally, is a particular kind of relationship. It could be a parent–child relationship or a romantic relationship, a relationship of allies or of adversaries, a relationship that feels safe or one that feels perilous. The variations are probably limitless, depending as they do upon the interaction of two unique individuals. . . .

> Enactments are the scenarios that arise at the intersection, so to speak, of the unconscious needs and vulnerabilities of the patient . . . and the therapist. . . .
>
> In an enactment, aspects of the therapist's representational world—the legacy of her original attachment experiences—are unconsciously activated and lived out. Exactly the same is true for the patient. . . .
>
> To the extent that enactments continue to unfold outside awareness, they usually impose limits on what can be experienced and understood; in this way they make the therapeutic dialogue less inclusive and less collaborative. To the extent that they can be made conscious, however, enactments have the potential to provide access to highly significant, as-yet-unrecognized facets of the patient and the therapist and the relationship that they share. (pp. 270–271)

Enactments can be repetitive, especially when their meaning remains unknown, unrecognized, and unexplored. They may involve full-fledged reenactments of traumatic experiences or more particular to the therapeutic dyad. As with other aspects of relationships, they can be identified, discussed, and used as reparative for what they represent from the past. Due to their role, therapists move from the position of participant to participant–observer as they attempt to discern a specific enactment and bring it to the client's attention for discussion and interpretation. It is in this way new information and new ways of being in relationship become open to the client.

Eight Common Transference–Countertransference Positions

Davies and Frawley (1994) identified

> eight relational positions, expressed within four relational matrices, alternately enacted by therapist and survivor in the transference and countertransference that repeatedly recur in psychoanalytic (and other forms of therapy) work with adult survivors of childhood sexual abuse. These positions include: *(1) the uninvolved non-abusing parent and the neglected child; (2) the sadistic abuser and the helpless, impotently enraged victim; (3) the idealized, omnipotent rescuer and the entitled child who demands to be rescued; and (4) the seducer and the seduced.* (p. 166; authors' italics)

These eight positions do not account for all possible manifestations of the transference or countertransference and they are likely to vary with other complex trauma subpopulations (e.g., refugees and survivors of political repression), yet they occur with sufficient regularity that the therapist treating complex trauma should be familiar with them. They are compatible with the attachment positions and manifestations described in Chapter 9 and with the transference themes discussed earlier in this chapter. Used together, they deepen the therapist's understanding of the client and of the relational "dance" they engage in over the course of treatment. We touch on their most pronounced manifestations here. For additional discussion, the reader is referred to Davies and Frawley (1991, 1994).

The Unseeing, Uninvolved Parent and the Unseen, Neglected Child

According to these authors, this transference–countertransference paradigm is often the first to emerge in the treatment of complex developmental trauma. As most child abuse and interpersonal traumatization are not recognized, "seen," or responded to, one aspect of the internal world of the abused child and later the adult is a relationship between a neglectful, unavailable, nonresponsive parent and an unseen, neglected and abused child. Within the transference–countertransference, the client sequentially enacts one or both sides of the relational scenario, as the therapist enacts the complementary role as the result of projective identification. At one pole, this client identifies with the parent and is withholding and distant from the therapist, who, in turn, feels unwanted, disconnected, and neglected. At the other pole, the client is the unseen, neglected child who responds to the therapist as he or she did to the parent and may have little or no compassion for him- or herself in replication of the parent's position. This may play out in the superficially compliant client who tries not to be seen as he or she seeks to please or take care of the therapist so as not to be further abandoned, while his or her needs go neglected.

The Sadistic Abuser and the Helpless, Impotently Enraged Victim

The ambivalence associated with attachment to a parent whose abuse alternates with care (attack-ment/disorganized attachment) is played out in this relational paradigm. In one position, the client identifies with the parent/abuser and invades or intrudes upon the therapist's physical and internal/psychological space, attempting to control the therapist by pushing boundaries. The therapist is likely to experience anxiety, discomfort, and dread in anticipation of sessions and to be overly involved in trying to please or placate the client or to be responsive to his or her needs, even those that are unrealistic and entitled. In this way, the therapist is attempting to please or offset the client's demands, much as the client did as a child to stave off abuse. Self-destructiveness may be another way of identifying with the perpetrator while sadistically terrifying and victimizing the therapist (some therapists describe being held hostage by their fear of the client's demands and potential for dysregulation and decompensation, and/or self-injury, suicidality, acting out, etc.). At the other end of the spectrum, the therapist may become aggressively reactive to the client. This involves a shift from the position of impotent victim to that of the sadistic abuser, a playing out of the sadomasochism that now involves identification with the powerful perpetrator rather than the powerless child. As described earlier, in some cases, this becomes a complete reenactment, resulting in sexual and coercive contact between client and therapist, in identification with the perpetrator and reenactment of the original victimization.

The Idealized, Omnipotent Rescuer and the Entitled Child

The therapist may feel a powerful pull to play the role of omnipotent rescuer to an idealizing and needy client. This response may be an honestly assumed role that comes with being a helping professional; however, it might also result from the therapist's overgratification at being needed and appreciated. It can also result in the therapist being overly intellectual or professional in working with the client in overly cognitive ways. If unrecognized or unaddressed, it can result in the vicarious indulgence described earlier that plays to and reinforces entitlement. In another variation, it might also mimic what the client did to placate the abuser as a child, or the client might reenact that scenario by taking care of the therapist and responding (or catering) to him or her, in this way becoming the rescuer and the therapist the rescued.

The Seducer and the Seduced

Clients (especially those who were abused after a relationship was developed (referred to in the literature as "grooming") may behave in kind in their interactions with the therapist, being highly pleasing, giving them special attention, or behaving seductively. The client is literally re-creating how he or she was drawn into the relationship and demonstrating what is known about how "to do" relationships. Therapists may find themselves responding in kind, looking forward to these clients' sessions, and becoming like the client, in a process of mutual seduction. With appropriate boundaries maintained, these feelings can be acknowledged and accepted as normal in human interactions; however, the client has the restorative opportunity to distinguish between situations in which they are used dishonestly to exploit and those in which they are authentic and benign. Both therapist and client can come to enjoy the positive regard and feelings of attraction they have for each other, similar to what occurs in healthy parent–child oedipal configurations. Its resolution allows healthy separation and individuation. Its expression and appreciation in a bounded and safe relationship is healing for the client and can be enormously satisfying for both members of the dyad, the benefit and reward of the hard work of complex trauma treatment.

CONCLUSION

Rarely are relational issues and paradigms so organized and linear as presented here. Real-life relationships and those inside the consulting room are much more diverse and complicated. Nevertheless, when transference, countertransference, enactments, and projective identifications such as those reviewed here come to light in the treatment, the therapist who has knowledge of them is more prepared to anticipate and manage them. As Chu so presciently wrote in his 1988 article on traps in trauma treatment, "Knowledge of them doesn't prevent them from happening but it does allow the therapist to know about them ahead of time, to not have as much anxiety about them and to get out of them much more quickly" (Chu, 1988, p. 26). So too with trauma- and attachment-based reactions and counterreactions, transference and countertransference, projective identification and enactments: The therapist who has foreknowledge of them has a means of anticipating and understanding them, may not be as likely to get mired in them, and may therefore be able to identify and interpret them earlier in the interest of the client's increased self-knowledge and symptom resolution.

Postscript

We didn't want to end this book without returning to the two individuals whose lives and treatment have brought a personal dimension to the technical information that we've covered. **Doris** and **Hector**, although fictional, are individuals whose histories and treatments closely parallel (and in fact are derived indirectly from) those of many real clients whom we have treated. No doubt, they bring to mind clients with whom you have interacted if you are a practicing therapist or people you have known regardless of which "side of the coffee table" you've been on—either as a client (or a family member or friend) of someone who has experienced complex trauma or as a therapist who has provided treatment to clients with complex trauma histories. You can understand, therefore, why we think of them with great respect and fondness because of their courage, resilience, and hard work in treatment.

As we conclude this book, both Doris and Hector are actively working on Phase 3 issues, having gone through the rigors of preparation and alliance building in Phase 1 and coming to terms with their memories and trauma-related distress and dysregulation in Phase 2. Neither has had a smooth or trouble-free life or therapy and both must occasionally go back to revisit old issues or to tune up specific skills. Their treatments are not yet complete, but their symptoms are more manageable and, most important, their lives are much more on the track and they each have regained hope for a better future. Although they are very different in many important respects, they have in common a new sense of having moved from being trapped in a revolving door of symptoms that they didn't understand or know how to cope with to being truly in recovery as whole human beings whose lives are affected—but no longer shattered—by past trauma.

Doris has made many significant changes in her personal outlook, self-concept, emotional regulation, and ability to interact well with others. Importantly, she has totally stopped drinking and that has helped her with her mood stability; her use of alcohol had been fueling her depression and lowering her inhibitions in interactions with others, creating other problems to contend with. Although her marriage needs ongoing attention, it is not at the crisis point it was at when she began treatment when her husband was threatening to leave. She and her husband are closer than they have been since the start of their relationship and they will begin couple therapy in several months, once Doris has completed group treatment, to build on the gains that have been achieved. She remains in individual therapy on a once-a-week basis and remains quite dependent on (and occasionally mistrustful of) her therapist. But she now is able to catch herself when she is "ratcheting up," and she has learned to question or discuss first rather than attack. She has also learned about relational repair and makes active use of the concept in therapy and in her interactions with her husband and others. Doris has repeatedly told her therapist of her appreciation that she stuck with her through some very difficult times and she has been able to internalize the idea that her therapist likes her and that she is liked by others as well. Her social network has grown and, with it, so have more emotional support and feelings of social success. She is much less lonely, isolated, and unsure of herself as a result.

Hector continues to have mood instability and occasional lapses into suicidality; however, he has been highly responsible in following his safety plan whenever his mood dips precariously. He uses what he learned in the service about being responsible for his buddies and applies it to himself and to his therapist. He now says that since it would not be fair to leave the therapist by committing suicide he won't, even though he still feels on some days that he would be better off dead. One reason for this is that his relationship with his parents remains lacking and he sees them only occasionally. Both parents (but especially his mother) remain disappointed that he did not enter the seminary and are not very sympathetic to his war injuries. Nor did they respond well to learning about the clergy abuse in his past; they preferred to believe that Hector exaggerated what happened with the parish priest, who was a frequent and revered guest in their home. As a result, Hector does not have much trust in his parents' capacity to really know and understand him; he keeps them at a distance and expects little or nothing from them. He has stated: "If I don't expect anything, I don't get disappointed." He has had more success in his interactions with his siblings who he feels are supportive of him and with whom he is developing increasingly close contacts. He was recently asked to be the godfather of a newly born nephew, something that makes him feel proud and honored. Hector is in a Veterans Administration–sponsored job-training program and is hopeful about finding a job once he completes it. He continues to work on his sobriety and is actively involved in AA and NA. He is dating casually and hopes to be able to marry and have a family of his own at some point in the future.

The therapists who treated these clients can share with them a well-deserved sense of pride and accomplishment. They did not provide "perfect" or “textbook” treatment—nor is that a realistic expectation for even the most skilled or experienced therapist—but they were able to “walk the walk” with these two clients by maintaining a consistent awareness of the guiding principles of sequenced (three-phase) and relationship-based treatment that are the core of this book. Although there were rocky times during the course of each client’s treatment, both therapists stayed the course by carefully sequencing, customizing, and individualizing treatment activities to help them recognize and build their capacities for finding security within themselves (self-regulation) and with other people (secure attachment working models). The therapists feel that they learned more about their own capacities and skills as they worked with Doris and Hector, which for them—as for most of us as therapists—is the greatest ancillary reward of helping clients to recover from the wounds of complex trauma.

References

Abramowitz, J. S., Deacon, B. J., & Whiteside, S. P. (2011). *Exposure therapy for anxiety disorders*. Cambridge, MA: Hogrefe & Huber.

Adams, R., Boscarino, J., & Figley, C. R. (2006). Compassion fatigue and psychological distress among social workers: A validation study. *American Journal of Orthopsychiatry*, *76*(1), 103–108.

Adults Surviving Child Abuse. (2012). *Practice guidelines for treatment of complex trauma and trauma-informed care and service delivery*. Kirribilli, Australia: Author.

Alexander, P., Neimeyer, R., Follete, V., Moore, M., & Harter, S. (1989). A comparison of group treatments of women sexually abused as children. *Journal of Consulting and Clinical Psychology*, *57*, 479–483.

Alexander, P. C., & Anderson, C. L. (1994). An attachment approach to psychotherapy with the incest survivor. *Psychotherapy: Theory, Research, Practice, Training*, *31*, 665–675.

Allen, J. (2005). *Coping with trauma: Hope through understanding* (2nd ed.). Washington, DC: American Psychiatric Press.

Allen, J. (2012). *Treating trauma with plain old therapy: Restoring mentalization in attachment relationships*. Washington, DC: American Psychiatric Publishing.

Allen, J., Fonagy, P., & Bateman, A. (2008). *Mentalizing in clinical practice*. Washington, DC: American Psychiatric Association.

American Psychiatric Association. (1980). *Diagnostic and statistical manual of mental disorders* (3rd ed.). Washington, DC: Author.

American Psychiatric Association. (1994). *Diagnostic and statistical manual of mental disorders* (4th ed.). Washington, DC: Author.

American Psychiatric Association. (2000). *Diagnostic and statistical manual of mental disorders* (4th ed., text rev.). Washington, DC: Author.

American Psychological Association. (1995). *Template for developing guidelines: Interventions for mental disorders and psychosocial aspects of physical disorders*. Washington, DC: Author.

Anda, B. , Butchart, A., Felitti, V. J., & Brown, D. W. (2010). Building a framework for global surveillance of the public health implications of adverse childhood experience. *American Journal of Preventive Medicine*, *39*, 93–98.

Armsworth, M. W. (1989). Therapy of incest survivors: Abuse or support? *Child Abuse and Neglect*, *13*(4), 549–562.

Arnold, C., & Fisch, R. (2011). *The impact of complex trauma on development.* New York: Aronson.

Arntz, A., Tiesema, M., & Kindt, M. (2007). Treatment of PTSD: A comparison of imaginal exposure with and without imagery rescripting. *Journal of Behavior Therapy and Experimental Psychiatry*, *38*(4), 345–370.

Baars, D. W., Van der Hart, O., Nijenhuis, E. R. S., Chu, J. A., Glas, G., & Draijer, N. (2011). Predicting stabilizing treatment outcomes for complex posttraumatic stress disorder and dissociative identity disorder: An expertise-based prognostic model. *Journal of Trauma and Dissociation*, *12*, 67–87.

Baker, J. A. H. (2003). Long-term responses to childhood sexual abuse: Life histories of Hispanic women in midlife. *Dissertation Abstracts International*, *64*(7-A), 2646.

Baker, S. (1997). Dancing the dance with dissociatives: Some thoughts on countertransference, projective identification and enactments in the treatment of dissociative disorders. *Dissociation*, *10*(4), 214–222.

Barach, P. M. (1991). Multiple personality disorder as an attachment disorder. *Dissociation: Progress in the Dissociative Disorders*, *4*(3), 117–123.

Barkham, M., Hardy, G. E., & Startup, M. (1996). The IIP-32: A short version of the Inventory of Interpersonal Problems. *British Journal of Clinical Psychology*, *35*(Pt. 1), 21–35.

Barrett, M. J. (2003, July/August). Constructing the third reality. *Psychotherapy Networking.*

Bartholomew, K. (1997). Adult attachment processes: Individual and couple perspectives. *British Journal of Medical Psychology*, *70*(Pt. 3), 249–263; discussion 281–290.

Bartholomew, K., & Horowitz, L. M. (1991). Attachment styles among young adults: A test of a four-category model. *Journal of Personality and Social Psychology*, *61*(2), 228–244.

Basham, K. K., & Miehls, D. (2004). *Transforming the legacy: Couple therapy with survivors of childhood abuse.* New York: Columbia University Press.

Bateman, A., & Fonagy, P. (2004a). Mentalization based treatment of borderline personality disorder. *Journal of Personality Disorders*, *18*, 36–51.

Bateman, A., & Fonagy, P. (2004b). *Psychotherapy for borderline personality disorder: Mentalization-based treatment.* New York: Oxford University Press.

Bateman, A., & Fonagy, P. (2006). *Mentalization based treatment: A practical guide.* Oxford, UK: Oxford University Press.

Beck, A. T., & Kovacs, M. (1979). Assessment of suicide intention: The Scale for Suicide Ideation. *Journal of Consulting and Clinical Psychology*, *47*(2), 343–352.

Beck, A. T., Brown, G. K., & Steer, R. A. (1997). Psychometric characteristics of the Scale for Suicide Ideation with psychiatric outpatients. *Behaviour Research and Therapy*, *33*(11), 1039–1046.

Beck, J., Coffey, S., Foy, D., Keane, T., & Blanchard, E. (2009). Group cognitive behavior therapy for chronic posttraumatic stress disorder: An initial randomized pilot study. *Behavior Therapy*, *40*(1), 82–92.

Beltran, R. O., Silove, D., & Llewellyn, G. M. (2009). Comparison of ICD-10 diagnostic guidelines and research criteria for enduring personality change after catastrophic experience. *Psychopathology*, *42*(2), 113–118.

Bennett, H., & Wells, A. (2010). Metacognition, memory disorganization and rumination in posttraumatic stress symptoms. *Journal of Anxiety Disorders*, *24*(3), 318–325.

Berger, D. (1984). On the way to empathic understanding. *American Journal of Psychotherapy*, *38*(1), 111–120.

Bernier, A., & Dozier, M. (2002). The client–counselor match and the corrective emotional experience: Evidence from interpersonal and attachment research. *Psychotherapy: Theory, Research, Practice, Training*, *39*(1), 32–43.

Bernstein, D. P., Fink, L., Handelsman, L., Foote, J., Lovejoy, M., Wenzel, K., et al. (1994). Initial reliability and validity of a new retrospective measure of child abuse and neglect. *American Journal of Psychiatry*, *151*(8), 1132–1136.

Berntsen, D., & Rubin, D. C. (2006). The Centrality of Event Scale: A measure of integrating a trauma into one's identity and its relation to post-traumatic stress disorder symptoms. *Behaviour Research and Therapy*, *44*(2), 219–231.

Bertran, R. O., & Silove, D. (1999). Expert opinions about the ICD-10 category of enduring personality change after catastrophic experience. *Comprehensive Psychiatry*, *40*(5), 396–403.

Betan, E., Heim, A. K., Conklin, C. Z., & Westen, D. (2005). Countertransference phenomena and personality pathology in clinical practice: An empirical investigation. *American Journal of Psychiatry*, *162*, 890–898.

Bichescu, D., Neuner, F., Schauer, M., & Elbert, T. (2007). Narrative exposure therapy for political imprisonment–related chronic posttraumatic stress disorder and depression. *Behavior Research and Therapy*, *45*(9), 2212–2220.

Black, C. (1981). *"It will never happen to me": Adult children of alcoholics*. Denver, CO: MAC.

Blake, D. D., Weathers, F. W., Nagy, L. M., Kaloupek, D. G., Gusman, F. D., & Charney, D. S., et al. (1995). The development of a clinician-administered PTSD scale. *Journal of Traumatic Stress*, *8*, 75–90.

Blank, A. S. (1994). Clinical detection, diagnosis, and differential diagnosis of posttraumatic stress disorder. *Psychiatric Clinics of North America*, *17*, 351–383.

Bloom, S. L. (2010). Organizational stress as a barrier to trauma-informed service delivery. In M. Becker & B. Levin (Eds.), *A public health perspective of women's mental health* (pp. 295–311). New York: Springer.

Bloom, S. L. (2011, August). *Destroying sanctuary: The crisis in human service delivery systems*. Invited address at the annual meeting of the American Psychological Association, Washington, DC.

Bloom, S. L., & Farragher, B. (2010). *Destroying sanctuary: The crisis in human service delivery systems*. New York: Oxford University Press.

Bloom, S. L. R. (1997). *Creating sanctuary: Toward the evolution of sane societies*. New York: Routledge.

Bollas, C. (1987). *The shadow of the object: Psychoanalysis of the unthought known*. New York: Columbia University Press.

Boniello, M. (1990). Grieving sexual abuse: The therapist's process. *Clinical Social Work Journal*, *18*(4), 367–379.

Boss, P. (2006). *Loss, trauma, and resilience: Therapeutic work with ambiguous loss*. New York: Norton.

Boston Change Project Study Group. (2010). *Change in psychotherapy: A unifying paradigm*. New York: W. W. Norton.

Bowlby, J. (1969). *Attachment and loss: Vol. 1. Attachment*. New York: Basic Books.

Bowlby, J. (1977a). The making and breaking of affectional bonds. I. Aetiology and psychopathology in the light of attachment theory. *British Journal of Psychiatry, 130*, 201–210.

Bowlby, J. (1977b). The making and breaking of affectional bonds. II. Some principles of psychotherapy. *British Journal of Psychiatry, 130*, 421–431.

Bowlby, J. (1988). *A secure base: Clinical applications of attachment theory*. London: Routledge.

Bradley, R., & Follingstad, D. (2003). Group therapy for incarcerated women who experienced interpersonal violence: A pilot study. *Journal of Traumatic Stress, 16*, 337–340.

Brady, K. T. (1997). Posttraumatic stress disorder and comorbidity: Recognizing the many faces of PTSD. *Journal of Clinical Psychiatry, 58*(Suppl. 9), 12–15.

Brand, S., Engel, S., Canfield, R., & Yehuda, R. (2006). The effect of maternal PTSD following *in utero* trauma exposure on behavior and temperament in the 9-month-old infant. *Annals of the New York Academy of Sciences, 1071*, 454–458.

Braun, B. G. (1986). *Treatment of multiple personality disorder*. Washington, DC: American Psychiatric Press.

Braun, B. G. (1988a). BASK model of dissociation. *Dissociation, 1*(1), 4–23.

Braun, B. G. (1988b). The BASK model of dissociation: Clinical applications. *Dissociation, 1*(2), 16–23.

Bridges, N. (1994). Meaning and management of attraction: Neglected aspects of psychotherapy training and practice. *Journal of Psychotherapy, 31*, 424–433.

Briere, J. (1989). *Therapy for adults molested as children: Beyond survival*. New York: Springer.

Briere, J. (1995). *Trauma Symptom Inventory (TSI)*. Odessa, FL: Psychological Assessment Resources.

Briere, J. (1996). *Therapy for adults molested as children: Beyond survival* (2nd ed.). New York: Springer.

Briere, J. (2000a). *Cognitive Distortions Scale (CDS)*. Odessa, FL: Psychological Assessment Resources.

Briere, J. (2000b). *Inventory of Altered Self-Capacities (IASC)*. Odessa, FL: Psychological Assessment Resources.

Briere, J. (2001). *Detailed Assessment of Posttraumatic Stress (DAPS)*. Odessa, FL: Psychological Assessment Resources.

Briere, J. (2002). *Multiscale Dissociation Inventory*. Odessa. FL: Psychological Assessment Resources.

Briere, J. (2004). *Psychological assessment of adult posttraumatic states: Phenomenology, diagnosis, and measurement* (2nd ed.). Washington, DC: American Psychological Association.

Briere, J. (2011). *Trauma Symptom Inventory–2 (TSI-2) Manual*. Odessa, FL: Psychological Assessment Resources.

Briere, J., & Elliott, D. M. (2003). Prevalence and psychological sequelae of self-reported childhood physical and sexual abuse in a general population sample of men and women. *Child Abuse and Neglect, 27*(10), 1205–1222.

Briere, J. N., & Lanktree, C. B. (2012). *Treating complex trauma in adolescents and young adults*. Thousand Oaks, CA: Sage.

Briere, J., & Scott, C. (2006). *Principles of trauma therapy: A guide to symptoms, evaluation, and treatment*. Thousand Oaks, CA: Sage.

Briere, J., & Spinazzola, J. (2005). Phenomenology and psychological assessment of complex posttraumatic states. *Journal of Traumatic Stress, 18*, 401–412.

Briere, J., & Spinazzola, J. (2009). Assessment of the sequelae of complex trauma:

Evidence-based measures. In C. A. Courtois & J. D. Ford (Eds.), *Treating complex traumatic stress disorders: An evidence-based guide* (pp. 104–123). New York: Guilford Press.

Briere, J., & Scott, C. (2012). *Principles of trauma therapy: A guide to symptoms, evaluation, and treatment* (2nd ed.). Thousand Oaks, CA: Sage.

Briere, J., Weathers, F. W., & Runtz, M. (2005). Is dissociation a multidimensional construct? Data from the Multiscale Dissociation Inventory. *Journal of Traumatic Stress, 18*(3), 221–231.

Briggs-Gowan, M. J., Ford, J. D., Fraleigh, L., McCarthy, K., & Carter, A. S. (2011). Prevalence of exposure to potentially traumatic events in a healthy birth cohort of very young children in the northeastern United States. *Journal of Traumatic Stress, 23*(6), 725–733.

Brisch, K. H. (2002). *Treating attachment disorders: From theory to therapy*. New York: Guilford Press.

Brockhouse, R., Msetfi, R. M., Cohen, K., & Joseph, S. (2011). Vicarious exposure to trauma and growth in therapists: The moderating effects of sense of coherence, organizational support, and empathy. *Journal of Traumatic Stress, 24*(6), 735–742.

Bromberg, P. M. (1993). Shadow and substance: A relational perspective on clinical process. *Psychoanalytic Psychology, 10*, 147–168.

Bromberg, P. M. (1995). A rose by any other name; Commentary on Lerner's "Treatment issues in a case of possible multiple personality disorder." *Psychoanalytic Psychology, 12*, 143–149.

Bromberg, P. M. (1998). *Standing in the spaces: Essays on clinical process, trauma, and dissociation*. Mahwah, NJ: Analytic Press.

Bromberg, P. M. (2003). Something wicked this way comes: Trauma, dissociation, and conflict: The space where psychoanalysis, cognitive science, and neuroscience overlap. *Psychoanalytic Psychology, 20*, 558–574.

Brown, D. (2009). Assessment of attachment and abuse history, and adult attachment style. In C. A. Courtois & J. D. Ford (Eds.), *Treating complex traumatic stress disorders: An evidence-based guide* (pp. 124–144). New York: Guilford Press.

Brown, L. S. (2008). *Cultural competence in trauma therapy: Beyond the flashback*. Washington, DC: American Psychological Association.

Brown, L. S. (2009). Cultural competence. In C. A. Courtois & J. D. Ford (Eds.), *Treating complex traumatic stress disorders: An evidence-based guide* (pp. 166–182). New York: Guilford Press.

Brown, L. S. (2012). *Your turn for care: Surviving the aging and death of adults who harmed you*. Available at *www.drlaurabrown.com*.

Bryant, R. A. (2010). The complexity of complex PTSD. *American Journal of Psychiatry, 167*, 879–881.

Bryant, R. A. (2012). Simplifying complex PTSD: Comment on Resick et al. (2012). *Journal of Traumatic Stress, 25*, 252–253.

Buss, A. H., & Durkee, A. (1957). An inventory for assessing different kinds of hostility. *Journal of Abnormal Social Psychology, 21*, 343–349.

Butler, R. W., Mueser, K. T., Sprock, J., & Braff, D. L. (1996). Positive symptoms of psychosis in posttraumatic stress disorder. *Biological Psychiatry, 39*(10), 839–844.

Cahill, S. P., Rothbaum, B. O., Resick, P., & Follette, V. (2009). Cognitive behavior therapy for adults. In E. B. Foa, T. M. Keane, M. J. Friedman, & J. A. Cohen (Eds.), *Effective treatments for PTSD* (2nd ed., pp. 139–222). New York: Guilford Press.

Calof, D. (1987). *Treating adult survivors of incest and child abuse.* Workshop presented at The Family Networker Symposium, Washington, DC.

Campanini, R. F., Schoedl, A. F., Pupo, M. C., Costa, A. C., Krupnick, J. L., & Mello, M. F. (2010). Efficacy of interpersonal therapy-group format adapted to post-traumatic stress disorder: An open-label add-on trial. *Depression and Anxiety, 27,* 72–77.

Cann, A., Calhoun, L. G., Tedeschi, R. G., Triplett, K. N., Vishnevsky, T., & Lindstrom, C. M. (2011). Assessing posttraumatic cognitive processes: The Event Related Rumination Inventory. *Anxiety Stress and Coping, 24*(2), 137–156.

Canning, M. (2008). *Lust, anger, love: Understanding sexual addiction and the road to healthy intimacy.* Naperville, IL: Sourcebooks.

Carey, T. A. (2011). Exposure and reorganization: The what and how of effective psychotherapy. *Clinical Psychology Review, 31*(2), 236–248.

Carlson, E. B. (1997). *Trauma assessments: A clinician's guide.* New York: Guilford Press.

Carlson, E. B., & Putnam, F. W. (1993). An update on the Dissociative Experiences Scale. *Dissociation: Progress in the Dissociative Disorders, 6*(1), 16–27.

Carmen, E. H., Rieker, P. R., & Mills, T. (1984). Victims of violence and psychiatric illness. *American Journal of Psychiatry, 143,* 378–383.

Carnes, P. J. (1991). *Don't call it love: Recovery from sex addiction.* New York: Bantam.

Carnes, P. J., & Delmonico, D. L. (1996). Childhood abuse and multiple addictions: Research findings in a sample of self-identified sexual addicts. *Sexual Addictions and Compulsivity, 3,* 258–268.

Catanzaro, S. J., & Mearns, J. (1990). Measuring generalized expectancies for negative mood regulation: Initial scale development and implications. *Journal of Personality Assessment, 54*(3–4), 546–563.

Catanzaro, S. J., Wasch, H. H., Kirsch, I., & Mearns, J. (2000). Coping-related expectancies and dispositions as prospective predictors of coping responses and symptoms. *Journal of Personality, 68*(4), 757–788.

Catherall, D. R. (1992). *Back from the brink: A family guide to overcoming traumatic stress.* New York: Bantam.

Catherall, D. R. (1998). Treating traumatized families. In C. R. Figley (Ed.), *Burnout in families: The systemic costs of caring* (pp. 187–215). Boca Raton, FL: CRC Press.

Catherall, D. R. (2004). *Handbook of stress, trauma, and the family.* New York: Brunner-Routledge.

Catherall, D. R. (2005). *Family stressors: Interventions for stress and trauma.* New York: Brunner-Routledge.

Caudill, B. O., Jr. (1977). Documentation: The therapist's shield. In L. E. Hedges, R. Hilton, V. S. Hilton, & B. O. Caudill, Jr., *Therapists at risk: Perils of the intimacy of the therapeutic relationship* (pp. 263–268). Northvale, NJ: Aronson.

Chefetz, R. A. (n.d.). *The erotic countertransference in the treatment of posttraumatic stress disorders.* Unpublished manuscript.

Chefetz, R. A. (1997). Special case transferences and countertransferences in the treatment of dissociative disorders. *Dissociation: Progress in the Dissociative Disorders, 10*(4), 255–265.

Chefetz, R. A., & Bromberg, P. M. (2004). Talking with "me" and "not-me": A dialogue. *Contemporary Psychoanalysis, 40*(3), 409–464.

Chemtob, C., Roitblat, H., Hamada, C. J., Carlson, J. G., & Twentyman, C. (1988). A cognitive action theory of PTSD. *Journal of Anxiety Disorders, 2,* 253–275.

Chemtob, C. M., Bauer, G. B., Hamada, R. S., Pelowski, S. R., & Muraoka, M. Y. (1989). Patient suicide: Occupational hazard for psychologists and psychiatrists. *Professional Psychology: Research and Practice*, *20*(5), 294–300.

Chu, J. A. (1988). Ten traps for therapists in the treatment of trauma survivors. *Dissociation*, *1*(4), 24–32.

Chu, J. A. (1992). The therapeutic roller coaster: Dilemmas in the treatment of childhood abuse survivors. *Journal of Psychotherapy Practice and Research*, *1*(4), 351–370.

Chu, J. A. (1998). *Rebuilding shattered lives: The responsible treatment of complex post-traumatic and dissociative disorders*. New York: Wiley.

Chu, J. A. (2011). *Rebuilding shattered lives: The responsible treatment of complex post-traumatic and dissociative disorders* (2nd ed.). Hoboken, NJ: Wiley.

Chu, J. A., Frey, L. M., Ganzel, B. L., & Matthews, J. A. (1999). Memories of childhood abuse: Dissociation, amnesia, and corroboration. *American Journal of Psychiatry*, *156*, 749–755.

Cicchetti, D., Rogosch, F. A., Howe, M. L., & Toth, S. L. (2010). The effects of maltreatment and neuroendocrine regulation on memory performance. *Child Development*, *81*(5), 1504–1519.

Classen, C., Koopman, C., Nevill-Manning, K., & Spiegel, D. (2001). A preliminary report comparing trauma-focused and present-focused group therapy against a wait-listed condition among childhood sexual abuse survivors with PTSD. *Journal of Aggression, Maltreatment and Trauma*, *4*, 265–288.

Cloitre, M., Cohen, L. R., & Koenen, K. C. (2006). *Treating survivors of childhood abuse: Psychotherapy for the interrupted life*. New York: Guilford Press.

Cloitre, M., Courtois, C. A., Charuvastra, A., Carapezza, R., Stolbach, B. C., & Green, B. L. (2011). Treatment of complex PTSD: Results of the ISTSS expert clinician survey on best practices. *Journal of Traumatic Stress*, *24*(6), 615–627.

Cloitre, M., & Koenen, K. (2001). The impact of borderline personality disorder on process group outcome among women with posttraumatic stress disorder related to childhood abuse. *International Journal of Group Psychotherapy*, *51*, 379–398.

Cloitre, M., Koenen, K., Cohen, L. R., & Han, H. (2002). Skills training in affective and interpersonal effectiveness in the treatment of women with PTSD. *Journal of Consulting and Clinical Psychology*, *70*, 1067–1074.

Cloitre, M., Stolbach, B. C., Herman, J. L., Van der Kolk, B., Pynoos, R., Wang, J., et al. (2009). Developmental approach to complex PTSD: Childhood and adult cumulative trauma as predictors of symptom complexity. *Journal of Traumatic Stress*, *22*, 399–408.

Cloitre, M., Stovall-McClough, K., Nooner, K., Zorbas, P., Cherry, S., Jackson, C. L., et al. (2010). Treatment for PTSD related to childhood abuse: A randomized controlled trial. *American Journal of Psychiatry*, *167*(8), 915–924.

Cloitre, M. K., Stovall-McClough, C., Miranda, R., & Chemtob, C. M. (2004). Therapeutic alliance, negative mood regulation, and treatment outcome in child abuse–related posttraumatic stress disorder. *Journal of Consulting and Clinical Psychology*, *72*(3), 411–416.

Cloitre, M., Miranda, R. Stovall-McClough, K. C., & Han, H. (2005). Beyond PTSD: Emotion regulation and interpersonal problems as predictors of functional impairment in survivors of childhood abuse. *Behavior Therapy*, *36*, 119–124.

Clum, G. (2008). Self-help. In G. Reyes, J. D. Elhai, & J. D. Ford (Eds.), *Encyclopedia of psychological trauma* (pp. 591–595). Hoboken, NJ: Wiley.

Cohen, E. (2008). Parenting in the throes of traumatic events. In D. Brom, R.

Pat-Horenczyk, & J. D. Ford (Eds.), *Treating traumatized children* (pp. 72–84). London: Routledge.

Cohen, J. A., Mannarino, A. P., & Iyengar, S. (2011). Community treatment of posttraumatic stress disorder for children exposed to intimate partner violence: A randomized controlled trial. *Archives of Pediatric and Adolescent Medicine, 165*(1), 16–21.

Cole, P., & Putnam, F. W. (1992). Effect of incest on self and social functioning: A developmental psychopathology perspective. *Journal of Consulting and Clinical Psychology, 60*, 174–184.

Collins, N. L., Ford, M. B., Guichard, A. C., & Allard, L. M. (2006). Working models of attachment and attribution processes in intimate relationships. *Personality and Social Psychology Bulletin, 32*(2), 201–219.

Cook, J., Schnurr, P. P., & Foa, E. B. (2004). Bridging the gap between posttraumatic stress disorder research and clinical practice: The example of exposure therapy. *Psychotherapy: Theory, Research, Practice, Training, 41*(4), 374–387.

Copeland, W. E., Keeler, G., Angold, A., & Costello, E. (2010). Posttraumatic stress without trauma in children. *American Journal of Psychiatry, 167*(9), 1059–1065.

Courtois, C. (2003, March). *Advances in trauma treatment.* Paper presented at the 26th annual Psychotherapy Networker Symposium, Washington, DC.

Courtois, C. A. (1988). *Healing the incest wound: Adult survivors in therapy.* New York: Norton.

Courtois, C. A. (1999). *Recollections of sexual abuse: Treatment principles and guidelines.* New York: Norton.

Courtois, C. A. (2004). Complex trauma, complex reactions: Assessment and treatment. *Psychotherapy: Theory, Research, Practice, and Training, 41*, 412–425.

Courtois, C. A. (2005). When one partner has been sexually abused as a child. In D. Catherall (Ed.), *Family stressors: Interventions for stress and trauma* (pp. 95–114). New York: Brunner/Routledge.

Courtois, C. A. (2010). *Healing the incest wound: Adult survivors in therapy* (2nd ed.). New York: Norton.

Courtois, C. A., & Ford, J. D. (Eds.). (2009). *Treating complex traumatic stress disorders: An evidence-based guide.* New York: Guilford Press.

Courtois, C. A., Ford, J. D., & Cloitre, M. (2009). Best practices in psychotherapy for adults. In C. A. Courtois & J. D. Ford (Eds.), *Treating complex traumatic stress disorders: An evidence-based guide* (pp. 82–103). New York: Guilford Press.

Courtois, C. A., & Gold, S. N. (2009). The need for inclusion of psychological trauma in the professional curriculum: A call to action. *Psychological Trauma: Theory, Research, Practice, and Policy, 1*(1), 3–23.

Cozolino, L. (2002). *The neuroscience of psychotherapy: Building and rebuilding the human brain.* New York: Norton.

Cozolino, L. (2004). *The making of a therapist: A practical guide for the inner journey.* New York: Norton.

Crittenden, P. M., & Landini, A. (2011). *Assessing adult attachment: A dynamic–maturational approach to discourse analysis.* New York: Norton.

Dalenberg, C. (2000). *Countertransference and the treatment of trauma.* Washington, DC: American Psychological Association.

Dalgleish, T. (2004). Cognitive theories of posttraumatic stress disorder: The evolution of multi-representational theorizing. *Psychological Bulletin, 130*, 228–260.

Danieli, Y. (1984). Psychotherapists' participation in the conspiracy of silence about the Holocaust. *Psychoanalytic Psychology, 1*, 23–42.

Davies, J. M., & Frawley, M. G. (1991). Dissociative processes and transference–countertransference paradigms in the psychoanalytically oriented treatment of adult survivors of childhood sexual abuse. *Psychoanalytic Dialogues*, *2*(1), 5–36.

Davies, J. M., & Frawley, M. G. (1994). *Treating the adult survivor of childhood sexual abuse: A psychoanalytic perspective*. New York: Basic Books.

Davis, L. (1991). *Allies in healing: When the person you love was sexually abused as a child*. New York: Harper Perennial.

Davis, L. (2002). *I thought we'd never speak again: The road from estrangement to reconciliation*. New York: Harper Collins.

Daviss, W. B., Mooney, D., Racusin, R., Ford, J. D., Fleischer, A., & McHugo, G. J. (2000). Predicting posttraumatic stress after hospitalization for pediatric injury. *Journal of the American Academy of Child and Adolescent Psychiatry*, *39*(5), 576–583.

Dell, P. F. (2006). Multidimensional Inventory of Dissociation (MID): A comprehensive measure of pathological dissociation. *Journal of Trauma and Dissociation*, *7*(2), 77–106.

Dell, P. F., & O'Neil, J. A. (Eds.). (2009). *Dissociation and the dissociative disorders: DSM-V and beyond*. New York: Routledge/Taylor & Francis Group.

Dennis, M. L., Chan, Y. F., & Funk, R. R. (2006). Development and validation of the GAIN Short Screener (GSS) for internalizing, externalizing and substance use disorders and crime/violence problems among adolescents and adults. *American Journal of Addictions*, *15*(Suppl. 1), 80–91.

Dennis, M. L., Funk, R., Godley, S. H., Godley, M. D., & Waldron, H. (2004). Cross-validation of the alcohol and cannabis use measures in the Global Appraisal of Individual Needs (GAIN) and Timeline Followback (TLFB; Form 90) among adolescents in substance abuse treatment. *Addiction*, *99*(Suppl. 2), 120–128.

DePrince, A. P., & Newman, E. (2011). The art and science of trauma-focused training and education. *Psychological Trauma: Theory, Research, and Policy*, *3*(3), 213–214.

Derogatis, L. R. (1977). *SCL-90: Administration, scoring and procedure manual-I for the R (revised) version*. Baltimore: Johns Hopkins University School of Medicine.

Derogatis, L. R., & Melisaratos, N. (1983). The Brief Symptom Inventory: An introductory report. *Psychological Medicine*, *13*(3), 595–605.

Derogatis, L. R., & Unger, R. (2010). Symptom Checklist–90—Revised. *Corsini Encyclopedia of Psychology*, 1–2.

Devilly, G., Wright, R., & Varker, T. (2009). Vicarious trauma, secondary traumatic stress or simply burnout? The effect of trauma therapy on mental health professionals. *Australian and New Zealand Journal of Psychiatry*, *43*(4), 373–385.

DeYoung, M. (1981). Case reports: The sexual exploitation of incest victims by helping professionals. *Victimology: An International Journal*, *67*(1–4), 91–101.

Doka, K. (1989). *Disenfranchised grief: Recognizing hidden sorrow*. Lexington, MA: Lexington Books.

Dolan, R., Arnkoff, D., & Glass, C. (1993). Client attachment style and the psychotherapist's interpersonal stance. *Psychotherapy*, *30*, 408–412.

Dozier, M. (1990). Attachment organization and treatment use for adults with serious psychopathological disorders. *Development and Psychopathology*, *2*, 47–60.

Dozier, M., Cue, K., & Barnett, L. (1994). Clinicians as caregivers: The role of attachment organization in treatment. *Journal of Consulting and Clinical Psychology*, *62*, 793–800.

Dozier, M., & Tyrrell, C. (1997). The role of attachment in therapeutic relationships. In J. A. Simpson & W. S. Rholes (Eds.), *Attachment theory and close relationships* (pp. 221–248). New York: Guilford Press.

Dozier, M., & Tyrell, C. (1999). *Foster parents' understanding of children's problematic attachment strategies: The need for therapeutic responsiveness.* Unpublished manuscript, University of Delaware.

Duckworth, M. P., & Follette, V. M. (2011). *Retraumatization: Assessment, treatment, and prevention.* New York: Routledge.

Ellason, J. W., & Ross, C. A. (1995). Positive and negative symptoms in dissociative identity disorder and schizophrenia: A comparative analysis. *Journal of Nervous and Mental Disease*, *183*(4), 236–241.

Elliott, D. M., Mok, D. S., & Briere, J. (2004). Adult sexual assault: Prevalence, symptomatology, and sex differences in the general population. *Journal of Traumatic Stress*, *17*(3), 203–211.

Elwood, L. S., Mott, J., Lohr, J. M., & Galovski, T. E. (2011). Secondary trauma symptoms in clinicians: A critical review of the construct, specificity, and implications for trauma-focused treatment. *Clinical Psychology Review*, *31*(1), 25–36.

Everson, R., & Figley, C. (2011). *Families under fire.* New York: Routledge.

Fairbank, J. A., Putnam, F. W., & Harris, W. W. (2007). The prevalence and impact of child traumatic stress. In M. J. Friedman, T. M. Keane, & P. A. Resick (Eds.), *Handbook of PTSD* (pp. 229–251). New York: Guilford Press.

Fallot, R. D., & Harris, M. (2002). The trauma recovery and empowerment model (TREM). *Community Mental Health Journal*, *38*, 475–485.

Fallot, R. D., & Harris, M. (2008). Trauma-informed approaches to systems of care. *Trauma Psychology Newsletter*, *3*(1), 6–7.

Farber, B. A., Lippert, R. A., & Nevas, D. B. (1995). The therapist as attachment figure. *Psychotherapy*, *32*, 204–212.

Farley, M. (2003). *Prostitution, trafficking, and traumatic stress.* New York: Haworth Press.

Felitti, V. J., Anda, R. F., Nordenberg, D., Williamson, D. F., Spitz, A. M., Edwards, V., et al. (1998). Relationship of childhood abuse and household dysfunction to many of the leading causes of death in adults: The Adverse Childhood Experiences (ACE) Study. *American Journal of Preventive Medicine*, *14*(4), 245–258.

Figley, C. E. (Ed.). (1985). *Trauma and its wake: The study and treatment of post-traumatic stress disorder.* New York: Brunner/Mazel.

Figley, C. R. (1989). *Helping traumatized families.* San Francisco: Jossey-Bass.

Figley, C. R. (1995). Compassion fatigue: Towards a new understanding of the costs of caring. In B. Stamm (Ed.), *Secondary traumatic stress: Self-care issues for clinicians researchers, and educators* (pp. 3–28). Lutherville, MD: Sidran.

Figley, C. R. (2002a). *Brief treatments for the traumatized: Special project of the Green Cross Foundation.* Connecticut: Westport.

Figley, C. R. (2002b). *Treating compassion fatigue.* New York: Brunner/Routledge.

Fine, C. G., & Madden, N. E. (2000). Group psychotherapy in the treatment of dissociative identity disorder and allied dissociative disorders. In R. H. Klein & V. L. Schermer (Eds.). *Group psychotherapy for psychological trauma* (pp. 298–325). New York: Guilford Press.

Finkelhor, D. (2007). Developmental victimology: The comprehensive study of childhood victimization. In R. C. Davis, A. J. Lurigio, & S. Herman (Eds.), *Victims of crime* (3rd ed., pp. 9–34). Thousand Oaks, CA: Sage.

Finkelhor, D. (2008). *Childhood victimization: Violence, crime, and abuse in the lives of young people*. New York: Oxford University Press.

Finklehor, D., Ormrod, R. K., Turner, H. A., & Hamby, S. L. (2005). The victimization of children and youth: A comprehensive, national survey. *Child Maltreatment*, *10*(1), 5–25.

Finkelhor, D., Turner, H. A., Ormrod, R. K., & Hamby, S. L. (2010). Trends in childhood violence and abuse exposure: Evidence from two national surveys. *Archives of Pediatrics and Adolescent Medicine*, *164*(3), 238–242.

First, M. B., Gibbon, M., Spitzer, R. L., Williams, J. B. W., & Benjamin, L. S. (1997). *Structured Clinical Interview for DSM-IV Axis II Personality Disorders (SCID-II)*. Washington, DC: American Psychiatric Press.

Fischman, Y. (1991). Interacting with trauma: Clinicians' responses to treating psychological aftereffects of political repression. *American Journal of Orthopsychiatry*, *61*(2), 179–185.

Fisher, J., & Ogden, P. (2009). Sensorimotor psychotherapy. In C. Courtois & J. D. Ford (Eds.), *Treating complex posttraumatic stress disorders: An evidence-based guide* (pp. 312–350). New York: Guilford Press.

Foa, E. B. (1995). *Posttraumatic Stress Diagnostic Scale*. Minneapolis, MN: National Computer Systems.

Foa, E. B., Ehlers, A., Clark, D. M., Tolin, D. F., & Orsillo, S. M. (1999). The Posttraumatic Cognitions Inventory (PTCI): Development and validation. *Psychological Assessment*, *11*(3), 303–314.

Foa, E. B., Hembree, E. A., & Rothbaum, B. O. (2007). *Prolonged exposure therapy for PTSD: Emotional processing of traumatic experiences: Therapist guide*. New York: Oxford University Press.

Foa, E. B., Johnson, K. M., Feeny, N. C., & Treadwell, K. R. (2001). The child PTSD Symptom Scale: A preliminary examination of its psychometric properties. *Journal of Clinical Child and Adolescent Psychology*, *30*(3), 376–384.

Foa, E. B., Keane, T. M., Friedman, M. J., & Cohen, J. A. (Eds.). (2009). *Effective treatments for PTSD: Practice guidelines from the International Society for Traumatic Stress Studies* (2nd ed.). New York: Guilford Press.

Foa, E. B., & Kozak, M. J. (1986). Emotional processing of fear: Exposure to corrective information. *Psychological Bulletin*, *99*(1), 20–35.

Foa, E. B., & Tolin, D. F. (2000). Comparison of the PTSD Symptom Scale—Interview Version and the Clinician-Administered PTSD scale. *Journal of Traumatic Stress*, *13*(2), 181–191.

Follette, V. M., Alexander, P., & Follette, W. (1991). Individual predictors of outcome in group treatment for incest survivors. *Journal of Consulting and Clinical Psychology*, *59*, 150–155.

Follette, V. M., Iverson, K. M., & Ford, J. D. (2009). Contextual behavior trauma therapy. In C. A. Courtois & J. D. Ford (Eds.), *Treating complex traumatic stress disorders: An evidence-based guide* (pp. 264–285). New York: Guilford Press.

Follette, V. M., La Bash, H. A., & Sewell, M. T. (2010). Adult disclosure of a history of childhood sexual abuse: Implications for behavioral psychotherapy. *Journal of Trauma and Dissociation*, *11*, 228–243.

Follette, V. M., Polusny, M. A., Bechtle, A. E., & Naugle, A. E. (1996). Cumulative trauma: The impact of child sexual abuse, adult sexual assault, and spouse abuse. *Journal of Traumatic Stress*, *9*, 25–35.

Follette, V. M., & Vijay, A. (2009). Mindfulness for trauma and posttraumatic stress disorder. *Clinical Handbook of Mindfulness*, *43*, 299–317.

Fonagy, P., Gergely, G., Jurist, E. L., & Target, M. (2002). *Affect regulation, mentalization, and the development of the self.* New York: Other Press.

Forbes, D., Creamer, M., Bisson, J. I., Cohen, J. A., Crow, B. E., Foa, E. B., et al. (2010). A guide to guidelines for the treatment of PTSD and related conditions. *Journal of Traumatic Stress, 23*(5), 537–552.

Ford, J. D. (2005). Treatment implications of altered neurobiology, affect regulation and information processing following child maltreatment. *Psychiatric Annals, 35*(5), 410–419.

Ford, J. D. (2009a). Dissociation in complex posttraumatic stress disorder or disorders of extreme stress not otherwise specified (DESNOS). In P. F. Dell & J. A. O'Neill (Eds.), *Dissociation and the dissociative disorders: DSM-V and beyond* (pp. 471–483). New York: Routledge.

Ford, J. D. (2009b). Neurobiological and developmental research: Clinical implications. In C. A. Courtois & J. D. Ford (Eds.), *Treating complex traumatic stress disorders: An evidence-based guide* (pp. 31–58). New York: Guilford Press.

Ford, J. D. (2009c). *Posttraumatic stress disorder: Scientific and professional dimensions.* Boston: Academic Press.

Ford, J. D. (2010). Complex adult sequelae of early life exposure to psychological trauma. In R. A. Lanius, E. Vermetten, & C. Pain (Eds.), *The impact of early life trauma on health and disease: The hidden epidemic* (pp. 69–76). New York: Cambridge University Press.

Ford, J. D. (2012). Enhancing affect regulation in psychotherapy with complex trauma survivors. In D. Murphy, S. Joseph, & B. Harris (Eds.), *Trauma, recovery, and the therapeutic relationship.* London: Oxford University Press.

Ford, J. D., & Courtois, C. A. (2009). Defining and understanding complex trauma and complex traumatic stress disorders. In C. A. Courtois & J. D. Ford (Eds.), *Treating complex traumatic stress disorders: An evidence-based guide* (pp. 13–30). New York: Guilford Press.

Ford, J. D., Courtois, C. A., Steele, K., Van der Hart, O., & Nijenhuis, E. R. (2005). Treatment of complex posttraumatic self-dysregulation. *Journal of Traumatic Stress, 18*(5), 437–447.

Ford, J. D., & DTD Field Trial Work Group. (2011). *Developmental Trauma Disorder Structured Interview (Version 10.4).* Farmington, CT: University of Connecticut Health Center.

Ford, J. D., Fallot, R., & Harris, M. (2009). Group therapy. In C. Courtois & J. D. Ford (Eds.), *Treating complex traumatic stress disorders: An evidence-based guide* (pp. 415–440). New York: Guilford Press.

Ford, J. D., & Kidd, P. (1998). Early childhood trauma and disorders of extreme stress as predictors of treatment outcome with chronic posttraumatic stress disorder. *Journal of Traumatic Stress, 11*(4), 743–761.

Ford, J. D., Racusin, R., Ellis, C. G., Daviss, W. B., Reiser, J., Fleischer, A., et al. (2000). Child maltreatment, other trauma exposure, and posttraumatic symptomatology among children with oppositional defiant and attention deficit hyperactivity disorders. *Child Maltreatment, 5*(3), 205–217.

Ford, J. D., & Russo, E. (2006). Trauma-focused, present-centered, emotional self-regulation approach to integrated treatment for posttraumatic stress and addiction: Trauma adaptive recovery group education and therapy (TARGET). *American Journal of Psychotherapy, 60*(4), 335–355.

Ford, J. D., & Saltzman, W. (2009). Family system therapy. In C. A. Courtois & J. D. Ford (Eds.), *Treating complex traumatic stress disorders: An evidence-based guide* (pp. 391–414). New York: Guilford Press.

Ford, J. D., & Smith, S. (2008). Complex posttraumatic stress disorder in trauma-exposed adults receiving public sector outpatient substance abuse disorder treatment. *Addiction Research and Theory, 16*(2), 193–203.

Ford, J. D., Steinberg, K., Hawke, J., Levine, J., & Zhang, W. (2012). Evaluation of trauma affect regulation: Guide for education and therapy (TARGET) with traumatized girls involved in delinquency. *Journal of Clinical Child and Adolescent Psychology, 41*(1), 27–37.

Ford, J. D., Steinberg, K., & Zhang, W. (2011). A randomized clinical trial comparing affect regulation and social problem solving psychotherapies for high risk mothers with PTSD. *Behavior Therapy, 42*(4), 560–578.

Forgays, D. G., Forgays, D. K., & Spielberger, C. D. (1997). Factor structure of the State–Trait Anger Expression Inventory. *Journal of Personality Assessment, 69*(3), 497–507.

Fosha, D. (2000). *The transforming power of affect: A model for accelerated change*. New York: Basic Books.

Fosha, D., Paivio, S. C., Gleiser, K., & Ford, J. D. (2009). Experiential and emotion-focused therapy. In C. A. Courtois & J. D. Ford (Eds.), *Treating complex traumatic stress disorders: An evidence-based guide* (pp. 286–311). New York: Guilford Press.

Fosha, D., Siegel, D. J., & Solomon, M. F. (Eds.). (2009). *The healing power of emotion: Affective neuroscience, development and clinical practice*. New York: Norton.

Foy, D. W. (2008). On the development of practice guidelines for evidence-based group approaches following disasters. *International Journal of Group Psychotherapy, 58*, 569–576.

Fradkin, H. (2012). *Joining forces: Empowering male survivors to thrive*. New York: Hay House.

Frank, J. (1973). *Persuasion and healing*. Baltimore: Johns Hopkins University Press.

Freyd, J. J. (1994). Betrayal trauma: Traumatic amnesia as an adaptive response to childhood abuse. *Ethics and Behavior, 4*(4), 307–329.

Friedman, M. J., & Davidson, J. R. T. (2007). Pharmacotherapy for PTSD. In M. J. Friedman, T. M. Keane, & P. A. Resick (Eds.), *Handbook of PTSD: Science and practice* (pp. 376–405). New York: Guilford Press.

Friedman, M. J., Davidson, J. R. T., & Stein, D. J. (2008). Pharmacotherapy for adults. In E. B. Foa, T. M. Keane, M. J. Friedman, & J. A. Cohen (Eds.), *Effective treatments for PTSD: Practice guidelines from the International Society for Traumatic Stress Studies* (pp. 245–278). New York: Guilford Press.

Friedman, M. J., & McEwen, B. S. (2004). Posttraumatic stress disorder, allostatic load, and medical illness. In P. P. Schnurr & B. L. Green (Eds.), *Trauma and health: Physical health consequences of exposure to extreme stress* (pp. 157–188). Washington, DC: American Psychological Association.

Gabbard, G. (Ed.). (1989). *Sexual exploitation in professional relationships*. Washington, DC: American Psychiatric Association.

Gabbard, G. O. (1993). An overview of countertransference with borderline patients. *Journal of Psychotherapy Practice and Research, 2*, 7–19.

Garner, D. M., & Garfinkel, P. E. (1979). The Eating Attitudes Test: An index of the symptoms of anorexia nervosa. *Psychological Medicine, 9*, 273–279.

Gartner, R. B. (1999). *Betrayed as boys: Psychodynamic treatment of sexually abused men*. New York: Guilford Press.

Gelinas, D. J. (1983). The persisting negative effects of incest. *American Journal of Psychiatry, 46*, 313–332.

Gelinas, D. J. (2003). Integrating EMDR into phase-oriented treatment for trauma. *Journal of Trauma and Dissociation*, *4*(3), 91–135.

Gendlin, E. T. (1982). *Focusing* (2nd ed.). New York: Bantam Books.

George, C., Kaplan, M., & Main, M. (1996). *Attachment interview for adults.* Unpublished manuscript, University of California, Berkeley.

Gold, S. N. (2000). *Not trauma alone: Therapy for child abuse survivors in family and social context.* Philadelphia: Brunner-Routledge.

Gold, S. N. (2009). Contextual therapy. In C. A. Courtois & J. D. Ford (Eds.), *Treating complex traumatic stress disorders: An evidence-based guide* (pp. 227–242). New York: Guilford Press.

Goodman, M. (2012). Complex PTSD is a distinct entity: Comment on Resick et al. (2012). *Journal of Traumatic Stress*, *25*(3), 254–255.

Greenson, R. (1967). *The technique and practice of psychoanalysis.* New York: International Universities Press.

Grunert, B. K., Weis, J. M., Smucker, M. R., & Christianson, H. F. (2007). Imagery rescripting and reprocessing therapy after failed prolonged exposure for post-traumatic stress disorder following industrial injury. *Journal of Behavior Therapy and Experimental Psychiatry*, *38*(4), 317–328.

Gutheil, T., & Brodsky, A. (2008). *Preventing boundary violations in clinical practice.* New York: Guilford Press.

Hahn, W. K. (2000). Shame: Countertransference identifications in individual psychotherapy. *Psychotherapy: Theory, Research, Practice, Training*, *37*(1), 10–21.

Halligan, S. L., Michael, T., Clark, D. M., & Ehlers, A. (2003). Posttraumatic stress disorder following assault: The role of cognitive processing, trauma memory, and appraisals. *Journal of Consulting and Clinical Psychology*, *71*(3), 419–431.

Hare-Mustin, R. T., Marecek, J., Kaplan, A. G., & Liss-Levinson, N. (1979). Rights of clients, responsibilities of therapists. *American Psychologist*, *34*(1), 3–16.

Harman, R., & Lee, D. (2010). The role of shame and self-critical thinking in the development and maintenance of current threat in post-traumatic stress disorder. *Clinical Psychology and Psychotherapy*, *17*(1), 13–24.

Harned, M. S., Jackson, S. C., Comtois, K. A., & Linehan, M. M. (2010). Dialectical behavior therapy as a precursor to PTSD treatment for suicidal and/or self-injuring women with borderline personality disorder. *Journal of Traumatic Stress*, *23*(4), 421–429.

Harney, P. A., & Harvey, M. R. (1999). Group psychotherapy: An overview. In B. H. Young & D. D. Blake (Eds.), *Group treatments for post-traumatic stress disorder* (pp. 1–14). New York: Brunner/Mazel.

Harris, M. (1998). *Trauma recovery and empowerment: A clinicians guide to working with women in groups.* New York: Simon & Schuster.

Harris, M., & Fallot, R. D. (2001). *Using trauma theory to design service systems.* San Francisco: Jossey-Bass.

Harvey, M. R. (1996). An ecological view of psychological trauma and trauma recovery. *Journal of Traumatic Stress*, *9*, 3–23.

Hathaway, S., & McKinley, J. C. (1989). *Minnesota Multiphasic Personality Inventory (MMPI-2).* Columbus, OH: Merrill/Prentice-Hall.

Hayes, S. C., Luoma, J. B., Bond, F. W., Masuda, A., & Lillis, J. (2006). Acceptance and commitment therapy: Model, processes and outcomes. *Behaviour Research and Therapy*, *44*(1), 1–25.

Hayes, S. C., Wilson, K. G., Gifford, E. V., Follette, V. M., & Strosahl, K. (1996). Experiential avoidance and behavioral disorders: A functional dimensional approach to diagnosis and treatment. *Journal of Consulting and Clinical Psychology, 64*(6), 1152–1168.

Hazan, C., & Shaver, P. R. (1987). Romantic love conceptualized as an attachment process. *Journal of Personality and Social Psychology, 52*, 511–524.

Hembree, E. A. (2008). Anxiety management training. In G. Reyes, J. D. Elhai & J. D. Ford (Eds.), *Encyclopedia of psychological trauma* (pp. 41–44). Hoboken, NJ: Wiley.

Hensel-Dittmann, D., Schauer, M., Ruf, M., Catani, C., Odenwald, M., Elbert, T., & Neuner, F. (2011). Treatment of traumatized victims of war and torture: A randomized controlled comparison of narrative exposure therapy and stress inoculation training. *Psychotherapy and Psychosomatics, 80*(6), 345–352.

Herman, J. L. (1992a). Complex PTSD: A syndrome in survivors of prolonged and repeated trauma. *Journal of Traumatic Stress, 3*, 377–391.

Herman, J. L. (1992b). *Trauma and recovery: The aftermath of violence—From domestic to political terror.* New York: Basic Books.

Herman, J. L. (2009). Forword. In C. A. Courtois & J. D. Ford (Eds.), *Treating complex traumatic stress disorders: An evidence-based guide* (pp. xiii–xvii). New York: Guilford Press.

Herman, J. L. (2012). CPTSD is a distinct entity: Comment on Resick et al. (2012). *Journal of Traumatic Stress, 25*(3), 256–257.

Herman, J. L., Cloitre, M., & Ford, J. D. (2009, February). *Proposal for adding complex PTSD as a new diagnosis to DSM-V.* Unpublished manuscript.

Hernandez, P., Gangsei, D., & Engstrom, D. (2007). Vicarious resilience: A new concept in work with those who survive trauma. *Family Process, 46*(2), 229–241.

Herzog, J. R., & Everson, R. B. (2007). The crisis of parental deployment in military service. In N. B. Webb (Ed.), *Play therapy with children in crisis: Individual, group, and family treatment* (3rd ed., pp. 228–248). New York: Guilford Press.

Hesse, E., & Main, M. (1999). Second-generation effects of unresolved trauma in nonmaltreating parents: Dissociated, frightened, and threatening parental behavior. *Psychoanalytic Inquiry, 19*(4), 481–540.

Hesse, E., & Main, M. (2000). Disorganized infant, child, and adult attachment: Collapse in behavioral and attentional strategies. *Journal of the American Psychoanalytic Association, 48*(4), 1097–1127.

Hien, D. A., Cohen, L. R., Litt, L. C., Miele, G. M., & Capstick, C. (2004). Promising empirically supported treatments for women with comorbid PTSD and substance use disorders. *American Journal of Psychiatry, 161*, 1426–1432.

Hien, D. A., Jiang, H., Campbell, A. N., Hu, M. C., Miele, G. M., Cohen, L. R., et al. (2010). Do treatment improvements in PTSD severity affect substance use outcomes? A secondary analysis from a randomized clinical trial in NIDA's Clinical Trials Network. *American Journal of Psychiatry, 167*(1), 95–101.

Higginson, S., Mansell, W., & Wood, A. M. (2011). An integrative mechanistic account of psychological distress, therapeutic change and recovery: The perceptual control theory approach. *Clinical Psychology Review, 31*(2), 249–259.

Horowitz, M., & Smit, M. (2008). Stress response syndromes. In G. Reyes, J. D. Elhai, & J. D. Ford (Eds.), *Encyclopedia of psychological trauma* (pp. 629–633). Hoboken, NJ: Wiley.

Horowitz, M. J. (1976). *Stress response syndromes.* New York: Aronson.

Horowitz, M. J. (1997). *Stress response syndromes: PTSD, grief, and adjustment disorders* (3rd ed.). Lanham, MD: Aronson.

Howell, E. F. (2005). *The dissociative mind.* New York: Analytic Press/Taylor & Francis Group.

Howell, E. F. (2011). *Understanding and treating Dissociative Identity Disorder: A relational approach.* New York: Routledge.

Hughes, D. A. (2007). *Attachment-focused family therapy.* New York: Norton.

Humeniuk, R., Ali, R., Babor, T. F., Farrell, M., Formigoni, M. L., Jittiwutikarn, J., et al. (2008). Validation of the Alcohol, Smoking and Substance Involvement Screening Test (ASSIST). *Addiction, 103*(6), 1039–1047.

International Society for the Study of Trauma and Dissociation. (2011). *Guidelines for treating dissociative identity disorder in adults.* McLean, VA: Author.

Janet, P. (1973). *L'automatisme psychologique.* Paris: Societe Pierre Janet. (Original work published 1889)

Janoff-Bulman, R. (1992). *Shattered assumptions: Towards a new psychology of trauma.* New York: Free Press.

Jehu, D. (1988). *Beyond sexual abuse: Therapy with women who were childhood victims.* New York: Wiley.

Jenkins, S., & Baird, S. (2002). Secondary traumatic stress and vicarious trauma: A validation study. *Journal of Traumatic Stress, 15,* 423–432.

Jennings, A. (2004). *Models for developing trauma-informed behavioral health systems and trauma-specific services.* Washington, DC: National Association of State Mental Health Program Directors and the National Technical Assistance Center for State Mental Health Planning.

Johnson, M. K. (2004). Psychology of false memories. In N. Smelser & P. B. Baltes (Eds.), *International encyclopedia of social and behavioral sciences* (pp. 5254–5259). London: Pergamon.

Johnson, S. M. (1989). Integrating marital and individual therapy for incest survivors: A case study. *Psychotherapy, 21*(6), 96–103.

Johnson, S. M. (2002). *Emotionally focused couple therapy with trauma survivors: Strengthening attachment bonds.* New York: Guilford Press.

Johnson, S. M., & Courtois, C. A. (2009). Couple therapy. In C. A. Courtois & J. D. Ford (Eds.), *Treating complex traumatic stress disorders: An evidence-based guide* (pp. 371–390). New York: Guilford Press.

Johnson, S. M., & Williams-Keeler, L. (1998). Creating healing relationships for couples dealing with trauma. *Journal of Marital and Family Therapy, 24,* 25–40.

Jordan, B. K., Marmar, C. R., Fairbank, J. A., Schlenger, W. E., Kulka, R. A., Hough, R. L., et al. (1992). Problems in families of male Vietnam veterans with posttraumatic stress disorder. *Journal of Consulting and Clinical Psychology, 60,* 916–926.

Joseph, S. (2008). *Trauma, recovery, and growth: Positive psychological perspectives on posttraumatic stress.* New York: Wiley.

Joseph, S. (2011). *What doesn't kill us: The new psychology of posttraumatic growth.* New York: Basic Books.

Joseph, S., & Linley, P. A. (Eds.). (2008). *Trauma, recovery, and growth: Positive psychological perspectives on posttraumatic stress.* Hoboken, NJ: Wiley.

Kaffman, A. (2009). The silent epidemic of neurodevelopmental injuries. *Biological Psychiatry, 66*(7), 624–626.

Kaltman, S., & Bonnano, G. A. (2003). Trauma and bereavement: Examining the impact of sudden and violent deaths. *Journal of Anxiety Disorders, 17*(2), 131–147.

Karam, E. G., Andrews, G., Bromet, E., Petukhova, M., Ruscio, A. M., Salamoun, M., et al. (2010). The role of criterion A2 in the DSM-IV diagnosis of posttraumatic stress disorder. *Biological Psychiatry, 68*(5), 465–473.

Kernberg, O. F. (1984). *Severe personality disorders: Psychotherapeutic strategies.* New Haven, CT: Yale University Press.

Kessler, R. C., Andrews, G., Colpe, L. J., Hiripi, E., Mroczek, D. K., Normand, S. L., et al. (2002). Short screening scales to monitor population prevalences and trends in non-specific psychological distress. *Psychological Medicine*, *32*(6), 959–976.

Kessler, R. C., Green, J. G., Gruber, M. J., Sampson, N. A., Bromet, E., Cuitan, M., et al. (2010). Screening for serious mental illness in the general population with the K6 screening scale: Results from the WHO World Mental Health (WMH) survey initiative. *International Journal of Methods in Psychiatric Research*, *19*(Suppl. 1), 4–22.

Kessler, R. C., Sonnega, A., Bromet, E., Hughes, M., & Nelson, C. B. (1995). Posttraumatic stress disorder in the National Comorbidity Survey. *Archives of General Psychiatry*, *52*(12), 1048–1060.

Kinsler, P. J. (1992). The centrality of relationship: What's not being said. *Dissociation*, *5*(5), 166–170.

Kinsler, P. J., Courtois, C. A., & Frankel, A. S. (2009). Therapeutic alliance and risk management. In C. A. Courtois & J. D. Ford (Eds.), *Treating complex traumatic stress disorders: An evidence-based guide* (pp. 183–201). New York: Guilford Press.

Kira, I. A. (2010). Etiology and treatment of post-cumulative traumatic stress disorders in different cultures. *Traumatology*, *16*(4), 128–141.

Kira, I. A., Alawneh, A. W. N., Aboumediane, S., Mohanesh, J., Ozkan, B., & Alamina, H. (2010). Identity salience and its dynamics in Palestinian adolescents. *Scientific Research*, *2*(8), 781–791.

Kira, I. A., Templin, T., Lewandowski, L., Ramaswamy, V., Ozcan, B., Abou-Mediane, S., et al. (2011). Cumulative tertiary appraisal of traumatic events across cultures: Two studies. *Journal of Loss and Trauma: International Perspectives on Stress and Coping*, *16*, 43–66.

Kiser, L. J., Donohue, A., Hodgkinson, S., Medoff, D., & Black, M. M. (2010). Strengthening family coping resources: The feasibility of a multi-family group intervention for families exposed to trauma. *Journal of Traumatic Stress*, *23*(6), 802–806.

Kislel, C., Pynoos, R., & Spinazzola, J. (2011). *Understanding complex patterns of trauma exposure and clinical needs among children and adolescents: Evidence from the large-scale core dataset of the National Child Traumatic Stress Network*. International Society for Traumatic Stress Studies, Annual Conference, Baltimore, MD.

Klein, R. H., & Schermer, V. L. (2000). *Group psychotherapy for psychological trauma*. New York: Guilford Press.

Kluft, R. P. (1984). Treatment of multiple personality disorder. *Psychiatric Clinics of North America*, *7*, 9–30.

Kluft, R. P. (Ed.). (1985). *Childhood antecedents of multiple personality*. Washington, DC: American Psychiatric Press.

Kluft, R. P. (1990a). Incest and subsequent re-victimization: The case of therapist–patient sexual exploitation with a description of "sitting-duck" syndrome. In R. P. Kluft (Ed.), *Incest-related syndromes of adult psychopathology* (pp. 263–288). Washington, DC: American Psychiatric Press.

Kluft, R. P. (1990b). *Incest-related syndromes of adult psychopathology*. Washington, DC: American Psychiatric Press.

Kluft, R. P. (1994a). Clinical observations on the use of the CSDS dimensions of therapeutic movement instrument (DTMI). *Dissociation*, *7*, 272–283.

Kluft, R. P. (1994b). Treatment trajectories in multiple personality disorder. *Dissociation*, *7*, 63–76.

Kluft, R. P. (1995). Natural history of multiple personality disorder. In R. P. Kluft (Ed.), *Childhood antecedents of multiple personality* (pp. 197–238). Washington, DC: American Psychiatric Press.

Kluft, R. P. (1999). An overview of the psychotherapy of dissociative identity disorder. *American Journal of Psychotherapy*, *53*, 289–319.

Kluft, R. P. (1999). An overview of the psychotherapy of dissociative identity disorder. *American Journal of Psychotherapy*, *53*, 289–319.

Kluft, R. P. (2000). The psychoanalytic psychotherapy of dissociative identity disorder in the context of trauma therapy. *Psychoanalytic Inquiry*, *53*, 289–339.

Kluft, R. P. (2011, January 11). Ramifications of incest. *Psychiatric Times*, *27*(12).

Kluft, R. P., & Fine, C. (Eds.). (1993). *Clinical perspectives on multiple personality disorder.* Washington, DC: American Psychiatric Press.

Knight, J. A., & Taft, C. T. (2004). Assessing neuropsychological concomitants of trauma and PTSD. In J. P. Wilson & T. M. Keane (Eds.), *Assessing psychological trauma and PTSD* (2nd ed., pp. 344–388). New York: Guilford Press.

Kohlenberg, R. J., & Tsai, M. (1991). *Functional analytic psychotherapy.* New York: Plenum.

Kohlenberg, R. J., & Tsai, M. (1998). Healing interpersonal trauma with the intimacy of the therapeutic relationship. In V. M. Follette, J. I., Ruzek, & F. R. Abueg (Eds.), *Cognitive behavioral therapies for trauma* (pp. 305–320). New York: Guilford Press.

Kohn, P. M., Kantor, L., DeCicco, T. L., & Beck, A. T. (2008). The Beck Anxiety Inventory—Trait (BAIT): A measure of dispositional anxiety not contaminated by dispositional depression. *Journal of Personality Assessment*, *90*(5), 499–506.

Kohut, H., & Wolf, E. S. (1978). The disorders of the self and their treatment: An outline. *International Journal of Psycho-Analysis*, *59*, 413–425.

Kopp, S. B. (1980). *Mirror, mask, and shadow: The risk and rewards of self-acceptance.* New York: Macmillan.

Korn, D. L., & Leeds, A. M. (2002). Preliminary evidence of efficacy for EMDR resource development and installation in the stabilization phase of treatment of complex PTSD. *Journal of Clinical Psychology*, *58*(12), 1465–1487.

Krakow, B., Hollifield, M., Johnston, L., Koss, M., Schrader, R., Warner, T. D., et al. (2001). Imagery rehearsal therapy for chronic nightmares in sexual assault survivors with PTSD: A randomized controlled trial. *Journal of the American Medical Association*, *286*(5), 537–545.

Kristof, N. D., & WuDunn, S. (2010). *Half the sky: Turning oppression into opportunity for women worldwide.* New York: Knopf.

Kubany, E. S., Abueg, F. R., Kilauano, W. L., Manke, F. P., & Kaplan, A. S. (1997). Development and validation of the Sources of Trauma-Related Guilt Survey—War-Zone Version. *Journal of Traumatic Stress*, *10*(2), 235–258.

Laddis, A. (2010). Outcome of crisis intervention for borderline personality disorder and posttraumatic stress disorder: A model for modification of the mechanism of disorder in complex posttraumatic syndromes. *Annals of General Psychiatry*, *9*, 19.

Laddis, A. (2011). Medication for complex traumatic disorders. *Journal of Aggression, Maltreatment, and Trauma*, *20*(6), 645–668.

Lanius, R. A., Brand, B. A., Vermetten, E., Frewen, P. A., & Spiegel, D. (2012). The dissociative subtype of posttraumatic stress disorder: Rational, clinical and neurobiological evidence, and implications. *Depression and Anxiety, 29*(8), 701–708.

Lanius, R. A., & Frewen, P. (2013). *Healing the traumatized self: Consciousness, neuroscience, and treatment.* New York: W. W. Norton.

Lanius, R. A., Vermetten, E., Loewenstein, R. J., Brand, B., Schmahl, C., Bremner, J., et al. (2010). Emotion modulation in PTSD: Clinical and neurobiological evidence for a dissociative subtype. *American Journal of Psychiatry, 167*(6), 640–647.

Lanius, R. A., Vermetten, E., & Pain, C. (2010). *The impact of early life trauma on health and disease: The hidden epidemic.* New York: Cambridge University Press.

Lanning, K., & Burgess, A. W. (1984). *Child pornography and sex rings.* New York: Wiley.

Lazowski, L. E., Miller, F. G., Boye, M. W., & Miller, G. A. (1998). Efficacy of the Substance Abuse Subtle Screening Inventory–3 (SASSI-3) in identifying substance dependence disorders in clinical settings. *Journal of Personality Assessment, 71,* 114–128.

Leehan, J., & Webb, L. (1996). *Group treatment for adult survivors of abuse: A manual for practitioners.* Thousand Oaks, CA: Sage.

Levine, P. A. (1997). *Waking the tiger, healing trauma: The innate capacity to transform overwhelming experiences.* Berkeley, CA: North Atlantic Books.

Levine, P. A. (2008). *Healing trauma: A pioneering program for restoring the wisdom of your body.* Boulder, CO: Sounds True.

Levitt, J. M. (2011). The wisdom project.

Levitt, H. M. (2011, June). *Principles of change used by expert therapists across psychotherapy orientations.* Keynote presentation at the 3rd International Psychotherapeutic Symposium, Masaryk University, Brno, Czech Republic.

Leyfer, O. T., Ruberg, J. L., & Woodruff-Borden, J. (2006). Examination of the utility of the Beck Anxiety Inventory and its factors as a screener for anxiety disorders. *Journal of Anxiety Disorders, 20*(4), 444–458.

Lindauer, R. J. L. (2012). Child maltreatment-Clinical PTSD diagnosis not enough?!: Comment on Resick et al. (2012). *Journal of Traumatic Stress, 25*(3), 258–259.

Linehan, M. M. (1993). *Cognitive-behavioral treatment of borderline personality disorder.* New York: Guilford Press.

Linehan, M. M., Heard, H. L., & Armstrong, H. E. (1993). Naturalistic follow-up of a behavioral treatment for chronically parasuicidal borderline patients. *Archives of General Psychiatry, 50*(12), 971–974.

Lineweaver, T. T., & Hertzog, C. (1998). Adults' efficacy and control beliefs regarding memory and aging: Separating general from personal beliefs. *Aging, Neuropsychology, and Cognition, 5*(4), 264–496.

Liotti, G. (1992). Disorganized/disoriented attachment in the etilogy of the dissociative disorders. *Dissociation: Progress in the Dissociative Disorders, 5*(4), 196–204.

Liotti, G. (1999). Understanding the dissociative processes: The contribution of attachment theory. *Psychoanalytic Inquiry, 19*(5), 757–783.

Loewenstein, R. J. (1991). An Office Mental Status Examination for Complex Chronic Dissociative Symptoms and Multiple Personality Disorder. *Psychiatric Clinics of North America, 14*(3), 567–604.

Loewenstein, R. J. (1993). Posttraumatic and dissociative aspects of transference and countertransference in the treatment of multiple personality disorder. In R. P. Kluft & S. C. Fine (Eds.), *Clinical perspectives on multiple personality disorder* (pp. 51–86). Washington, DC, American Psychiatric Association Press.

Loewenstein, R. J., & Welzant, V. (2010). Pragmatic approaches to stage-oriented treatment for early life trauma-related complex post-traumatic stress and dissociative disorders. In R. A. Lanius, E. Vermetten, & C. Pain (Eds.), *The impact of early life trauma on health and disease: The hidden epidemic* (pp. 257–267). London: Cambridge University Press.

Long, M. E., Hammons, M. E., Davis, J. L., Frueh, B. C., Khan, M. M., Elhai, J. D., et al. (2011). Imagery rescripting and exposure group treatment of post traumatic nightmares in veterans with PTSD. *Journal of Anxiety Disorders, 25*(4), 531–535.

Lubin, H., & Johnson, D. (2008). *Trauma-centered group psychotherapy for women.* New York: Routledge.

Lubin, H., Loris, M., Burt, J., & Johnson, D. R. (1998). Efficacy of psychoeducational group therapy in reducing symptoms of posttraumatic stress disorder among multiply traumatized women. *American Journal of Psychiatry, 155,* 1172–1177.

Luyten, P., & Blatt, S. J. (2011). Integrating theory-driven and empirically derived models of personality development and psychopathology: A proposal for DSM V. *Clinical Psychology Review, 31*(1), 52–68.

Lyons-Ruth, K. (2008). Contributions of the mother–infant relationship to dissociative, borderline, and conduct symptoms in young adulthood. *Infant Mental Health Journal, 29*(3), 203–218.

Lyons-Ruth, K., Dutra, L., Schuder, M. R., & Bianchi, I. (2006). From infant attachment disorganization to adult dissociation: Relational adaptations or traumatic experiences? *Psychiatric Clinics of North America, 29*(1), 63–86.

Lyons-Ruth, K., Melnick, S., Patrick, M., & Hobson, R. P. (2007). A controlled study of hostile–helpless states of mind among borderline and dysthymic women. *Attachment and Human Development, 9*(1), 1–16.

Main, M., & Goldwyn, R. (1994). *Adult attachment classification system.* Unpublished manuscript, University of California, Berkeley.

Main, M., Goldwyn, R., & Hesse, E. (2002). *Adult attachment scoring and classification systems, Version 7.1.* Unpublished manuscript, University of California, Berkeley.

Main, M., & Goldwyn, T. (1994). *The Adult Attachment interview.* Berkeley, CA: University of California.

Main, M., & Hesse, E. (1990). Parent's unresolved traumatic experiences are related to infant disorganized attachment status: Is frightened and/or frightening parental behavior the linking mechanism? In M. Greenberg, D. Cicchetti, & M. Cummings (Eds.), *Attachment in the preschool years* (pp. 161–182). Chicago: University of Chicago Press.

Maltz, W. (2012). *The sexual healing journey: A guide for survivors of child sexual abuse* (3rd ed.). New York: HarperCollins.

Maltz, W., & Maltz, L. (2008). *The porn trap: The essential guide to overcoming problems caused by pornography.* New York: HarperCollins.

Marmar, C. R., Foy, D., Kagan, B., & Pynoos, R. S. (1994). An integrated approach for treating posttraumatic stress. In R. Pynoos (Ed.), *Posttraumatic stress disorder: A clinical review* (pp. 99–132). Baltimore: Sidran.

Marotta, S. A. (2003). Unflinching empathy: Counselors and tortured refugees. *Journal of Counseling and Development, 81,* 111–114.

Marx, B. P., Forsyth, J. P., Gallup, G. G., Fuse, T., & Lexington, J. M. (2008). Tonic immobility as an evolved predator defense: Implications for sexual assault survivors. *Clinical Psychology: Science and Practice, 15*(1), 74–90.

Matsakis, A. (1998). *Trust after trauma: A guide to relationship for survivors and those who love them.* Oakland, CA: New Harbinger.

McCann, I. L., & Pearlman, L. A. (1990). Vicarious traumatization: A framework for understanding the psychological effects of working with victims. *Journal of Traumatic Stress*, *3*(1), 131–149.

McCann, I. L., & Pearlman, L. A. (1992). Constructivist self-development theory: A theoretical framework for assessing and treating traumatized college students. *Journal of the American College Health Association*, *40*(4), 189–196.

McCullough, L., Kuhn, N., Andrews, S., Kaplan, A., Wolf, J., & Hurley, C. A. (2003). *Treating affect phobia: A manual for short-term dynamic psychotherapy*. New York: Guilford Press.

McCullough-Vaillant, L. (1994). *Changing character: Short-term anxiety-regulating psychotherapy for restructuring defenses*. New York: Basic Books.

McDonagh-Coyle, A., Friedman, M., McHugo, G., Ford, J. D., Mueser, K., Descamps, M., et al. (2005). Psychometric outcomes of a randomized clinical trial of psychotherapies for PTSD-SA. *Journal of Consulting and Clinical Psychology*, *73*, 515–524.

McDonald, S. D., & Calhoun, P. S. (2010). The diagnostic accuracy of the PTSD checklist: A critical review. *Clinical Psychology Review*, *30*(8), 976–987.

McMackin, R. A., Newman, E., Fogler, J. M., & Keane, T. M. (Eds.). (2012). *Trauma therapy in context: The science and craft of evidence-based practice*. Washington, DC: American Psychological Association Press.

McNally, R. J. (2003). *Remembering trauma*. Cambridge, MA: Belknap Press.

Meeks, T. W., & Jeste, D. V. (2009). Neurobiology of wisdom: A literature overview. *Archives of General Psychiatry*, *66*(4), 355–365.

Meichenbaum, D., & Novaco, R. (1985). Stress inoculation: A preventative approach. *Issues in Mental Health Nursing*, *7*(1–4), 419–435.

Meichenbaum, D. (1985). *Stress inoculation training*. New York: Penguin.

Meichenbaum, D. (1994). *A clinical handbook/practical therapist manual for assessing and treating adults with posttraumatic stress disorder (PTSD)*. Waterloo, Ontario, Canada: Institute Press.

Meiser-Stedman, R. A., Yule, W., Dalgleish, T., Smith, P., & Glucksman, E. (2006). The role of the family in child and adolescent posttraumatic stress following attendance at an emergency department. *Journal of Pediatric Psychology*, *31*, 397–402.

Mendelsohn, M., Lewis, J. L., Schatzow, E., Coco, M., Kallivayalil, D., & Levitan, J. (2011). *The trauma recovery group: A guide for practitioners*. New York: Guilford Press.

Mendelsohn, M., Zachary, R. S., & Harney, P. A. (2007). Group therapy as an ecological bridge to new community for trauma survivors. *Journal of Aggression, Maltreatment and Trauma*, *14*, 227–243.

Mendes, D., Mello, M. F., Ventura, P., Passarela, C. M., & Mari Jde, J. (2008). A systematic review on the effectiveness of cognitive behavioral therapy for posttraumatic stress disorder. *International Journal of Psychiatry in Medicine*, *38*(3), 241–259.

Merrit, R. D., & You, S. (2008). Is there really a dissociative taxon on the dissociative experiences scale? *Journal of Personality Assessment*, *90*(2), 201–203.

Miller, G. D., & Baldwin, D. C. (1987). Implications of the wounded-healer paradigm for the use of the self in therapy. In M. Baldwin & V. Satir (Eds.), *The use of self in therapy* (pp. 130–151). New York: Haworth Press.

Miller, J. B., & Stiver, I. P. (1997). *The healing connection: How women form relationships in therapy and in life*. Boston: Beacon Press.

Miller, W. R., & Rollnick, S. (2009). Ten things that motivational interviewing is not. *Behavioral and Cognitive Psychotherapy*, *37*(2), 129–140.

Miller, W. R., & Rollnick, S. (2012). *Motivational interviewing: Helping people change*. New York: Guilford Press.

Millon, T. (1987). *Millon Clinical Multiaxial Inventory–II: Manual for the MCMI-II*. Minneapolis, MN: National Computer Systems.

Modestin, J., & Erni, T. (2004). Testing the dissociative taxon. *Psychiatric Research, 126*(1), 77–82.

Monson, C. M., & Fredman, S. J. (2012). *Cognitive-behavioral conjoint therapy for PTSD: Harnessing the healing power of relationships*. New York: Guilford Press.

Moore, B. A., & Krakow, B. (2007). Imagery rehearsal therapy for acute posttraumatic nightmares among combat soldiers in Iraq. *American Journal of Psychiatry, 164*, 683–684.

Morey, L. C. (1991). *Personality Assessment Inventory professional manual*. Odessa, FL: Psychological Assessment Resources.

Morey, L. C. (2007). *Personality Assessment Inventory professional manual* (2nd ed.). Lutz, FL: Psychological Assessment Resources.

Morrissey, J., Jackson, E., Ellis, A., Amaro, H., Brown, V., & Najavits, L. (2005). Twelve-month outcomes of trauma-informed interventions for women with co-occurring disorders. *Psychiatric Services, 56*, 1213–1222.

Muller, R. T. (2009). Trauma and dismissing (avoidant) attachment: Intervention strategies in individual psychotherapy. *Psychotherapy Theory, Research, Practice, Training, 46*, 68–81.

Muller, R. T. (2010). *Trauma and the avoidant client: Attachment-based strategies for healing*. New York: Norton.

Nader, K., Pynoos, R., Fairbanks, L., & Frederick, C. (1990). Children's PTSD reactions one year after a sniper attack at their school. *American Journal of Psychiatry, 147*, 1526–1530.

Najavits, L. (2002a). *Seeking Safety: A treatment manual for PTSD and substance abuse*. New York: Guilford Press.

Najavits, L. (2002b). *A women's addiction workbook: Your guide to in-depth healing*. Oakland, CA: New Harbinger.

Najavits, L. M., Gallop, R. J., & Weiss, R. D. (2006). Seeking safety therapy for adolescent girls with PTSD and substance use disorder: A randomized controlled trial. *Journal of Behavioral Health Services Research, 22*, 453–463.

Neimeyer, R. A. (Ed.). (2001). *Meaning reconstruction and the experience of loss*. Washington, DC: American Psychological Association Press.

Neumann, D. A., & Gamble, S. J. (1995). Issues in the professional development of psychotherapists: Countertransference and VT in the new trauma therapist. *Psychotherapy: Theory, Research, Practice, Training, 32*, 341–347.

Neuner, F., Schauer, M., Klaschik, C., Karunakara, U., & Elbert, T. (2004). A comparison of narrative exposure therapy, supportive counseling, and psychoeducation for treating posttraumatic stress disorder in an African refugee settlement. *Journal of Consulting and Clinical Psychology, 72*(4), 579–587.

Nijenhuis, E. R. S. (2004). *Somatoform dissociation: Phenomena, measurement, and theoretical issues*. New York: Norton.

Nijenhuis, E. R. S., Spinhoven, P., Van Dyck, R., Van der Hart, O., & Vanderlinden, J. (1996). The development and the psychometric characteristics of the Somatoform Dissociation Questionnaire (SDQ-20). *Journal of Nervous and Mental Disease, 184*, 688–694.

Nijenhuis, E. R. S., & Van der Hart, O. (2011). Defining dissociation in trauma. *Journal of Trauma and Dissociation, 12*, 469–473.

Nijenhuis, E. R. S., van Dyck, R., Spinhoven, P., Van der Hart, O., Chatrou, M.,

Vanderlinden, J., et al. (1999). Somatoform dissociation discriminates among diagnostic categories over and above general psychopathology. *Australian and New Zealand Journal of Psychiatry, 33*, 511–520.

Nijenhuis, E. R. S., van Dyck, R., Ter Kuile, M., Mourits, M., Spinhoven, P., & Van der Hart, O. (1999). *Evidence for associations between somatoform dissociation, psychological dissociation, and reported trauma in chronic pelvic pain patients.* In E. R. S. Nijenhuis (Ed.), *Somatoform dissociation: Phenomena, measurement, and theoretical issues* (pp. 146–160). Ossen, Netherlands: Van Gorcum.

Nijenhuis, E. R. S., Van Engen, A., Kusters, I., & Van der Hart, O. (2001). Peritraumatic somatoform and psychological dissociation in relation to recall of childhood sexual abuse. *Journal of Trauma and Dissociation, 2*(3), 49–68.

Noll, J. G. (2005). Does childhood sexual abuse set in motion a cycle of violence against women? *Journal of Interpersonal Violence, 20*(1), 155–162.

Norcross, J. C., & Guy, J. D. (2007). *Leaving it at the office: A guide to therapist self-care.* New York: Guilford Press.

Norcross, J. C., & Lambert, M. J. (2011). Psychotherapy relationships that work: II. *Psychotherapy Theory, Research, Practice, Training, 48*(1), 4–8.

Obegi, J. H. (2008). The development of the client–therapist bond through the lens of attachment theory. *Psychotherapy: Theory, Research, Practice, Training, 45*(4), 431–446.

Ochberg, F. M. (1988). Post-traumatic therapy and victims of violence. In F. M. Ochberg (Ed.), *Post-traumatic therapy and victims of violence* (pp. 3–19). Philadelphia: Brunner/Mazel.

O'Donnell, M. L., Creamer, M., McFarlane, A. C., Silove, D., & Bryant, R. A. (2010). Should A2 be a diagnostic requirement for posttraumatic stress disorder in DSM-V? *Psychiatry Research, 176*(2–3), 257–260.

Ogden, P., Minton, K., & Pain, C. (2006). *Trauma and the body: A sensorimotor approach to psychotherapy.* New York: Norton.

Ogden, P., & Fisher, J. (2013). *The body as resource: A therapist's manual for sensorimotor psychotherapy.* New York: W. W. Norton.

Olio, K., & Cornell, W. (1993). The therapeutic relationship as the foundation for treatment with adult survivors of sexual abuse. *Psychotherapy: Theory, Research, Practice, Training, 30*, 512–523.

Omaha, J. (2004). *Psychotherapeutic interventions for emotion regulation.* New York: Norton.

Opler, L. A., Grennan, M. S., & Ford, J. D. (2009). Pharmacotherapy. In C. A. Courtois & J. D. Ford (Eds.), *Treating complex traumatic stress disorders: An evidence-based guide* (pp. 329–349). New York: Guilford Press.

Orr, S. P., Metzger, L. J., Miller, M. W., & Kaloupek, D. G. (2004). Psychophysiological assessment of PTSD. In J. P. Wilson & T. M Keane (Eds.), *Assessing psychological trauma and PTSD* (2nd ed., pp. 289–343). New York: Guilford Press.

Osman, A., Gutierrez, P. M., Smith, K., Fang, Q., Lozano, G., & Devine, A. (2010). The Anxiety Sensitivity Index-3: Analyses of dimensions, reliability estimates, and correlates in nonclinical samples. *Journal of Personality Assessment, 92*(1), 45–52.

Osterman, J. E., & Chemtob, C. M. (1999). Emergency intervention for acute traumatic stress. *Psychiatric Services, 50*(6), 739–740.

Paivio, S. C., Jarry, J. L., Chagigiorgis, H., Hall, I., & Ralston, M. (2010). Efficacy of two versions of emotion-focused therapy for resolving child abuse trauma. *Psychotherapy Research, 20*(3), 353–366.

Paivio, S. C., & Nieuwenhuis, J. (2001). Efficacy of emotion focused therapy for adult survivors of child abuse: A preliminary study. *Journal of Traumatic Stress*, *14*(1), 115–133.

Paivio, S. C., & Pascual-Leone, A. (2010). *Emotion-focused therapy for complex trauma: An integrative approach*. Washington, DC: American Psychological Association.

Panksepp, J. (1998). *Affective neuroscience: The foundations of human and animal emotions*. New York: Oxford University Press.

Panksepp, J., & Bivens, L. (2012). *The archeology of mind: Neuroevolutionary origins of human emotions*. New York: W. W. Norton.

Parker, A., Fourt, A., Langmuir, J. I., Dalton, E. J., & Classen, C. C. (2007). The experience of trauma recovery: A qualitative study of participants in the Women Recovering from Abuse Program (WRAP). *Journal of Child Sexual Abuse*, *16*(2), 55–77.

Parker, G. (1989). The Parental Bonding Instrument: Psychometric properties reviewed. *Psychiatry and Development*, *7*(4), 317–335.

Pat-Horenczyk, R., Rabinowitz, M., Rice, A., & Tucker-Levin, A. (2008). The search for risk and protective factors in childhood PTSD. In D. Brom, R. Pat-Horenczyk, & J. D. Ford (Eds.), *Treating traumatized children* (pp. 51–71). London: Routledge.

Pearlman, L. (1999). Self-care for trauma therapists: Ameliorating vicarious traumatization. In B. H. Stamm (Eds.), *Secondary traumatic stress: Self-care issues for clinicians, researchers, and educators* (2nd ed.). Lutherville, MD: Sidran.

Pearlman, L. A. (2001). Treatment of persons with complex PTSD and other trauma-related disruptions of the self. In M. J. Friedman, T. M. Keane, & P. A. Resick (Eds.), *Treating psychological trauma and PTSD* (pp. 205–236). New York: Guilford Press.

Pearlman, L. A. (2003). *Trauma and Attachment Belief Scale (TABS) manual*. Los Angeles: Western Psychological Services.

Pearlman, L. A., & Caringi, J. (2009). Living and working self-reflectively to address vicarious trauma. In C. A. Courtois & J. D. Ford (Eds.), *Treating complex traumatic stress disorders: An evidence-based guide* (pp. 202–224). New York: Guilford Press.

Pearlman, L. A., & Courtois, C. A. (2005). Clinical applications of the attachment framework: Relational treatment of complex trauma. *Journal of Traumatic Stress*, *18*(5), 449–459.

Pearlman, L. A., & MacIan, P. S. (1995). Vicarious traumatization: An empirical study of the effects of trauma work on trauma therapists. *Professional Psychology: Research and Practice*, *26*, 558–566.

Pearlman, L. A., & Saakvitne, K. W. (1995). *Trauma and the therapist: Countertransference and vicarious traumatization in psychotherapy with incest survivors*. New York: Norton.

Pelcovitz, D., Van der Kolk, B. A., Roth, S., Mandel, F. S., Kaplan, S., & Resick, P. A. (1997). Development of a criteria set and a structured interview for disorders of extreme stress (SIDES). *Journal of Traumatic Stress*, *10*, 3–17.

Pennebaker, J. W. (1990). *Opening up: The healing power of expressing emotion*. New York: Guilford Press.

Pennebaker, J. W. (2004). *Writing to heal: A guided journal for recovering from trauma and emotional upheaval*. Oakland, CA: New Harbinger.

Perlman, S. D. (1999). *The therapist's emotional survival: Dealing with the pain of exploring trauma*. Northvale, NJ: Aronson.

Perls, F. S. (1973). *The Gestalt approach and eyewitness to therapy*. New York: Bantam Books.

Perry, B. D. (1993a). Neurodevelopment and the neurophysiology of trauma: I. Conceptual considerations for clinical work with maltreated children. *APSAC Advisor, 6*(1), 14–18.

Perry, B. D. (1993b). Neurodevelopment and the neurophysiology of trauma: II. Clinical work along the alarm–fear–terror continuum. *APSAC Advisor, 6*(2), 14–20.

Perry, B. D. (1994). Neurobiological sequelae of childhood trauma: PTSD in children. In M. M. Murburg (Ed.), *Catecholamine function in PTSD: Emerging concepts* (pp. 233–255). Washington, DC: American Psychiatric Association.

Perry, B. D. (1995). Childhood trauma, the neurobiology of adaptation, and "use-dependent" development of the brain: How "states" become "traits." *Infant Mental Health Journal, 16*(4), 271–291.

Perry, B. D. (2007). *The boy who was raised as a dog*. New York: Basic Books.

Perry, R. J., Rosen, H. R., Kramer, J. H., Beer, J. S., Levenson, R. L., & Miller, B. L. (2001). Hemispheric dominance for emotions, empathy, and social behavior: Evidence from right and left-handers with frontotemporal dementia. *Neurocase, 7*, 145–160.

Perry, A. E., & Gilbody, S. (2009). Detecting and predicting self-harm behaviour in prisoners: A prospective psychometric analysis of three instruments. *Social Psychiatry and Psychiatric Epidemiology, 44*(10), 853–861.

Piazza-Bonin, E., & Levitt, H. M. (2011, September). *Developing wisdom in psychotherapy trainees*. Paper presented at the North American Society for Psychotherapy Research Conference, Banff, Canada.

Pine, D. S., Costello, J., & Masten, A. (2005). Trauma, proximity, and developmental psychopathology: The effects of war and terrorism on children. *Neuropsychopharmacology, 30*(10), 1781–1792.

Piper, W., Ogrodniczuk, J., Joyce, A., Weideman, R., & Rosie, J. (2007). Group composition and therapy for complicated grief. *Journal of Consulting and Clinical Psychology, 75*, 116–125.

Pope, K., & Vasquez, M. J. (2005). *How to survive and thrive as a therapist: Information, ideas, and resources for psychologists*. Washington, DC: American Psychological Association.

Pope, K. S. (1990). Therapist–patient sexual involvement: A review of the research. *Clinical Psychology Review, 10*, 477–490.

Pope, K. S. (1994). *Sexual involvement with therapists: Patient assessment, subsequent therapy, forensics*. Washington, DC: American Psychological Association.

Pope, K. S., & Bouhoutsos, J. (1986). *Sexual intimacies between therapists and patients*. New York: Praeger.

Pope, K. S., & Keith-Spiegel, P. (2008). A practical approach to boundaries in psychotherapy: Making decisions, bypassing blunders, and mending fences. *Journal of Clinical Psychology, 64*(5), 638–652.

Pope, K. S., Sonne, J. L., & Holroyd, J. (1993). *Sexual feelings in psychotherapy: Explorations for therapists and therapists-in-training*. Washington, DC: American Psychological Association.

Porges, S. W. (2011). *The polyvagal theory: Neurophysiological foundations of emotions, attachment, communication, and self-regulation*. New York: Norton.

Porges, S. W. (2013). *Clinical insights from the polyvagal theory: The transformative power of feeling safe*. New York: W. W. Norton.

Powers, M. B., Halpern, J. M., Ferenschak, M. P., Gillihan, S. J., & Foa, E. B. (2010). A meta-analytic review of prolonged exposure for posttraumatic stress disorder. *Clinical Psychology Review, 30*(6), 635–641.

Prochaska, J. O., & DiClemente, C. C. (1992). Stages of change in the modification of problem behaviors. *Progress in Behavior Modification*, *28*, 183–218.

Putnam, F. W. (1989). *Diagnosis and treatment of multiple personality disorder.* New York: Guilford Press.

Putnam, F. W. (1997). *Dissociation in children and adolescents: A developmental perspective.* New York: Guilford Press.

Putnam, F. W. (2009). Taking the measure of dissociation. *Journal of Trauma and Dissociation*, *10*(3), 233–236.

Rando, T. (1993). *Treatment of complicated mourning.* Chicago: Research Press.

Ravitz, P., Maunder, R., Hunter, J., Sthankiya, B., & Lancee, W. (2010). Adult attachment measures: A 25-year review. *Journal of Psychosomatic Research*, *69*(4), 419–432.

Read, J. (1997). Child abuse and psychosis: A literature review and implications for professional practice. *Professional Psychology: Research and Practice*, *28*(5), 448–456.

Ready, D. J., Thomas, K. R., Worley, V., Backscheider, A. G., Harvey, L. A., Baltzell, D., et al. (2008). A field test of group-based exposure therapy with 102 veterans with war-related PTSD. *Journal of Traumatic Stress*, *21*, 150–157.

Renshaw, D. (1982). *Incest: Understanding and treatment.* Boston: Little, Brown.

Resick, P. A., Bovin, M., Calloway, A. L., Dick, A. M., King, M. W., Mitchell, K. S., et al. (2012). A critical evaluation of the complex PTSD literature: Implications for DSM-5. *Journal of Traumatic Stress*, *25*(3), 241–251.

Resick, P. A., Galovski, T. E., O'Brien Uhlmansiek, M., Scher, C. D., Clum, G. A., & Young-Xu, Y. (2008). A randomized clinical trial to dismantle components of cognitive processing therapy for posttraumatic stress disorder in female victims of interpersonal violence. *Journal of Consulting and Clinical Psychology*, *76*(2), 243–258.

Resick, P. A., Nishith, P., & Griffin, M. G. (2003). How well does cognitive-behavioral therapy treat symptoms of complex PTSD? An examination of child sexual abuse survivors within a clinical trial. *CNS Spectrums*, *8*, 340–342, 351–355.

Resick, P. A., Nishith, P., Weaver, T. L., Astin, M. C., & Feuer, C. A. (2002). A comparison of cognitive processing therapy, prolonged exposure, and a waiting condition for the treatment of posttraumatic stress disorder in female rape victims. *Journal of Consulting and Clinical Psychology*, *70*, 867–879.

Resick, P. A., & Schnicke, M. K. (1993). *Cognitive processing therapy for rape victims: A treatment manual.* Thousand Oaks, CA: Sage.

Resick, P. A., Wolf, E. J., Stirman, S., Wells, S. Y., Suvak, M. K., Mitchell, K. S., et al. (2012). Advocacy through science: Reply to comments on Resick et al. (2012). *Journal of Traumatic Stress*, *25*(3), 260–263.

Reynolds, W. M. (1991). Psychometric characteristics of the Adult Suicidal Ideation Questionnaire in College Students. *Journal of Personality Assessment*, *56*, 289–307.

Riggs, D. (2000). Marital and family therapy. In E. B. Foa, T. M. Keane, & M. J. Friedman (Eds.), *Effective treatments for PTSD* (pp. 280–301). New York: Guilford Press.

Riley, W. T., & Trieber, F. A. (1989). The validation of multidimensional self-report anger and hostility. *Journal of Clinical Psychology*, *45*, 397–404.

Rorschach, H. (1981). *Psychodiagnostics: A diagnostic test based upon perception.* New York: Grune & Stratton. (Original work published 1921)

Ross, C. A. (1996). *Dissociative identity disorder: Diagnosis, clinical features, and treatment of multiple personality* (2nd ed.). Hoboken, NJ: Wiley.

Ross, C. A. (1989). *Multiple personality disorder: Diagnosis, clinical features, and treatment.* Oxford, UK: Wiley.

Ross, C. A., Heber, S., Norton, G., Anderson, D., Anderson, G., & Barchet, P. (1989). The Dissociative Disorders Interview Schedule: A structured interview. *Dissociation: Progress in the Dissociative Disorders*, *2*(3), 169–189.

Ross, C. A., Joshi, S., & Currie, R. (1990). Dissociative experiences in the general population. *American Journal of Psychiatry*, *147*, 1547–1552.

Rothschild, B. (2000). *The body remembers: The psychophysiology of trauma and trauma treatment.* New York: Norton.

Rothschild, B. (2003). *The body remembers: Casebook unifying methods and models in the treatment of trauma and PTSD.* New York: Norton.

Rothschild, B. (with Rand, M.). (2006). *Help for the helper: The psychophysiology of compassion fatigue and vicarious trauma.* New York: Norton.

Ruden, R. A. (2011). *When the past is always present: Emotional traumatization, causes, and cures.* New York: Routledge.

Ruf, M., Schauer, M., Neuner, F., Catani, C., Schauer, E., & Elbert, T. (2010). Narrative exposure therapy for 7- to 16-year-olds: A randomized controlled trial with traumatized refugee children. *Journal of Traumatic Stress*, *23*(4), 437–445.

Ruf, M., Schauer, M., Neuner, F., Schauer, E., Catani, C., et al. (2007, June). *KIDNET: A highly effective treatment approach for traumatized refugee children.* Paper presented at the European Conference on Traumatic Stress, Opatja, Croatia.

Ruscio, A. M., Weathers, F. W., King, L. A., & King, D. W. (2002). Male war-zone veterans' perceived relationships with their children. *Journal of Traumatic Stress*, *15*, 351–357.

Saakvitne, K. W., Gamble, S. G., Pearlman, L. A., & Lev, B. T. (2000). *Risking connection: A training curriculum for working with survivors of childhood abuse.* Lutherville, MD: Sidran.

Saakvitne, K. W., & Pearlman, L. A. (1996). *Transforming the pain: A workbook on vicarious traumatization.* New York: Norton.

Sable, P. (2000). *Attachment and adult psychotherapy.* Northvale, NJ: Aronson.

Sanness, K. J. (2011). *Complex posttraumatic stress disorder: Conceptualizations and effective interventions.* Dissertation, George Washington University.

Santa Mina, E. E., Gallop, R., Links, P., Heslegrave, R., Pringle, D., Wekerle, C., et al. (2006). The Self-Injury Questionnaire: The evaluation of the psychometric properties in a clinical population. *The Journal of Psychiatric and Mental Health Nursing*, *13*, 221–227.

Saunders, T., Driskell, J. E., Johnston, J. H., & Salas, E. (1996). The effect of stress inoculation training on anxiety and performance. *Journal of Occupational Health Psychology*, *1*(2), 170–186.

Schaal, S., Elbert, T., & Neuner, F. (2009). Narrative exposure therapy versus interpersonal psychotherapy: A pilot randomized controlled trial with Rwandan genocide orphans. *Psychotherapy and Psychosomatics*, *78*(5), 298–306.

Scheeringa, M. S., & Zeanah, C. H. (2001). A relational perspective on PTSD in early childhood. *Journal of Traumatic Stress*, *14*(4), 799–815.

Schmidt, S.J. (2009). *The developmental needs meeting strategy: An ego state therapy for healing adults with childhood trauma and attachment wounds.* San Antonio, TX: DMNS Institute.

Schnurr, P. P., Friedman, M. J., Foy, D. W., Shea, M. T., Hsieh, F. Y., Lavori, P. W., et al. (2003). Randomized trial of trauma-focused group therapy for PTSD:

Results from a Department of Veterans Affairs cooperative study. *Archives of General Psychiatry*, *60*, 481–489.

Schnurr, P. P., & Green, B. L. (2004). *Trauma and health: Physical health consequences of exposure to extreme stress*. Washington, DC: American Psychological Association.

Schore, A. N. (1994). *Affect regulation and the origin of the self*. Mahwah, NJ: Erlbaum.

Schore, A. N. (2001). The effects of early relational trauma on right brain development, affect regulation, and infant mental health. *Infant Mental Health Journal*, *22*(1–2), 201–269.

Schore, A. N. (2002). Dysregulation of the right brain: A fundamental mechanism of traumatic attachment and the psychogenesis of posttraumatic stress disorder. *Australian and New Zealand Journal of Psychiatry*, *36*, 9–30.

Schore, A. N. (2003a). *Affect dysregulation and disorders of the self*. New York: Norton.

Schore, A. N. (2003b). *Affect regulation and the repair of the self*. New York: Norton.

Schore, A. N. (2003c). Early relational trauma, disorganized attachment, and the development of a predisposition to violence. In M. F. Solomon & D. J. Siegel (Eds.), *Healing trauma: Attachment, mind, body, and brain* (pp. 107–167). New York: Norton.

Schore, A. N. (2009). Relational trauma and the developing right brain. *Annals of the New York Academy of Sciences*, *1159*, 189–203.

Schore, A. N. (2013). *The science of the art of psychotherapy*. New York: W. W. Norton.

Schwartz, H. L. (2000). *Dialogues with forgotten voices: Relational perspective on child abuse trauma and treatment of dissociative disorders*. New York: Basic Books.

Schwartz, R. C., Schwartz, M. F., & Galperin, L. (2009). Internal family system therapy. In C. A. Courtois & J. D. Ford (Eds.), *Treating complex traumatic stress disorders: An evidence-based guide* (pp. 353–370). New York: Guilford Press.

Scott, W. (1999). Group therapy for survivors of severe childhood abuse: Repairing the social contract. *Journal of Child Sexual Abuse*, *7*, 35–54.

Seidler, G. H., & Wagner, F. E. (2006). Comparing the efficacy of EMDR and trauma-focused cognitive-behavioral therapy in the treatment of PTSD: A meta-analytic study. *Psychological Medicine*, *36*(11), 1515–1522.

Selvini, M. P., Boscolo, L., Cecchin, G., & Prata, G. (1980). Hypothesizing–circularity–neutrality: Three guidelines for the conductor of the session. *Family Process*, *19*(1), 3–12.

Selzer, M. L. (1971). The Michigan Alcoholism Screening Test: The quest for a new diagnostic instrument. *American Journal of Psychiatry*, *127*, 1653–1658.

Shapiro, F. (2001). *Eye movement desensitization and reprocessing: Basic principles, protocols, and procedures* (2nd ed.). New York: Guilford Press.

Shapiro, F. (2002). EMDR 12 years after its introduction: Past and future research. *Journal of Clinical Psychology*, *58*, 1–22.

Shapiro, R. (2010). *The trauma treatment handbook: Protocols across the spectrum*. New York: W. W. Norton.

Shapiro, F. (2012). *Getting past your past: Take control of your life with self-help techniques from EMDR therapy*. New York: Rodale.

Shapiro, F., & Solomon, R. M. (2010). Eye movement desensitization and reprocessing. *Corsini Encyclopedia of Psychology, (4th ed.)*, *2*, 1–3.

Shapiro, R. (Ed.). (2005). *EMDR solutions: Pathways to healing.* New York: Norton.

Shea, M. T., McDevitt-Murphy, M., Ready, D. R., & Schnurr, P. P. (2009). Group therapy. In E. B. Foa, T. M. Keane, M. Friedman, & J. A. Cohen (Eds.), *Effective treatments for PTSD* (2nd ed., pp. 306–326). New York: Guilford Press.

Siegel, D. J. (2001). Toward an interpersonal neurobiology of the developing mind: Attachment relationships, "mindsight," and neural integration. *Infant Mental Health Journal, 22*(1–2), 67–94.

Siegel, D. J. (2007). *The mindful brain.* New York: Norton.

Siegel, D. J. (2010). *Mindsight: The new science of personal transformation.* New York: Bantam Books.

Siegel, D. J. (2010). *The mindful therapist: A clinician's guide to mindsight and neural integration.* New York: W. W. Norton.

Siegel, D. J. (2012b). *Pocket guide to interpersonal neurobiology: An integrative handbook of the mind.* New York: W. W. Norton.

Siegel, D. J. (2012a). *The developing mind: How relationships and the brain interact to shape who we are* (2nd ed.). New York: Guilford Press.

Siegel, D. J., & Hartzell, M. (2003). *Parenting from the inside out: How a deeper self-understanding can help you raise children who thrive.* New York: Tarcher/Penguin.

Smucker, M. R., Dancu, C., Foa, E. B., & Niederee, J. L. (2002). Imagery rescripting: A new treatment for survivors of childhood sexual abuse suffering from posttraumatic stress. In R. L. Leahy & E. T. Dowd (Eds.), *Clinical advances in cognitive psychotherapy: Theory and application* (pp. 294–310). New York: Springer.

Sneath, L., & Rheem, K. D. (2011). The use of emotionally focused couples therapy with military couples coping with PTSD. In R. B. Everson & C. R. Figley (Eds.), *Families under fire: Systemic therapy with military families* (pp. 127–151). New York: Routledge.

Snyder, C. R., Hoza, B., Pelham, W. E., Rapoff, M., Ware, L., Danovsky, M., et al. (1997). The development and validation of the Children's Hope Scale. *Journal of Pediatric Psychology, 22*(3), 399–421.

Snyder, C. R., Sympson, S. C., Ybasco, F. C., Borders, T. F., Babyak, M. A., & Higgins, R. L. (1996). Development and validation of the State Hope Scale. *Journal of Personality and Social Psychology, 70*(2), 321–335.

Snyder, D. K., & Monson, C. M. (2012). *Couple based interventions for military and veteran families: A practitioner's guide.* New York: Guilford Press.

Solomon, E. P., & Heide, K. M. (1999, June). *Levels of psychological trauma: Implications for diagnosis and treatment.* Paper presented at the 24th International Congress on Law and Mental Health, Toronto, Canada.

Solomon, M. F. (2003). Connection, disruption, repair: Treating the effects of attachment trauma on intimate relationships. In M. F. Solomon & D. Siegel (Eds.), *Healing trauma: Attachment, trauma, the brain, and the mind* (pp. 322–346). New York: Norton.

Solomon, M. F., & Siegel, D. J. (2003). *Healing trauma: Attachment, mind, body, and brain.* New York: Norton.

Solomon, M., & Tatkin, S. (2010). *Love and war in intimate relationships: Connection, disconnection, and mutual regulation in couple therapy.* New York: Norton.

Spermon, D., Darlington, Y., & Gibney, P. (2010). Psychodynamic psychotherapy for complex trauma: Targets, focus, applications, and outcomes. *Psychology Research and Behavior Management, 3*, 119–127.

Spiegel, D. (1986). Dissociation, double binds, and posttraumatic stress in multiple personality disorder. In B. G. Braun (Ed.), *Treatment of multiple personality disorder* (pp. 61–79). Washington, DC: American Psychiatric Press.

Spielberger, C. D., Reheiser, E. C., & Sydeman, S. J. (1995). Measuring the experience, expression, and control of anger. *Issues in Comprehensive Pediatric Nursing, 18*(3), 207–232.

Spielberger, C. D., & Vagg, P. R. (1984). Psychometric properties of the STAI: A reply to Ramanaiah, Franzen, and Schill. *Journal of Personality Assessment, 48*(1), 95–97.

Spitzer, R. L., Kroenke, K., Williams, J. B., & the Patient Health Questionnaire Primary Care Study Group. (1999). Validation and utility of a self-report version of PRIME-MD: The PHQ primary care study. *Journal of the American Medical Association, 282*(18), 1737–1744.

Stangier, U., Von Consbruch, K., Schramm, E., & Heidenreich, T. (2010). Common factors of cognitive therapy and interpersonal psychotherapy in the treatment of social phobia. *Anxiety, Stress, and Coping, 23*(3), 289–301.

Steele, H., & Steele, M. (Eds.). (2008). *Clinical applications of the Adult Attachment Interview.* New York: Guilford Press.

Steele, K., & Van der Hart, O. (2009). Treating dissociation. In C. A. Courtois & J. D. Ford (Eds.), *Treating complex traumatic stress disorders: An evidence-based guide* (pp. 145–165). New York: Guilford Press.

Steele, K., Van der Hart, O., & Nijenhuis, E. R. S. (2001). Dependency in the treatment of complex posttraumatic stress disorder and dissociative disorders. *Journal of Trauma and Dissociation, 2*(4), 79–116.

Steele, K., Van der Hart, O., & Nijenhuis, E. R. S. (2005). Phase-oriented treatment of structural dissociation in complex traumatization: Overcoming trauma-related phobias. *Journal of Trauma and Dissociation, 6*(3), 11–53.

Steer, R. A., Ball, R., Ranieri, W. F., & Beck, A. T. (1997). Further evidence for the construct validity of the Beck Depression Inventory–II with psychiatric outpatients. *Psychological Reports, 80*(2), 443–446.

Steer, R. A., Ball, R., Ranieri, W. F., & Beck, A. T. (1999). Dimensions of the Beck Depression Inventory–II in clinically depressed outpatients. *Journal of Clinical Psychology, 55*(1), 117–128.

Steinberg, M. (1994). *Structured Clinical Interview for DSM-IV Dissociative Disorders—Revised (SCID-D-R).* Washington, DC: American Psychiatric Press.

Stewart, S. H. (1996). Alcohol abuse in individuals exposed to trauma: A critical review. *Psychological Bulletin, 120*(1), 83–112.

Stovall-McClough, K. C., Cloitre, M., & McClough, J. F. (2008). Adult attachment and posttraumatic stress disorder in women with histories of childhood abuse. In H. Steele & M. Steele (Eds.), *Clinical applications of the Adult Attachment Interview* (pp. 320–340). New York: Guilford Press.

Straus, M. A., & Douglas, E. M. (2004). A short form of the Revised Conflict Tactics Scales and typologies for severity and mutuality. *Violence and Victimology, 19*(5), 507–520.

Straus, M. A., Hamby, S. L., Finkelhor, D., Moore, D. W., & Runyan, D. (1998). Identification of child maltreatment with the Parent–Child Conflict Tactics Scales: Development and psychometric data for a national sample of American parents. *Child Abuse and Neglect, 22*(4), 249–270.

Tangney, J. P., Wagner, P., Fletcher, C., & Gramzow, R. (1992). Shamed into anger? The relation of shame and guilt to anger and self-reported aggression. *Journal of Personality and Social Psychology, 62*(4), 669–675.

Taylor, J. E., & Harvey, S. T. (2010). A meta-analysis of the effects of psychotherapy with adults sexually abused in childhood. *Clinical Psychology Review, 30*, 749–767.

Taylor, S., Zvolensky, M. J., Cox, B. J., Deacon, B., Heimberg, R. G., Ledley, D. R., et al. (2007). Validation of the Anxiety Sensitivity Index–3. *Psychological Assessment, 19*(2), 176–188.

Tedeschi, R. G., & Calhoun, L. G. (1995). *Trauma and transformation: Growing in the aftermath of suffering.* Thousand Oaks, CA: Sage.

Tedeschi, R. G., & Calhoun, L. G. (2004). Posttraumatic growth: Conceptual foundations and empirical evidence. *Psychological Inquiry, 15*(1), 1–18.

Teicher, M. H., Samson, J. A., Polcari, A., & McGreenery, C. E. (2006). Sticks, stones, and hurtful words: Relative effects of various forms of childhood maltreatment. *American Journal of Psychiatry, 163*(6), 993–1000.

Terr, L. (1991). Childhood traumas: An outline and overview. *American Journal of Psychiatry, 148*, 10–20.

Thornberry, T. P., Henry, K. L., Ireland, T. O., & Smith, C. A. (2010). The causal impact of childhood-limited maltreatment and adolescent maltreatment on early adult adjustment. *Journal of Adolescent Health, 46*(4), 359–365.

Travis, L., Binder, J., Bliwise, N., & Horne-Moyer, L. (2001). Changes in clients' attachment styles over the course of time-limited psychotherapy. *Psychotherapy, 38*(2), 149–159.

Trickett, P. K., Kurtz, D. A., & Noll, J. G. (2005). The consequences of child sexual abuse for female Development. In D. Bell, S. L. Foster, & E. J. Mash (Eds.), *Handbook of behavioral and emotional problems in girls* (pp. 357–379). New York: Kluwer Academic/Plenum Publishers.

Tull, M. T., Barrett, H. M., McMillan, E. S., & Roemer, L. (2007). A preliminary investigation of the relationship between emotion regulation difficulties and posttraumatic stress symptoms. *Behavior Therapy, 38*(3), 303–313.

Tull, M. T., Jakupcak, M., McFadden, M. E., & Roemer, L. (2007). The role of negative affect intensity and the fear of emotions in posttraumatic stress symptom severity among victims of childhood interpersonal violence. *Journal of Nervous and Mental Disease, 195*(7), 580–587.

Van der Hart, O., Bolt, H., & Van der Kolk, B. A. (2005). Memory fragmentation in dissociative identity disorder. *Journal of Trauma and Dissociation, 6*(1), 55–70.

Van der Hart, O., Brown, P., & Van der Kolk, B. A. (1989). Pierre Janet's treatment of post-traumatic stress. *Journal of Traumatic Stress, 2*(4), 379–395.

Van der Hart, O., Nijenhuis, E. R. S., & Steele, K. (2006). *The haunted self: Structural dissociation and the treatment of chronic traumatization.* New York: Norton.

Van der Hart, O., Steele, K., Nijenhuis, E. R. S., & De Soir, E. (2009). Souvenirs traumatiques: Leur traitement selon le modele de la dissociation structurelle de la personalite. *Revu Francophone du Stress et du Trauma, 9*(2), 81–92.

Van der Hart, O., van Ochten, J. M., van Son, M. J. M., Steele, K., & Lensvelt-Mulders, G. (2008). Relations among peritraumatic dissociation and posttraumatic stress: A critical review. *Journal of Trauma and Dissociation, 9*(4), 481–505.

Van der Kolk, B. A. (1996). Trauma and memory. In B. A. Van der Kolk, A. C. McFarlane, & L. Weisaeth (Eds.), *Traumatic stress: The effects of overwhelming experience on mind, body, and society* (pp. 279–302). New York: Guilford Press.

Van der Kolk, B. A. (2005). Developmental trauma disorder: Toward a rational diagnosis for children with complex trauma histories. *Psychiatric Annals, 35*(5), 401–408.

Van der Kolk, B. A., Roth, S., Pelcovitz, D., Sunday, S., & Spinazzola, J. (2005). Disorders of extreme stress: The empirical foundation of a complex adaptation to trauma. *Journal of Traumatic Stress*, *18*(5), 389–399.

Veysey, B., & Clark, C. (2004). *Responding to physical and sexual abuse in women with alcohol and other drug and mental disorders*. Binghamton, NY: Haworth Press.

Vrouva, I. Fonagy, P., Fearon, P. R., & Roussow, T. (2010). The risk-taking and self-harm inventory for adolescents: Development and psychometric evaluation. *Psychological Assessment*, *22*(4), 852–865.

Vujanovic, A. A., Youngwirth, N. E., Johnson, K. A., & Zvolensky, M. J. (2009). Mindfulness-based acceptance and posttraumatic stress symptoms among trauma-exposed adults without axis I psychopathology. *Journal of Anxiety Disorders*, *23*(2), 297–303.

Wachtel, P. L. (2008). *Relational theory and the practice of psychotherapy*. New York: Guilford Press.

Waelde, L. C., Silvern, L., Carlson, E., Fairbank, J. A., & Kletter, H. (2009). Dissociation in PTSD. In P. F. Dell & J. A. O'Neill (Eds.), *Dissociation and the dissociative disorders: DSM-V and beyond* (pp. 447–456). New York: Routledge/Taylor & Francis Group.

Wagner, A. W., Rizvi, S. L., & Harned, M. S. (2007). Applications of dialectical behavior therapy to the treatment of complex trauma-related problems: When one case formulation does not fit all. *Journal of Traumatic Stress*, *20*(4), 391–400.

Wallin, D. J. (2007). *Attachment in psychotherapy*. New York: Guilford Press.

Wampold, B. E., Imel, Z. E., Laska, K. M., Benish, S., Miller, S. D., Fluckiger, C., et al. (2010). Determining what works in the treatment of PTSD. *Clinical Psychology Review*, *30*, 923–933.

Warner, S. (2009). *Understanding the effects of child sexual abuse: Feminist revolutions in theory, research and practice*. New York: Routledge/Taylor & Francis Group.

Way, I., VanDeusen, K., & Cottrell, T. (2007). Vicarious trauma: Predictors of clinicians' disrupted cognitions about self-esteem and self-intimacy. *Journal of Child Sexual Abuse*, *16*(4), 81–98.

Way, I., VanDeusen, K. M., Martin, G., Applegate, B., & Jandle, D. (2004). Vicarious trauma: A comparison of clinicians who treat survivors of sexual abuse and sexual offenders. *Journal of Interpersonal Violence*, *19*(1), 49–71.

Weathers, F. W., Keane, T. M., & Davidson, J. R. T. (2001). Clinician-Administered PTSD Scale: A review of the first ten years of research. *Depression and Anxiety*, *13*(3), 132–156.

Weiss, D. S. (2004). The Impact of Event Scale—Revised. In J. P. Wilson & T. M. Keane (Eds.), *Assessing psychological trauma and PTSD: A practitioner's handbook* (2nd ed., pp. 168–189). New York: Guilford Press.

Weiss, K. (2002). Authority as coercion: When authority figures abuse their positions to perpetrate child sexual abuse. *Journal of Child Sexual Abuse*, *11*(1), 27–52.

Weissman, M. M., Olfson, M., Gameroff, M. J., Feder, A., & Fuentes, M. (2001). A comparison of three scales for assessing social functioning in primary care. *American Journal of Psychiatry*, *158*(3), 460–466.

Werdel, M. B., & Wicks, R. J. (2012). *Primes on posttraumatic growth: An introduction and guide*. New York: Wiley.

Westen, D., Thomas, C., Nakash, O., & Bradley, R. (2006). Clinical assessment of attachment patterns and personality disorder in adolescents and adults. *Journal of Consulting and Clinical Psychology*, *74*, 1065–1085.

White, M. (2011). *Narrative practice: Continuing the conversation*. New York: W. W. Norton.

White, J. W., Koss, M. P., & Kazdin, A. E. (2011). *Violence against women and children: Vol. 1. Mapping the terrain*. Washington, DC: American Psychological Association.

Wicks, R. J. (2008). *The resilient clinician*. New York: Oxford University Press.

Widom, C. S., Czaja, S. J., & Dutton, M. A. (2008). Childhood victimization and lifetime revictimization. *Child Abuse and Neglect*, *32*(8), 785–796.

Wilkinson, M. (2009). *Changing minds in therapy: Emotion, attachment, trauma, and neurobiology*. New York: Norton.

Willer, J. (2009). *The beginning psychotherapist's companion*. Lanham, MD: Rowman & Littlefield.

Wilson, J. P., Drozdek, B., & Turkovic, S. (2006). Posttraumatic shame and guilt. *Trauma, Violence, and Abuse*, *7*(2), 122–141.

Wilson, J. P., & Keane, T. M. (Eds.). (2004). *Assessing psychological trauma and PTSD* (2nd ed.). New York: Guilford Press.

Wilson, J. P., & Lindy, J. (Eds.). (1994). *Countertransference in the treatment of PTSD*. New York: Guilford Press.

Wilson, J. P., & Thomas, R. B. (2004). *Empathy in the treatment of trauma and PTSD*. New York: Brunner/Routledge.

Winnicott, D. (1971). *Playing and reality*. London: Tavistock.

Winnicott, D. W. (1963). The development of the capacity for concern. *Bulletin of the Menninger Clinic*, *27*, 167–176.

Wolfsdorf, B. A., & Zlotnick, C. (2001). Affect management in group therapy for women with posttraumatic stress disorder and histories of childhood sexual abuse. *Journal of Clinical Psychology*, *57*(2), 169–181.

World Health Organization. (2005). *International classification of diseases and related health problems* (10th rev.). Geneva, Switzerland: Author.

Young, B. H., & Blake, D. D. (1999). *Group treatments for posttraumatic stress disorder*. Philadelphia: Brunner/Mazel.

Young, J. E. (1999). *Cognitive therapy for personality disorders: A schema-focused approach* (rev. ed.). Sarasota, FL: Professional Resources Press.

Young, J. E., & Brown, G. (2001). *Young schema questionnaire (Short Form, Version 3)*. New York: Schema Therapy Institute.

Young, J. E., Klosko, J. S., & Weishaar, M. E. (2003). *Schema therapy: A practitioner's guide*. New York: Guilford Press.

Zayfert, C., & DeViva, J. C. (2011). *When someone you love suffers from posttraumatic stress: What to expect and what you can do*. New York: Guilford Press.

Zlotnick, C., Capezza, N., & Parker, D. (2011). An interpersonally based intervention for low-income pregnant women with intimate partner violence: A pilot study. *Archives of Women's Mental Health*, *14*(1), 55–65.

Zlotnick, C., Johnson, J., & Najavits, L.M. (2009). Randomized controlled pilot study of cognitive-behavioral therapy in a sample of incarcerated women with substance use disorder and PTSD. *Behavior Therapy*, *40*, 325–336.

Index

Page numbers followed by *t* refer to tables.

Abuse, 100, 223–224
Accelerated Experiential–Dynamic Psychotherapy (AEDP), 164
Acceptance and commitment therapy (ACT), 127–130
Acknowledgement, 154–155
Acting-out behaviors, 19–20
Active stance, 278–279
Acute stress disorder (ASD), 11, 12–13
Adaptations, 8–9, 55–58, 193*t*
Addictions. *see also* Substance use
  adolescent trauma and, 19–20
  assessment instruments and inventories and, 112*t*
  contraindications to membership in group treatment, 193*t*–194*t*
  goals for treatment and, 90
  group treatment and, 210
  overview, 24*t*, 26
  as secondary elaborations, 4
Addictions and Trauma Recovery (ATRIUM), 210
Adolescence, 19–21, 23, 41–42. *see also* Childhood trauma
Adulthood, 21–22, 33
Affective disorders, 31, 145. *see also* Depression
Affective intensity, 167–169
Aggression
  assessment instruments and inventories and, 111*t*
  contraindications to membership in group treatment, 193*t*–194*t*
  couple therapy and, 216, 217
  crises and, 172
  family therapy and, 223–224
  goals for treatment and, 90, 93
  informed consent and refusal and, 82–83
  overview, 24*t*
Alcohol use. *see* Addictions; Substance use
Alexithymia, 238, 240
Alienation
  complex trauma histories and, 4
  goals for treatment and, 90–91, 93
  overview, 24*t*, 239–240
Allostatis, 97–98
American Association for Marriage and Family Therapy Code of Ethics, 70*t*–74*t*. *see also* Ethical considerations
American Psychological Association Ethical Principles of Psychologists and Code of Conduct: 2010 Amendments, 76*t*–77*t*. *see also* Ethical considerations
Amnesia, 262–263
Analgesia, 33
Anger
  adolescent trauma and, 19–20
  assessment instruments and inventories and, 111*t*
  complex PTSD/DESNOS and, 48
  complex trauma histories and, 4
  couple therapy and, 215–216
  group treatment and, 207
  overview, 24*t*
  phase 2 of psychotherapy and, 145
  posttraumatic emotional dysregulation and, 146–150
  posttraumatic stress disorder (PTSD) and, 45–46
  reactions to complex trauma and, 31–32
  stabilization and, 127–130
  therapeutic relationship and, 135, 285–287
  transference and, 310–311
Anguish, 93, 178–179
Anhedonia, 45–46, 127–130
Anxiety
  anxiety disorders, 31–32
  assessment and, 99
  childhood trauma and, 17, 18
  complex trauma and, 4, 31
  goals for treatment and, 93, 95

medication and, 85
phase 2 of psychotherapy and, 145, 153
posttraumatic emotional dysregulation and, 146–150
posttraumatic stress disorder (PTSD) and, 44
safety and, 126
stabilization and, 127–130, 129–130

"Apparently normal personality" (ANP)
assessment and, 103
discontinuity and, 249–250
overview, 36
structural dissociation and, 252–253
transference and, 305–306, 309–310

Appraisals, 109*t*

Arousal states. *see also* Hyperarousal; Hypoarousal
goals for treatment and, 93
group treatment and, 193*t*
mind–body integration and, 97–98
posttraumatic emotional dysregulation and, 146–150
preparing the client for trauma and emotion processing, 167–169

Assertiveness, 35–36, 217

Assessment
contraindications to membership in group treatment, 207, 208*t*–209*t*, 209–210
crisis presentation and, 104–105
group treatment and, 203*t*
instruments and inventories used in, 108–118, 109*t*–112*t*
issues and approaches, 98–108
overview, 119
pacing of, 102

Assumptions, 140–142

Attachment
assessment instruments and inventories and, 110*t*, 114
childhood trauma and, 17–18
complex trauma in childhood and, 14–15
discontinuity and, 250–251
dissociation and, 255–256
emotional processing and, 151–152
family therapy and, 223–224
goals for treatment and, 90–91
phase 1 of psychotherapy, 122
phase 3 of psychotherapy and, 181
posttraumatic themes in treatment and, 258–259
reactions to complex trauma and, 38, 39
rights and responsibilities of clients and therapists and, 74
therapeutic relationship and, 64, 275, 276–277, 286
therapists and, 298–299
transference–countertransference positions and, 324–326
traumatic transference and, 301–302

Attachment styles
overview, 24*t*, 297
therapeutic relationship and, 63, 270
transference and, 299
treatment and, 287–297

Attachment-based treatments, 164

Attendance, 86, 141, 197*t*

Attentional functioning, 24*t*, 49, 85, 95, 261–262

Attributions, 309–310

Attunement, 63–64, 280–282

Authority figures, 11–12, 135–136

Autonomy, 89, 91–93

Avoidance
assessment instruments and inventories and, 109*t*
countertransference and, 315
discontinuity and, 249–251
goals for treatment and, 90–91, 93
phase 2 of psychotherapy and, 145, 153–154
posttraumatic emotional dysregulation and, 146–150
preparing the client for trauma and emotion processing, 165
SAFER strategies and, 154–155
therapeutic exposure and, 150

B

BASK model, 251–252

Behavioral functioning, 18, 49, 91, 134

Behavioral-analytic interventions, 128–129

Beliefs
phase 2 of psychotherapy and, 153
phase 3 of psychotherapy and, 186–187
posttraumatic stress disorder (PTSD) and, 45–46
readiness for change and, 132
transference and, 312

Beliefs about oneself, 36–37, 45, 134, 186–187

Bereavement, 24*t*, 178–179, 318

Betrayal, 135–136, 303–305

Binge eating, 19–20, 24*t*

Biological assessment, 114–115. *see also* Assessment

Body areas, 33–34, 97–98, 193*t*, 274–275. *see also* Physical effects

Borderline personality disorder (BPD), 47, 127–130, 207

Boundaries
attachment styles and, 289–290
group treatment and, 197*t*–198*t*
posttraumatic themes in treatment and, 257
sexual involvement with clients, 320–322
therapeutic relationship and, 135, 136, 282–284
treatment and, 54

Brain functioning, 146–150, 250–251

Bulimarexia, 24*t*

Bulimia, 24*t*
Burnout, vicarious trauma and, 273–274

C

Caregivers, 11, 15, 64, 136
Caretaking behaviors, 40, 307, 308–310
Change, 130–134, 193*t*–194*t*, 271
Chaos, 127–130
Child maltreatment, 11–12, 82–83
Childhood trauma, 3, 11–19, 23, 34–35, 49. *see also* Abuse; Adolescence
Child-rearing, 186
Choice, 67*t*, 133, 139, 150
Client education, 130–134, 140
Clients. *see also* Therapeutic relationship
  attachment styles and, 294–297
  group treatment and, 204*t*
  impact of assessment on, 102
  rights and responsibilities of, 65–87, 66*t*–68*t*, 69*t*, 70*t*–74*t*, 76*t*–77*t*, 78*t*–79*t*, 204*t*
Cognitions, 109*t*, 153
Cognitive errors, 148, 153, 265–266. *see also* Distortions
Cognitive functioning, 91
Cognitive processing therapy (CPT), 158
Cognitive-behavioral therapy (CBT), 127–130, 129–130, 148
Collaboration, 35–36, 132, 139
Collateral assessment, 115–116
Communication, 138, 199*t*, 225–226, 284–285
Comorbidities, 110*t*, 172, 210; *see also* Co-ocurring disorders
Compartmentalization, 240–246
Compassion fatigue, 270, 271
Competence, 67*t*, 68–69, 72*t*, 81
Complex posttraumatic reactions, 8–9
Complex PTSD, 46–49, 50, 89–90, 118, 252–253. *see also* Posttraumatic stress disorder (PTSD)
Complex PTSD/DESNOS, 48, 50, 89–90, 118
Complex trauma
  during adolescence, 19–21
  during adulthood, 21–22
  in childhood, 11–19
  countertransference and, 313–322
  defining, 9–10
  diagnosis and, 118
  history of, 3–4, 5–9
  overview, 27
  transference and, 299–313
  treatment and, 23–27, 24*t*
Complex trauma-sequenced model, 120–122, 142–143. *see also* Phase 1; Phase 2; Phase 3; Treatment
Complex traumatic stress disorders, 89–90, 118. *see* Disorders
Compulsive behaviors, 18, 24*t*, 90, 127–130, 153
Concentration problems, 44
Conduct disorders, 24*t*, 31
Confidence, 153
Confidentiality
  group treatment and, 195, 196, 203*t*–204*t*
  phase 1 of psychotherapy and, 141–142
  rights and responsibilities of clients and therapists and, 66*t*, 71*t*–72*t*
Conflict, 199*t*, 284–285
Conflict of interests, 72*t*
Confrontation, 291–292
Confusion, 4, 17, 93
Consent to services. *see* Informed consent and refusal
Consolidating therapeutic gains, 180–182. *see also* Phase 3
Control
  assessment instruments and inventories and, 110*t*
  goals for treatment and, 94
  informed consent and refusal and, 81–83
  loss and mourning and, 179
  reactions to complex trauma and, 40
  readiness for change and, 133
  transference and, 309
Co-occuring disorders, 110*t*, 172, 210; *see also* Comorbidities
Coping mechanisms
  complex trauma histories and, 4
  dissociation and, 255–256
  emptiness feelings and, 240–246
  goals for treatment and, 93, 97–98
  group treatment and, 199*t*
  phase 2 of psychotherapy and, 145
  phase 3 of psychotherapy and, 182
  posttraumatic stress disorder (PTSD) and, 44
  safety and, 124–125
  symptoms as, 55–58
  therapeutic relationship and, 137–138
Cotherapists, 199*t*–200*t*, 200, 210–214. *see also* Therapist
Countertransference
  crises and, 173
  dissociative/posttraumatic transference field and, 256–267
  empathic attunement and, 281–282
  overview, 298–299, 299–300, 314, 326–327
  rights and responsibilities of clients and therapists and, 75, 80
  themes, issues and reactions, 313–322
  transference–countertransference positions and, 324–326
Couple therapy, 190, 214–222, 230–231. *see also* Systemic therapy; Treatment
Crisis
  assessment and, 104–105
  attachment styles and, 293–294
  group treatment and, 210

preventing and managing, 172–177
transference and, 304
Cumulative trauma, 12

D

Danger seeking, 126; *see also* High-risk behavior
Decompensation, 172–177
Defenses
complex trauma histories and, 4
goals for treatment and, 97–98
posttraumatic emotional dysregulation and, 146–150
readiness for change and, 132
therapeutic relationship and, 137–138
Delusions, 127–130
Denial, 193*t*–194*t*, 315
Dependency, 24*t*, 38, 92, 135, 137
Depression
assessment and, 99
childhood trauma and, 18
complex trauma histories and, 4
goals for treatment and, 95
medication and, 85
overview, 24*t*
posttraumatic stress disorder (PTSD) and, 44
safety and, 126
stabilization and, 127–130
Depressive reactions in complex trauma, 31
Despair, 17, 24*t*, 178–179
Detached/dismissive/avoidant attachment style, 287, 290–292. *see also* Dismissive attachment style; Insecure attachment style
Detachment from others
goals for treatment and, 97–98
overview, 24*t*, 26
posttraumatic stress disorder (PTSD) and, 45–46
reactions to complex trauma and, 39, 40
safety and, 124–125
traumatic transference and, 302
Developmental factors, 49–50, 54, 64
Developmental perspective, 124
Developmental trauma disorder (DTD), 48–49
Diagnosis
assessment and, 98–99
complex PTSD and, 46–49
defining complex trauma and, 9–10
overview, 30–43, 42–50, 118
posttraumatic stress disorder (PTSD) and, 9
Diagnostic and Statistical Manual of Mental Disorders (DSM-5), 9–10, 43, 44–46, 47–48
Diagnostic and Statistical Manual of Mental Disorders (DSM-IV), 45–49
Diagnostic and Statistical Manual of Mental Disorders (DSM-IV-TR), 9, 11, 118
Dialectical behavior therapy (DBT), 163, 207
Disclosure of past abuse and trauma
assessment and, 100, 105–108
contraindications to membership in group treatment, 193*t*–194*t*
couple therapy and, 217, 218
failure to disclose, 106–108
group treatment and, 200–201
preparing the client for trauma and emotion processing, 166–167
Disconfirmation of self, 304–305
Disconnection from others, 240, 276–277. *see also* Emptiness feelings
Discontinuity, 247–251
Disempowerment, 21–22, 95, 132. *see also* Power
Disenfranchised grief, 178–179
Disgust, 316–317
Disillusionment, 303–305
Dismissive attachment style, 39, 92–93. *see also* Attachment; Detached/dismissive/avoidant attachment style
Disorders. *see also individual disorders*
assessment instruments and inventories and, 112–113
conceptualizing and diagnosing, 42–50
crises and, 172
diagnosis and, 118
goals for treatment and, 94–95
overview, 8–9, 30–42
phase 2 of psychotherapy and, 145
Disorganized/unresolved/dissociative attachment style. *see also* Attachment; Insecure attachment style
dissociation and, 255–256
goals for treatment and, 92–93
overview, 287, 292–294, 296–297
posttraumatic themes in treatment and, 258–259
reactions to complex trauma and, 39
therapeutic relationship and, 276–277
Disparity, 150–151; *see also* Emotion processing
Dissociation. *see also* Self-integration
assessment and, 103, 111*t*, 112–113
attachment styles and, 292–294
case examples of, 175–177, 251–252
childhood trauma and, 18
contraindications to membership in group treatment, 193*t*–194*t*
crises and, 172
discontinuity and, 247–251
emptiness feelings and, 240–246
focusing on needs of others as a form of, 40
as a form of coping with emotion dysregulation, 255–256
goals for treatment and, 90, 90–91, 93, 95, 97–98
group treatment and, 191, 209–210, 210
models of, 251–256

Dissociation (*continued*)
overview, 24*t*
phase 2 of psychotherapy and, 145
posttraumatic emotional dysregulation and, 146–150
reactions to complex trauma and, 33, 36–39
safety and, 124–125, 126
stabilization and, 127–130
treatment and, 256–267
Dissociative identity disorder (DID), 36, 193*t*–194*t*, 210, 253, 293
Distance–closeness dance, 282–284
Distortions, 18, 45–46, 265–266
Distrust, 4, 43, 60–62. *see also* Mistrust of others; Trust
Documentation, 284. *see also* Record keeping
Domestic abuse. *see* Family violence
Double bind communication, 303–304
Drug use. *see* Substance use
Duration of treatment, 83–84, 86
Dysphoria, 18, 45, 93

E

Eating disorders, 24*t*, 26, 95
Ecological model of trauma treatment, 192
Economic status, 100–101. *see also* Financial considerations; Financial mismanagement and chaos
Education, client, 130–134, 140
Emotion dysregulation. *see also* Emotion regulation
case examples of, 175–177
complex PTSD/DESNOS and, 46–47
contraindications to membership in group treatment, 193*t*–194*t*
developmental trauma disorder (DTD) and, 49
dissociation and, 255–256
goals for treatment and, 91
overview, 28, 35–36
phase 2 of psychotherapy and, 145, 146–150
posttraumatic stress disorder (PTSD) and, 45–46
therapeutic exposure and, 150–156
Emotion processing
evidence-based treatments and, 156–165
phase 2 of psychotherapy and, 144–145, 165–177
phase 3 of psychotherapy and, 182–183
preparing the client for, 165–177
when to stop, 171–172
Emotion regulation. *see also* Emotion dysregulation
assessment instruments and inventories and, 111*t*
childhood trauma and, 17
emotional processing and, 152
goals for treatment and, 89
group treatment and, 193*t*
overview, 54
phase 3 of psychotherapy and, 182
rights and responsibilities of clients and therapists and, 75, 77
Emotional expression, 155
Emotional functioning, 91
Emotional lability, 126
"Emotional personality" (EP), 36, 103, 252–253, 305–306
Emotional processing, 150–156, 173–177, 202
Emotional reactions, 18–19, 24*t*, 44, 255–256
Emotion-based therapies, 128, 159, 164
Emotions, 4, 17, 33, 240–246; *see also* Affective intensity
Empathic attunement, 64, 280–282. *see also* Attunement
Empathic errors, 281–282
Empathic mindfulness, 276–277. *see also* Mindfulness interventions
Empathic mirroring, 275–277
Empathic strain, 271, 281–282
Empathy
adolescent trauma and, 20–21
attachment styles and, 291–292
group treatment and, 193*t*
reactions to complex trauma and, 38, 42
therapeutic relationship and, 59–60, 64, 280–282
treatment and, 56–57
Employment problems, 99, 109*t*, 185–187
Empowerment, 81–83, 95, 139
Emptiness feelings
case examples of, 242–246, 249, 251–252
as described by complex trauma survivors, 236–246
discontinuity and, 247–251
impact of on therapists, 267
models of dissociation and, 251–256
overview, 235, 268
posttraumatic stress disorder (PTSD) and, 44
treatment and, 256–267
working in the posttraumatic and dissociative field, 256–267
Enactments, 80, 323–324, 326–327
Ending treatment. *see* Termination of treatment
Engagement in therapy, 132, 169–170, 210
Enslavement, 22
Entrancement of the therapist, 264–265
Environmental factors, 124–125, 139, 218
Erotized transference, 258–259, 302–303. *see also* Transference
Estrangement, 44, 44–45, 93
Ethical considerations
rights and responsibilities of clients and therapists and, 65–87, 66*t*–68*t*, 69*t*, 70*t*–74*t*, 76*t*–77*t*, 78*t*–79*t*
sexual involvement with clients, 320–322
therapeutic relationship and, 135
Evidence-based treatments, 156–165

Existential issues, 44, 186–187
Expectations
  group treatment and, 195–210, 197*t*–200*t*, 203*t*–207*t*, 208*t*–209*t*
  phase 1 of psychotherapy, 140–142
  posttraumatic stress disorder (PTSD) and, 44–45
  posttraumatic themes in treatment and, 257
  reactions to complex trauma and, 41
  readiness for change and, 131, 132
Expectations of others, 289
Experiential awareness, 155
Experiential treatment, 128–129, 150–156, 92*t*
Exploitation, 303–305
Exposure, therapeutic. *see* Therapeutic exposure
Eye movement desensitization and reprocessing (EMDR) therapy, 159–160, 171–172, 175–177

F

Family therapy, 190, 223–230, 230–231. *see also* Systemic therapy; Treatment
Family violence. *see also* Interpersonal violence; Violence
  complex trauma and, 12, 16
  couple therapy and, 216
  safety and, 125–126
  sexual behavior and, 41–42
Fear
  of intimacy, 24*t*
  phase 2 of psychotherapy and, 153–154
  posttraumatic emotional dysregulation and, 146–150
  posttraumatic stress disorder (PTSD) and, 44–45
  safety and, 126
  stabilization and, 129–130
  therapeutic relationship and, 135, 136
  transference and, 312
Fees, 203*t*–207*t*. *see* Financial considerations
"Fight–flight–freeze" response, 132. *see also* Defenses
Financial considerations, 73*t*, 86, 140–142, 203*t*–207*t*
Financial mismanagement and chaos, 26, 100–101. *see also* Economic status; Shopping addiction; Spending problems
Flashbacks, 215–216, 257, 259–260, 266–267
Focused attention, 128–129, 261–262. *see also* Attentional functioning
Forgetting, 103–104. *see also* Memory
FREEDOM acronym, 162–163
Frequency of sessions, 84, 86
Functioning, 94–95, 95–96, 155

G

Goals for treatment, 88–98, 108–118, 109*t*–112*t*, 119, 133
Graduated exposure, 157–158. *see also* Therapeutic exposure
Grief
  childhood trauma and, 17
  complex trauma histories and, 4
  countertransference and, 318
  loss and mourning and, 178–179
  transference and, 311–312
Group treatment. *see also* Systemic therapy; Treatment
  benefits of, 193*t*
  case examples of, 210–214
  contraindications to membership in, 193*t*–194*t*, 207, 208*t*–209*t*, 209–210
  expectations and ground rules, 195–210, 197*t*–200*t*, 203*t*–207*t*, 208*t*–209*t*
  overview, 190, 191–214, 193*t*–194*t*, 197*t*–200*t*, 203*t*–207*t*, 208*t*–209*t*, 230–231
  types of groups, 192
Guilt
  childhood trauma and, 17, 18
  countertransference and, 316–317
  overview, 24*t*
  phase 2 of psychotherapy and, 145
  posttraumatic stress disorder (PTSD) and, 44–45
  transference and, 307, 309

H

Hallucinations, 24*t*, 127–130, 264–265
Health, 33–34, 114–115, 145. *see also* Medical issues
Helplessness, 24*t*, 89, 95, 317
High-risk behavior, 19–20, 24*t*
Holding environment, 59–60. *see also* Secure base; Therapeutic relationship
Homicide, 5, 82–83, 193*t*–194*t*, 293–294
Honesty, 191, 285–287
Hopelessness
  complex PTSD/DESNOS and, 48
  couple therapy and, 215–216
  overview, 24*t*
  posttraumatic stress disorder (PTSD) and, 43
  readiness for change and, 131
  safety and, 124–125
  stabilization and, 127–130
  therapeutic relationship and, 135
Horror, 45, 90–91, 315
Hospitalization, 84–86, 99, 283
Hyperarousal
  assessment instruments and inventories and, 109*t*
  goals for treatment and, 90–91, 93
  overview, 24*t*
  posttraumatic emotional dysregulation and, 146–150
  preparing the client for trauma and emotion processing and, 170

Hypermnesia, 262–263
Hyperresilience, 308–310
Hypervigilance
assessment instruments and inventories and, 109*t*
childhood trauma and, 18
crises and, 172
emptiness feelings and, 241–242
reactions to complex trauma and, 38
traumatic transference and, 300–301
Hypoarousal
goals for treatment and, 90–91, 93
overview, 24*t*
phase 2 of psychotherapy and, 145
posttraumatic emotional dysregulation and, 146–150
preparing the client for trauma and emotion processing and, 170

I

Identification with the perpetrator, 20–21
Identity issues, 4, 16, 22, 93–94, 178–179
Imagery rehearsal/rescripting therapy (IRT), 160–161
Immobility, 132–133
Impulsivity
adolescent trauma and, 19–20
attachment styles and, 289
goals for treatment and, 90, 93, 95
overview, 24*t*
posttraumatic stress disorder (PTSD) and, 44
posttraumatic themes in treatment and, 257, 260
safety and, 126
In vivo exposure, 157, 158, 169. *see also* Therapeutic exposure
Incoherence, 24*t*, 263–264
Indifference, 124–125
Ineffectiveness, 24*t*, 89
Infancy, 15–16. *see also* Childhood trauma
Information gathering, 115–116
Information-processing problems, 24*t*
Informed consent and refusal
group treatment and, 203*t*–207*t*
phase 1 of psychotherapy and, 140–142
preparing the client for trauma and emotion processing, 167
rights and responsibilities of clients and therapists and, 81–83
therapeutic exposure and, 150
Insecure attachment style. *see also* Attachment; Detached/dismissive/avoidant attachment style; Disorganized/unresolved/dissociative attachment style; Preoccupied attachment style
family therapy and, 223–224
goals for treatment and, 91
overview, 287
reactions to complex trauma and, 39–40
therapeutic relationship and, 276–277
Insurance. *see* Financial considerations
Intake interview, 98, 203*t*, 207, 208*t*–209*t*, 209–210. *see also* Assessment
Intentionality, 278–279
Interdependency, 35, 185–187
Internal working models, 63. *see also* Working models
International Classification of Diseases, 10th edition (ICD-10), 43, 43–44, 118
Interpersonal functioning, 91, 109*t*, 155–156, 239–240, 303–307. *see also* Relationship problems
Interpersonal violence, 99, 172, 178–179, 216. *see also* Family violence; Violence
Intersubjective perspective, 279–280
Interviews, 115–116. *see also* Structured interviews
Intimacy. *see also* Relationship problems
couple therapy and, 217–218
fear of, 24*t*
overview, 24*t*
phase 3 of psychotherapy and, 185–187
posttraumatic stress disorder (PTSD) and, 44
transference and, 305–307
"Into the breach", 235, 256–267, 268. *see also* Emptiness feelings
Intrusive reexperiencing, 109*t*, 247–248
Inventories, 108, 112–113. *see also* Assessment
Irritability, 44, 145

L

Language use, countertransference and, 319–320
Learning problems, 44, 95
Legal factors, 141–142, 218
Lifespan, 21–22. *see also* Adolescence; Adulthood; Childhood trauma; Infancy
Limit setting, 257, 282–284, 289–290, 320–322. *see also* Boundaries
Living situation, 100–101, 124–125, 185–187
Loathing of self or others, 90–91. *see also* Self-loathing
Loneliness, 4
Loss, 17, 178–179, 311–312
Love, transference, 302–303. *see also* Transference

M

Mania, 24*t*, 145
Meaning, systems of, 48, 186–187
Measurement tools, 108–118, 109*t*–112*t*. *see also* Assessment
Medical issues. *see also* Health
assessment and, 114–115
complex PTSD/DESNOS and, 48
overview, 5, 24*t*
phase 2 of psychotherapy and, 145
reactions to complex trauma and, 33–34

Medication, 85–86, 120–121, 127–130, 149
Meditative approaches, 128
Memory
assessment and, 103–104
couple therapy and, 215–216
disclosure of past abuse and trauma and, 107–108
evidence-based treatments and, 156–165
goals for treatment and, 95
group treatment and, 202
phase 2 of psychotherapy and, 144–145
phase 3 of psychotherapy and, 180–181, 182–183
posttraumatic themes in treatment and, 262–263
preparing the client for trauma and emotion processing, 165–177
prolonged exposure (PE) and, 156–158
therapeutic exposure and, 150–156
"Me–not-me" dialogues, 254. *see also* Dissociation
Mental health status, 5, 210
Mentalization approaches, 148, 250, 276–277, 286–287
Metagoals, 90–98
Mind–body connection, 97–98, 274–275; *see also* Somatic problems
Mindfulness interventions
overview, 129
posttraumatic emotional dysregulation and, 148
readiness for change and, 132–133
therapeutic relationship and, 274–275, 276–277, 286–287
Minimizing, 290–291, 319
Mirroring, 276–277
Miscommunication, 284–285. *see also* Communication
Mistrust of others. *see also* Distrust; Trust
case examples of, 60–62
informed consent and refusal and, 83
overview, 24*t*
reactions to complex trauma and, 38, 40–41
therapeutic relationship and, 135–136
transference and, 303–305
Modeling, 276–277
Mood disorders, 85. *see also* Depression
Motivated suppression, 103–104. *see also* Memory
Motivation, 138, 170, 193*t*–194*t*
Motivational enhancement, 133–134
Mourning, 178–179, 318
Munchausen, 34

N

Narcissistic/borderline personality, 193*t*–194*t*
Narrative exposure therapy (NET), 161–162
National Association of Social Workers, 78*t*–79*t*
National Child Traumatic Stress Network (NCTSN), 49–50
Neediness, 38, 39, 289
Negative thinking, 148, 153
Neglect, 12, 15
Neurobiological perspective, 146–150
Neurological assessment, 114–115. *see also* Assessment
Neurophysiologically based treatments, 164
Numbing
assessment instruments and inventories and, 109*t*
childhood trauma and, 18
crises and, 172
discontinuity and, 247–248
emptiness feelings and, 240
goals for treatment and, 93
posttraumatic stress disorder (PTSD) and, 44, 45–46

O

Obsessions, 145, 153
Obsessive rumination, 18, 127–130. *see also* Rumination
Obsessive–compulsive disorder, 129–130
Oppositional defiant disorder, 24*t*, 31
Outrage, 310–311
Overreporting, 102–104
Overwork, 24*t*. *see also* Workaholism

P

Panic, 18, 145
Panic attacks, 127–130
Paradoxical prescription, 133
Paranoid personality, 193*t*–194*t*
Parentified behaviors, 40, 307, 308–310
Parenting issues, 186, 218, 223–224
Parents, complex trauma in childhood and, 11
Participation expectations, 197*t*–198*t*. *see also* Attendance
Passivity, 24*t*, 44, 132; *see also* Helplessness
Patients. *see* Clients
Payment for services. *see* Financial considerations
Perceptual distortions, 18, 44, 48, 264–265
Perfectionism, 40–41
Personal dimensions, 274–275
Personal discourse, 263–264
Personality, 98–99
Personality disorder, 26, 47, 193*t*–194*t*
Personality type, 314–315
Phase 1. *see also* Complex trauma-sequenced model; Treatment
adapting phase 1 interventions to phase 3, 182
couple therapy and, 216
overview, 121–122, 122, 142–143
practical arrangements for, 138–142
readiness for change and, 130–134

Phase 1 (*continued*)
returning to, 183–185
safety and, 123–127
stabilization and, 127–130
therapeutic working alliance and, 134–138
Phase 2. *see also* Complex trauma-sequenced model; Treatment
adapting phase 2 interventions to phase 3, 182–183
case examples of, 173–177
couple therapy and, 216–217
crises and, 172–177
evidence-based treatments and, 156–165
loss and mourning as special issues in, 178–179
overview, 122, 144–145, 189
posttraumatic emotional dysregulation and, 146–150
preparing the client for trauma and emotion processing, 165–177
returning to, 183–185
technical considerations in, 166–167
therapeutic exposure and, 150–156
Phase 3. *see also* Complex trauma-sequenced model; Treatment
adapting phase 1 interventions to, 182
adapting phase 2 interventions to, 182–183
case examples of, 187–189, 329–331
couple therapy and, 217–218
issues in, 185–187
overview, 122–123, 144, 180–182
returning to phase 1 or 2, 183–185
Phase-oriented models, 194–195; *see also* Sequenced model
Phobias, 18, 33–34, 129–130, 153
Physical abuse, 12, 16, 41–42
Physical arousal, 167–169. *see also* Arousal states
Physical effects, 33. *see also* Health; Medical issues
Pity, 316–317
Planning skills, 38
Posttraumatic emotional dysregulation, 146–150. *see also* Emotion dysregulation
Posttraumatic growth, 38–39, 272–273
Posttraumatic reactions, 4–5, 30–43
Posttraumatic stress disorder (PTSD)
cognitive processing therapy and, 158
complex PTSD, 46–49
complex trauma in childhood and, 11, 12–13
diagnosis and, 118
Diagnostic and Statistical Manual of Mental Disorders (DSM-5) and, 44
discontinuity and, 247–251
goals for treatment and, 88–89
group treatment and, 193*t*
International Classification of Diseases, 10th edition (ICD-10) and, 43–44
medication and, 85
overview, 9, 30, 50
prolonged exposure (PE) and, 156–158
Posttraumatic symptoms, 24*t*, 215–216
Post-traumatic therapy (PTT), 53–54
Power, 11–12, 21–22. *see also* Disempowerment
Powerlessness, 124–125; *see also* Helplessness
Preoccupied attachment style, 39, 258–259, 287, 288–290. *see also* Attachment; Insecure attachment style
PRIDE acronym, 54. *see also* Developmental factors; Emotion regulation; Relational working models; Self-identity
Privacy, 191, 195, 196, 285
Privileged voyeurism, 320
Problem-solving skills, 193*t*
Processing therapies, 148, 164–165, 202
Procrastination, 26
Professional training/development, 68–69, 273–274
Prognostic indicators, 116–118
Projective identification, 298–299, 322–323, 326–327
Prolonged exposure (PE), 156–158, 173–174, 200–201. *see also* Therapeutic exposure
Prosody, 64
Pseudo-psychotic symptoms, 127–130, 264–265
Psychiatric symptoms, 172
Psychic dimensions, 274–287
Psychodynamic psychotherapy, 170–171
Psychogenic amnesia, 45–46
Psychological withdrawal, 42. *see also* Withdrawal
Psychophysiological assessment, 114–115. *see also* Assessment
Psychosis, 24*t*, 108, 193*t*–194*t*
Psychosocial evaluation, 98. *see also* Assessment
Psychotherapy. *see* Complex trauma-sequenced model; Phase 1; Phase 2; Phase 3; Treatment
Psychotic symptoms, 85, 127–130
Psychotic-like experiences, 24*t*
Purpose of life, 186–187

R

Racing thoughts, 127–130
Rage; *see also* Anger
childhood trauma and, 17
countertransference and, 317–318
couple therapy and, 217
loss and mourning and, 178–179
phase 2 of psychotherapy and, 145
reactions to complex trauma and, 32
transference and, 310–311
Reactive depression, 145. *see also* Depression
Reactivity, 147, 257, 260
Realization, 165

Recall difficulties, 18
Reciprocity, 309
Record keeping, 72*t*, 142, 204*t*, 284
Record review, 115–116
Reenactments
  goals for treatment and, 90, 95–97
  group treatment and, 200
  rights and responsibilities of clients and therapists and, 80
  traumatic transference and, 301–302
Reexperiencing trauma, 150–156, 167
Refusal of services. *see* Informed consent and refusal
Relational aggression, 172. *see also* Aggression; Interpersonal violence
Relational breaches, 284–285
Relational working models, 54
Relationship problems. *see also* Couple therapy; Interpersonal functioning; Intimacy
  assessment and, 99
  complex PTSD/DESNOS and, 46–47
  couple therapy and, 216
  developmental trauma disorder (DTD) and, 49
  goals for treatment and, 95
  overview, 24*t*, 28
  phase 3 of psychotherapy and, 185–187
  preparing the client for trauma and emotion processing, 166
  reactions to complex trauma and, 39–43
  therapeutic relationship and, 134–135
  transference and, 305–307
Relationships, 131, 156
Religious beliefs, 186–187
Resilience, 89, 193*t*, 272–273, 319
Resistance, 83, 134
Resources, 98–99, 138, 166
Respect, 20–21, 191
Responsibility, 20–21, 307
Restructuring of reality, 304–305
Retraumatization, 4, 110*t*
Revictimization, 44, 56–57, 289
Risk assessment, 99, 123–124, 125–126. *see also* Assessment
Risk factors, 4, 9–10, 110*t*
Risk management perspective, 142
Risk taking, 126, 193*t*–194*t*; *see also* Danger seeking
"Risking Connection" curriculum, 270
Risky behavior, 172
Ritualized behaviors, 18
Role models, 134
Role reversal, 307
"Roll with resistance", 134
Rules, 195–210, 197*t*–200*t*, 203*t*–207*t*, 208*t*–209*t*
Rumination, 129, 145, 146–150, 153. *see also* Obsessive rumination

S

Sadness, 178–179. *see also* Depression
SAFER (Self-care and symptom control, Acknowledgement, Functioning, Expression, and Relationships) strategies, 154–156
Safety
  attachment styles and, 293–294
  couple therapy and, 215–216, 218
  goals for treatment and, 95
  group treatment and, 191, 210
  overview, 120–121
  phase 1 of psychotherapy, 122, 123–127, 139, 142–143
  phase 3 of psychotherapy and, 182
  therapeutic relationship and, 59–65, 135, 283
  traumatic transference and, 301–302
  treatment and, 54, 59
Secondary PTSD, 271
Secondary secrets, 307–308
Secondary trauma, 269–270, 271
Secrets, secondary, 307–308
Secure attachment. *see also* Attachment
  discontinuity and, 250–251
  goals for treatment and, 90–91
  overview, 287
  phase 3 of psychotherapy and, 181
  therapeutic relationship and, 275, 276–277
  treatment and, 288, 294–297
Secure base, 275
Security, 139. *see also* Safety
Seeking Safety (SS), 163, 210
Self psychology, 170–171
Self-anesthesia, 33–34
Self-awareness, 90, 170–171
Self-blame, 19–20, 24*t*
Self-capacities, 98–99
Self-care, 154, 182
Self-compassion, 181
Self-concept, 89, 181
Self-confidence, 289
Self-defeating behavior, 172
Self-destructiveness, 47
Self-determination, 89, 91–93
Self-disclosure by therapist, 285
Self-disregard, 93
Self-dysregulation, 49
Self-efficacy, 94, 110*t*
Self-empathy, 181
Self-esteem
  complex trauma histories and, 4
  loss and mourning and, 178–179
  overview, 24*t*
  posttraumatic stress disorder (PTSD) and, 44
  structural dissociation and, 252–253
  therapeutic relationship and, 277
Self-estrangement, 32
Self-forgiveness, 181

Self-fragmentation, 172
Self-harm, 90, 99, 111*t*, 126
Self-identity, 54
Self-injury, 4, 24*t*, 126, 193*t*–194*t*
Self-integration, 35–38. *see also* Dissociation
Self-integrity, 14–15, 28, 35–38
Self-knowledge, 181
Self-loathing, 4, 93. *see also* Loathing of self or others
Self-management skills, 129–130
Self-medicating behavior, 26
Self-mutilation, 19–20, 172
Self-perception, 48. *see also* Perceptual distortions
Self-preservation, 255–256
Self-protection, 257–258
Self-reflexivity, 148
Self-regulation, 14–15, 75, 77, 90, 246
Self-sacrificing behavior, 309
Self-soothing, 4, 26, 193*t*–194*t*
Self-sufficiency, 24*t*, 39, 40
Self-void, 236–238. *see also* Emptiness feelings
Sense of self, 17, 93–94
Sensitivity to others, 38–39
Sensorimotor psychotherapy interventions, 97–98, 128–129, 164, 169–170
Separation, 312
Sequenced model of treatment, 120–121
Sexual abuse, 12, 16, 42–43, 148
Sexual behavior
  adolescent trauma and, 19–20
  assessment and, 99
  erotic transference and, 302–303
  family therapy and, 223–224
  overview, 26
  phase 3 of psychotherapy and, 185–187
  reactions to complex trauma and, 42–43
  transference and, 308
Sexual enslavement, 22
Sexual intimacy, 217–218. *see also* Intimacy
Sexualized countertransference, 320–322. *see also* Countertransference
Sexualized transference, 302–303. *see also* Transference
Sexualizing, 24*t*
Sexually reactive children, 41
Shame
  childhood trauma and, 17, 18
  complex trauma histories and, 4
  countertransference and, 316–317
  group treatment and, 193*t*
  overview, 24*t*
  posttraumatic stress disorder (PTSD) and, 45–46
  transference and, 309
Shopping addiction, 24*t*, 26. *see also* Financial mismanagement and chaos; Spending problems
"Sick" role, 136–137
Skill development
  couple therapy and, 217
  goals for treatment and, 90–91
  group treatment and, 192, 193*t*, 199*t*
  posttraumatic themes in treatment and, 259–260
  stabilization and, 129–130
Skill Training for Affect and Interpersonal Regulation (STAIR), 163–164, 170
Sleep disturbances, 18, 95, 145
Social anxiety, 127–130
Social isolation, 24*t*
Social justice, 78*t*–79*t*
Social problems, 24*t*, 99
Social skills, 24*t*, 192, 239–240
Social support
  assessment and, 98–99
  family therapy and, 224
  group treatment and, 191–192
  phase 1 of psychotherapy and, 131
  phase 3 of psychotherapy and, 185–187
  preparing the client for trauma and emotion processing, 166
Sociopathic/antisocial personality, 193*t*–194*t*
Somatic dimensions, 274–287
Somatic dysregulation, 34, 35, 46, 49
Somatic problems. *see also* Health; Physical effects, mind–body
  complex PTSD/DESNOS and, 48
  goals for treatment and, 93
  phase 2 of psychotherapy and, 145
  posttraumatic stress disorder (PTSD) and, 44
  reactions to complex trauma and, 34
  stabilization and, 127–130
Somatic tactics, 169–170
Somatic void, 238. *see also* Emptiness feelings
Somatoform disorders, 34
Spending problems, 24*t*, 26. *see also* Financial mismanagement and chaos; Shopping addiction
Spirituality, 24*t*, 186–187
Splitting, 241–247
Stabilization, 126–130, 135, 154
Stages of change, 131–134
Stance, 278–279
Strengths, 38, 98–99, 124, 138
Stress, 75, 146–150, 193*t*
Structural dissociation, 252–254. *see also* Dissociation
Structured interviews, 108, 112–113. *see also* Assessment
Substance use. *see also* Addictions
  adolescent trauma and, 19–20
  assessment and, 99
  contraindications to membership in group treatment, 193*t*–194*t*
  family therapy and, 223–224
  group treatment and, 210
  overview, 24*t*
  safety and, 124–125

Suicidality
  adolescent trauma and, 19–20
  assessment and, 99, 111*t*
  attachment styles and, 293–294
  case examples of, 173–174
  contraindications to membership in group treatment, 193*t*–194*t*
  crises and, 172
  informed consent and refusal and, 82–83
  overview, 5, 24*t*
  safety and, 126
  as secondary elaborations, 4
  transference and, 307
Supportive neutrality, 101
Survival tactics, 14, 137–138, 147, 199*t*
Survivor guilt, 44, 307
"Survivor missions", 38
Survivor perspective, 319
Suspicion of others, 24*t*, 135
Symptoms. *see also individual symptoms*
  assessment instruments and inventories and, 112–113
  childhood trauma and, 18–19
  as coping skills and adaptations, 55–58
  crises and, 172
  group treatment and, 193*t*
  list of, 24*t*
  SAFER strategies and, 154
  stabilization and, 127–130
  treatment and, 23–27, 24*t*, 54
Systemic therapy, 188–189, 190–191, 230–231. *see also* Couple therapy; Family therapy; Group treatment; Treatment

T

Task-by-stage (or phase) model, 192
Tension, 19–20, 284–285
Termination of treatment, 82–83, 187, 201–202
Terror, 17, 90–91
Themes in treatment, 257–267. *see also* Treatment
Theory of mind, 171
Therapeutic exposure, 150–156, 156–165, 173–177, 200–201. *see also* Prolonged exposure (PE)
Therapeutic relationship. *see also* Clients; Countertransference; Therapist; Transference
  attachment styles and, 287–297
  case examples of, 60–62
  discontinuity and, 250–251
  goals for treatment and, 89, 92–93
  overview, 59–65, 269–270, 297
  phase 1 of psychotherapy, 134–138
  posttraumatic emotional dysregulation and, 148
  safety and, 54, 125–126
  therapist's use of self and, 274–287
  transference–countertransference positions and, 324–326
  vicarious trauma and, 273–274
Therapist. *see also* Countertransference; Therapeutic relationship; Transference
  attachment styles and, 294–297
  crises and, 173
  dissociation and, 267
  group treatment and, 199*t*, 200, 210–214
  impact of assessment on, 102
  overview, 298–299
  posttraumatic themes in treatment and, 267
  preparing the client for trauma and emotion processing and, 168–169
  self-awareness and, 171
  use of self by, 274–287
  vicarious trauma and, 80, 270–274
Therapist self-care, 75, 80, 273–274
Therapists
  goals for treatment and, 92–93
  introduction of himself or herself and the therapy by, 140
  rights and responsibilities of, 65–87, 66*t*–68*t*, 69*t*, 70*t*–74*t*, 76*t*–77*t*, 78*t*–79*t*
Toddlerhood, 16–19. *see also* Childhood trauma
Training, professional, 68–69, 273–274
Trance-like phenomena, 264–265
Transference
  dissociative/posttraumatic transference field and, 256–267
  overview, 298–299, 326–327
  rights and responsibilities of clients and therapists and, 80
  safety and, 124
  themes, issues and reactions, 299–313
  therapeutic relationship and, 63
  transference–countertransference positions and, 324–326
  traumatic transference, 300–302
  vicarious trauma and, 271
Transparency, 285–287
Trauma Affect Regulation: Guide for Education and Therapy (TARGET), 162–163, 170
Trauma bonding, 12, 17–18, 307
Trauma Recovery and Empowerment (TREM), 192, 210
Trauma-related memories. *see* Memory
Trauma-specific assessment instruments, 108. *see also* Assessment
Traumatic brain injuries (TBI), 114–115
Traumatic transferences, 300–302. *see also* Transference
Treatment. *see also* Complex trauma-sequenced model; Phase 1; Phase 2; Phase 3; Systemic therapy
  assessment for, 120–121
  attachment styles and, 287–297
  case examples of, 57–58, 60–62, 329–331

Treatment (*continued*)
- challenges of, 54–65
- defining complex trauma and, 10
- dissociation and, 256–267
- duration of, 83–84
- emotion dysregulation and, 34–35
- emptiness feelings and, 256–267
- foundations of, 53–54
- frequency of sessions, 84
- goals for complex traumatic stress disorders and, 89–90
- goals for PTSD treatment, 88–89
- metagoals for, 90–98
- mind–body integration and, 97–98
- overview, 23–27, 24*t*, 87, 119
- rights and responsibilities of clients and therapists and, 65–87, 66*t*–68*t*, 69*t*, 70*t*–74*t*, 76*t*–77*t*, 78*t*–79*t*
- sequenced model, 120–121
- therapeutic relationship and, 59–65
- therapist's use of self and, 274–287

Triggers, 25–26, 75

Trust. *see also* Mistrust of others
- couple therapy and, 215–216
- phase 3 of psychotherapy and, 185–187
- posttraumatic themes in treatment and, 257, 260
- therapeutic relationship and, 60, 135–136, 275, 285–287
- transference and, 303–305
- traumatic transference and, 301–302

Trustworthiness, 139

Type I trauma, 11–12

Type II trauma, 11–19

Type III trauma, 22

Type IV trauma, 22

U

Underreporting of trauma, 102–104

Unfinished business, void of, 238–239. *see also* Emptiness feelings

Unpredictability, 127–130

V

Validation, 55, 166

Vicarious trauma, 80, 269–270, 270–274, 271–272

Victim perspective, 319

Victim role, 131, 136–137

Victimization, repeated, 39–40

Victimization of others, 20–21

Victims of Violence program at Cambridge Hospital, 192

Violence. *see also* Family violence; Interpersonal violence
- adulthood trauma and, 22
- assessment and, 100
- complex trauma in childhood and, 11–12
- complex trauma in infancy and, 16
- couple therapy and, 216
- crises and, 172
- family therapy and, 223–224
- safety and, 125–126

Vocational problems, 99, 109*t*, 185–187

Void of the self, 236–238. *see also* Emptiness feelings

Voyeurism, privileged, 320

W

Wisdom, 38–39, 81

Wish for a cure through love and nurturance, 257, 258–259

Withdrawal, 26, 38, 41–42, 44, 302

Witnessing trauma, 22, 23, 42–43

Women Recovering from Abuse Program (WRAP) at Women's Hospital in Toronto, 195, 201–202

Workaholism, 24*t*, 26, 252–253

Working alliance. *see* Therapeutic relationship

Working models, 38, 110*t*, 171, 276–277, 278–279. *see also* Internal working models

Work-related problems, 99, 109*t*, 185–187

Worry, 18, 146–150